MW01141291

All rights reserved. No part of this book may be reproduced or transmitted in any form or by any means, electronic or mechanical, including photocopying, recording, or by any information storage and retrieval system, without permission in writing from the publisher.

Special First Edition
Printed 2016

Copyright ©2000 Life Science Publishing
1-800-336-6308 • DiscoverLSP.com

ISBN 0-9966364-5-2

Printed in the United States of America

Disclaimer: The information contained in this book is for educational purposes only. It is not provided to diagnose, prescribe, or treat any condition of the body. The information in this book should not be used as a substitute for medical counseling with a health professional. Neither the author nor publisher accepts responsibility for such use.

ESSENTIAL OILS
DESK REFERENCE

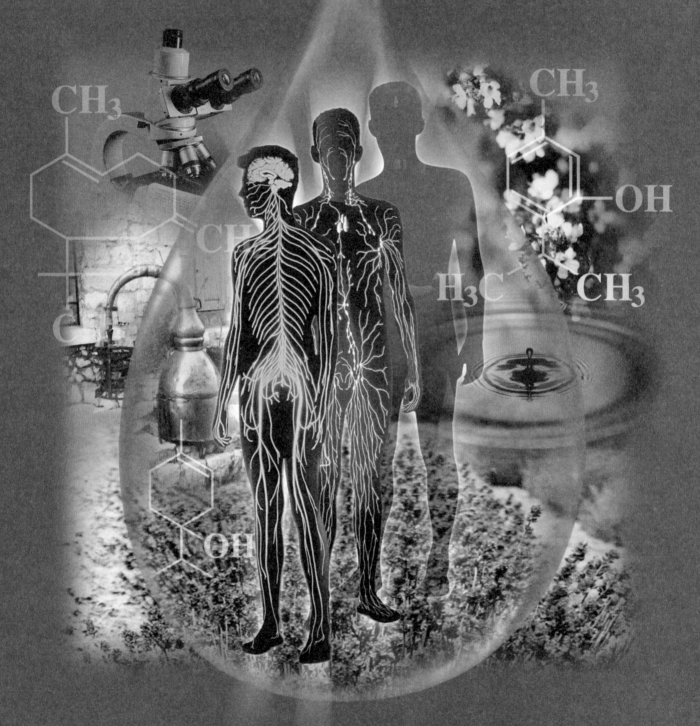

Compiled by Life Science Publishing

Special First Edition

To all those who seek truth, light and wisdom.
After all, it is their hearts that turn to
the information in this book.

Table of Contents

SECTION 1

Preface

Essential oils are the oldest and some of the most powerful therapeutic agents known. They have enjoyed a millennium-long history of use in healing and anointing throughout the ancient world. Oils, like frankincense, are cited repeatedly in many Judeo-Christian religious texts and were used to cure every ailment "from gout to a broken head." Myrrh, lotus, and sandalwood oils were widely used in ancient Egyptian purification and embalming rituals. Other oils like clove and lemon were highly valued as antiseptics hundreds of years before the discovery of chemical germkillers.

With the advent of modern industrial biochemicals during the last two centuries, natural therapeutic agents, like essential oils, have been largely forgotten. It has been only during the last 20 years that essential oils have enjoyed a resurgence in popularity as their broad-spectrum antibacterial and therapeutic action has been rediscovered by many health-care professionals. Essential oils are some of the most concentrated natural extracts known, exerting significant antiviral, anti-inflammatory, antibacterial, hormonal, and psychological effects. Essential oils have the ability to penetrate cell membranes, travel throughout the blood and tissues, and enhance electrical frequencies. As we watch an essential oil work, it becomes clear that the powerful life force inherent in many essential oils gives them an unmatched ability to communicate and interact with cells in the human body.

After using them, there is no doubt that essential oils were ordained as the medicine for mankind and will be held as the medicine of our future: the missing link of modern medicine, where allopathic and holistic medicine join together for the leap into the 21st century.

Acknowledgements

We wish to acknowledge D. Gary Young, N.D., for his tremendous contribution to the rebirth of essential oils in North America. One of the pioneers in researching, cultivating, and distilling essential oils in North America, he has spent decades conducting clinical research on the ability of essential oils to combat disease and improve health. He has also developed new methods of application from which thousands of people have benefited, especially his integration of essential oils with dietary supplements and personal care products. He is certainly one of the first, if not the first, to create these types of products.

Growing up as a farmer and rancher in Idaho, Gary has a passion for the land that has driven him to become one of the leading organic growers and distillers of essential oils in North America. With over 2,000 acres of land under cultivation in North America, he has set new standards for excellence that are redefining how therapeutic-grade essential oils are produced throughout the world.

Gary's roles as a grower, distiller, researcher, and alternative care practitioner not only give him an unsurpassed insight into essential oils but also make him an ideal spokesperson and educator on therapeutic properties of essential oils. Few people have as comprehensive a knowledge as he does. Gary regularly travels throughout the world lecturing on the powerful potential of essential oils and how to produce therapeutic-grade essential oils that can consistently deliver results.

Much of the material contained in the book is derived from his research, lectures, and workshops, as well as the work of other practitioners and physicians who are at the forefront of understanding the clinical potential of essential oils to treat disease. To these researchers, the publishers are deeply indebted.

CHAPTER 1

Essential Oils:
The Missing Link in Modern Medicine

Yesterday's Wisdom, Tomorrow's Destiny

Plants not only play a vital role in the ecological balance of our planet, but they have also been intimately linked to the physical, emotional, and spiritual well-being of people since the beginning of time.

The plant kingdom is still the subject of an enormous amount of research and discovery. About 25% of prescription drugs in the United States are based on naturally-occurring compounds from plants. Each year, millions of dollars are allocated to universities searching for new therapeutic agents that lie undiscovered in the bark, roots, and foliage of jungle canopies, river bottoms, forests, hillsides, and vast wilderness regions throughout the world.

As the most powerful part of the plant, essential oils and plant extracts have been woven into history since time immemorial. Essential oils have been used medicinally to kill bacteria, fungi, and viruses. They provide exquisite fragrances to balance mood, lift spirits, dispel negative emotions, and create a romantic atmosphere. They can stimulate the regeneration of tissue or stimulate nerves. They can even act to oxygenate and carry nutrients into the cells.

Today, it has become evident that we have not yet found permanent solutions for dreaded diseases, such as the Ebola virus and hantavirus, as well as new strains of tuberculosis and influenza. Essential oils may assume an increasingly important role in combating new mutations of bacteria, viruses, and fungi. More and more researchers are undertaking serious clinical studies on the use of essential oils to combat these types of diseases.

The research that Gary Young has conducted at Weber State University as well as other documented research indicates that most viruses, fungi, and bacteria cannot live in the presence of many essential oils, especially those high in phenols, carvacrol, thymol, and terpenes. This perhaps offers a modern explanation why the Old Testament prophet Moses used aromatic substances to protect the Israelites from the plagues that decimated the ancient Egyptians. It may also help us understand why a notorious group of thieves, reputed to be spice traders and perfumers, was protected from the black plague as they robbed the bodies of the dead during the 15th century.

A vast body of anecdotal evidence (testimonials) suggests that those who use essential oils are less likely to contract infectious diseases. Moreover, oil users who do contract an infectious illness tend to recover faster than those using antibiotics.

Essential oils are, without question, substances that definitely deserve the respect of proper education. Users need to be fully versed in the chemistry and safety of the oils. However, this knowledge is not taught at universities in the United States. There is a disturbing lack of institutional information, knowledge, and training on essential oils, a science commonly known as aromatherapy. Only in Europe, which has a far longer history of using natural products and botanical extracts, can one obtain adequate instruction.

The European communities have a tight framework of controls and standards concerning botanical extracts and who may administer them. Only practitioners with proper training and certification can practice aromatherapy. However, in the United States, the regulatory agencies have not recognized these disciplines or mandated the type and degree of training required to distribute and apply essential oils. This means that individuals can bill themselves as "aromatherapists" after a brief class in essential oils and apply oils to people—even though they may not have the experience or training to properly administer them. This may not only undermine and damage the credibility of the entire discipline of aromatherapy, but it can be dangerous.

Essential oils are not simple substances. They are mosaics of hundreds—or even thousands—of different chemicals. The average essential oil may contain anywhere from 80 to 200 chemical constituents. An essential oil like lavender can contain even more, many occurring in minute quantities but all contributing to the oil's therapeutic effects to some degree. To understand these constituents and their activity and function requires years of study.

Even though an essential oil may be labeled as "basil" and have the botanical name *Ocimum basilicum*, it can have widely different therapeutic actions, depending on its chemistry. For example, basil high in linalool or fenchol is primarily used for its antiseptic properties. However, basil high in methyl chavicol is more anti-inflammatory than antiseptic. A third type, basil high in eugenol, has both anti-inflammatory and antiseptic effects.

Moreover, essential oils can be processed in different ways that may have dramatic effects on their chemistry and medicinal action. Oils that are redistilled two or three times are obviously not as potent as oils that are distilled only once. Also, oils that are subjected to high heat and pressure processing will have a distinctly simpler and inferior profile of chemical constituents, since excessive heat and temperature will fracture and break down many of the delicate aromatic compounds within the oil—some of which are responsible for its therapeutic action. In addition, oils that are steam distilled are far different from those that are solvent extracted.

Of even greater concern is the fact that some oils are adulterated or "extended" with the use of synthetic chemicals. Oftentimes pure frankincense is extended by the addition of colorless, odorless solvents, such as diethylphthalate or dipropylene glycol. The only way to distinguish the authentic from the adulterated is to subject it to rigorous analytical testing using state-of-the-art gas chromatography and mass spectroscopy.

Different Schools of Application

Therapeutic treatment using essential oils follows three different models or frameworks: the French, German, and English.

The English model advocates diluting a small amount of essential oil in a vegetable oil and massaging the body for the purpose of relaxation and relieving stress.

The French prefer the ingestion of therapeutic-grade essential oils. A common form of internal use is to add several drops of an essential oil to a sugar cube or a piece of bread. Many French practitioners have found that taking the oils internally yields excellent benefits.

The German model recommends inhalation of the essential oil. Research has shown that the effect of fragrance and aromatic compounds on the sense of smell can exert strong effects on the brain—especially on the hypothalamus (the hormone command center of the body) and limbic system (the seat of emotions). Some essential oils high in sesquiterpenes, such as myrrh and frankincense, can dramatically increase oxygenation and activity in the brain. This may directly improve the function of many systems of the body.

Together, these three models show how versatile and powerful essential oils may be. By integrating all three techniques in conjunction with Vita Flex, auricular technique, contact therapy, spinal touch, lymphatic massage, and Raindrop Technique, the best possible results may be obtained.

In some cases, inhalation of essential oils might be preferred over topical application if the goal is to increase growth hormone secretion, induce weight loss, or balance mood and emotions. Sandalwood, lavender, and fir oil would be outstanding used this way. In other cases, however, topical application of essential oils would produce better results, particularly in the case of spinal or muscle injuries or defects. Topically applied, rosemary is excellent for muscles, lemongrass for ligaments, and birch for bones. For indigestion, peppermint oil taken orally may be very effective. However, this does not mean that peppermint cannot produce the same results when massaged on the stomach. In some cases, all three methods of application (topical, inhalation, and ingestion) are interchangeable and may produce the similar benefits.

The ability of essential oils to act both on the mind and body is what makes them truly unique among natural therapeutic agents. The fragrance of an essential oil may be very stimulating—both psychologically and physically. Similarly, the fragrance of the same essential oil may also be calming and sedating, helping to overcome anxiety or hyperactivity. On a physiological level, essential oils may stimulate immune function and regenerate damaged tissue. Essential oils may also combat infectious disease by killing viruses, bacteria, and other pathogens.

During the last 15 years, there has been extensive research conducted worldwide at many universities to expand the knowledge of essential oils and their history.

The two most effective methods of essential oil application are cold-air diffusing and neat (undiluted) topical application. By incorporating essential oils into the disciplines of reflexology, Vita Flex, acupressure, and acupuncture, the healing response is greatly enhanced. Essential oils produce phenomenal results that, in many cases, can never be achieved by acupuncture or reflexology alone. Only one to three drops of an essential oil applied to an acupuncture meridian or Vita Flex point on the hand or foot may produce dramatic effects—sometimes within minutes.

Many practitioners doubt that essential oils can produce these types of results—even though research has shown that essential oils can magnify the benefits of healing modalities like acupuncture, by two to ten times.

Several years ago at a university in Europe, a professor very well known throughout the field of aromatherapy commented that anyone who claims to cure diseases using essential oils is a quack. However, there are many people who are living proof that essential oils can be used to engineer cures and recoveries from serious illness. Essential oils have been pivotal in helping many people live pain-free after many years of suffering intense pain. Many people have also witnessed firsthand how essential oils have corrected scoliosis and restored hearing in those who are born deaf.

A woman from Palisades Park, California, developed scoliosis as a result of surviving polio as a teenager. Over 22 years ago she had fallen and dislocated her shoulder. Suffering pain and immobility, she had traveled extensively in a fruitless

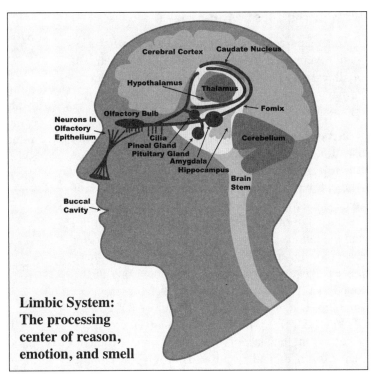

Limbic System: The processing center of reason, emotion, and smell

search to locate a practitioner who could permanently reset her shoulder. She topically applied the oils of Valor, helichrysum, and birch to the shoulder. Within a short time she became pain free as the shoulder relocated. She was able to raise her arm over her head for the first time in 22 years.

When one sees such dramatic recoveries, it is difficult to discredit the value and the power of essential oils and the potential they hold.

What Is an Essential Oil?

Essential oils are subtle, volatile liquids distilled from shrubs, flowers, trees, roots, bushes, and seeds. They are oxygenating and help transport nutrients to the cells of our body. Without oxygen, nutrients cannot be assimilated; so the oxygenating essential oils can help us maintain our health.

Essential oils are chemically very complex, consisting of hundreds of different chemical compounds. Moreover, they are highly concentrated and far more potent than dried herbs. The distillation of an entire plant may produce only a single drop of essential oil.

Essential oils are also different from vegetable oils, such as corn oil, peanut oil, and olive oil. They are not greasy and do not clog the pores like vegetable oils can.

Mankind's First Medicine

For many centuries essential oils and other aromatics were used for religious rituals, the treatment of illness, and other physical and spiritual needs. Perhaps the people of ancient times had a greater understanding of essential oils than we have today.

Records dating back to 4500 B.C. describe the use of balsamic substances with aromatic properties for religious rituals and medical applications. Ancient writings tell of scented barks, resins of spices, and aromatic vinegars, wines, and beers that were used in rituals, temples, astrology, embalming, and medicine. The Egyptians were masters in using essential oils and other aromatics in the embalming process. Historical records describe how one of the founders of "pharaonic" medicine was the architect Imhotep, who was the Grand Vizier of King Zeser (2780 - 2720 B.C.). Imhotep is often given credit for ushering in the use of oils, herbs, and aromatic plants for medicinal purposes. Hieroglyphics on the walls of Egyptian temples depict the blending of oils and describe hundreds of oil recipes. A sacred room in the temple of Isis on the island of Philae depicts a ritual called "Cleansing the Flesh and Blood of Evil Deities." This emotional clearing required three days of cleansing using essential oils.

The translation of ancient papyrus found in the Temple of Edfu reveals the medicinal formulas and perfume recipes used by the alchemist and high priest in blending aromatic substances for rituals.

The Egyptians were the first to discover the potential of fragrance. They created various aromatic blends for both personal use and for the ceremonies performed in the temples and pyramids. Many Egyptian temple carvings and reliefs describe how essential oils were used by priests and physicians in ancient ceremonies. Well before the time of Christ, the ancient Egyptians collected essential oils and placed them in alabaster vessels. These vessels were specially carved and shaped for housing scented oils. In 1922, when King Tut's tomb was opened, 350 liters of oils were discovered in alabaster jars. Plant waxes had solidified into a thickened residue around the inside of the container openings, leaving the liquefied oil in excellent condition.

In 1817, the Ebers Papyrus, a medical scroll over 870 feet long, was discovered. Dating back to 1500 B.C., the scroll included over 800 different herbal prescriptions and remedies. Other scrolls described a high success rate in treating 81 different diseases. Many mixtures contained myrrh and honey. Myrrh is still recognized for its ability to help with infections of the skin and throat and to regenerate skin tissue. Because of its effectiveness in preventing bacterial growth, myrrh was used for embalming.

The physicians of Ionia, Attia, and Crete came to the cities of the Nile to increase their knowledge. At this time, the school of Cas was founded and was attended by Hippocrates (460 to 377 B.C.), whom the Greeks, with perhaps some exaggeration, named the "Father of Medicine."

The Romans purified their temples and political buildings by diffusing essential oils. They also used aromatics in their steam baths to both invigorate the flesh and ward off disease.

Early History of Essential Oil Extraction

Ancient cultures found that aromatic essences or oils could be extracted from the plant by a variety of methods. One of the oldest and crudest forms of extraction was known as enfleurage. Raw plant material (usually stems, foliage, bark, or roots) was crushed and steeped with olive oil. In the case of cedar, the bark was stripped from the trunk and branches, ground fairly fine, soaked with olive oil, and wrapped in a wool cloth. The cloth was then burned. The heat would pull the essential oil out of the bark into the olive oil. The wool cloth was then pressed to extract the essential oil. By placing petals in goose or goat fat, the essential oil molecules would be pulled into the fat. The oil was then separated from the fat. This ancient technique was among the most primitive forms of essential oil extraction.

Many extraction techniques were used throughout ancient cultures. Some of these included:

- Soaking plant parts in boiling water
- Pressing flower petals, roots, and leaves into fat ("enfleurage" from the French, meaning to saturate with the perfume of flowers)

- Cold-pressing

- Soaking in alcohol

- Steam distillation by passing steam through the plant material and condensing the steam to separate the oil from the plant.

Many ancient cosmetic formulas were created from a base of goat fat. The ancient Egyptians formulated eyeliners, eyeshadows, and other cosmetics. They also stained their hair and nails with a variety of ointments and perfumes. They probably used the same aromatic oils that were used in the temples. Such temple oils were commonly poured into evaporation dishes for fragrancing the chambers associated with sacred rituals and religious rites.

The ancient Arabians were another early culture that developed and refined a process of distillation. They perfected the extraction of rose oils and rose water, which were popular in the Middle East during the Byzantine Empire (330 A.D. - 1400 A.D.).

Biblical and Ancient References to Essential Oils

There are over 200 references to aromatics, incense, and ointments throughout the Old and New Testaments of the Bible. Aromatics, such as frankincense, myrrh, galbanum, cinnamon, cassia, rosemary, hyssop, and spikenard, were used for anointing and healing the sick. In Exodus, the Lord gave the following recipe to Moses for a holy anointing oil:

Myrrh	"five hundred shekels" (about 1 gallon)
Cinnamon	"two hundred and fifty shekels"
Calamus	"two hundred and fifty shekels"
Cassia	"five hundred shekels"
Olive Oil	"an hin" (about 1 1/3 gallons)

Psalms 133:2 speaks of the sweetness of brethren dwelling together in unity: "*It is like the precious ointment upon the head, that ran down the beard, even Aaron's beard: that went down to the skirts of his garments.*" Another scripture that refers to anointing and the overflowing abundance of precious oils is Ecclesiastes 9:8: "*Let thy garments be always white; and let thy head lack no ointment.*"

The Bible also lists an incident where an incense offering by Aaron stopped a plague. Numbers 16:46-50 records that Moses instructed Aaron to take a censer, add burning coals and incense, and to "go quickly into the congregation to make an atonement for them: for there is a wrath gone out from the Lord; the plague is begun." The Bible records that Aaron stood between the dead and the living and the plague was stayed. It is significant that according to the biblical and Talmudic recipes for incense, three varieties of cinnamon were included. Cinnamon is known to be highly antimicrobial, anti-infectious and antibacterial. The incense ingredient listed as "stacte" is believed to be a sweet, myrrh-related spice, which would make it anti-infectious and antiviral as well. Whether the antibacterial nature of the incense played a part in stopping the plague or not, 14,700 Israelites died of the plague before Aaron brought forth the incense.

The New Testament records that wise men presented the Christ child with frankincense and myrrh. There is another precious aromatic, spikenard, described in the anointing of Jesus: "*And being in Bethany in the house of Simon the leper, as he sat at meat, there came a woman having an alabaster box of ointment of spikenard very precious; and she brake the box, and poured on his head*" (Mark 14:3). The anointing of Jesus is also referred to in John 12:3: "*Then took Mary a pound of ointment of spikenard, very costly, and anointed the feet of Jesus, and wiped his feet with her hair: and the house was filled with the odour of the ointment.*"

Other Historical References

Throughout world history, fragrant oils and spices played a prominent role in everyday life. One of the Dead Sea Scrolls on display in Israel at the Shrine of the Book Museum contains this intriguing phrase: "and he will know his children by their scent."

Napoleon is reported to have liked a cologne water made of neroli and other ingredients so much that he ordered 162 bottles of it. After conquering Jerusalem, one of the things the Crusaders brought back to Europe was solidified essence of roses.

And the 12th century mystic, Hildegard of Bingen, used herbs and oils extensively in healing. This Benedictine nun founded her own convent and was the author of numerous works. Her book, *Physica*, has more than 200 chapters on plants and their uses in healing.

The Rediscovery

The reintroduction of essential oils into modern medicine first became evident during the late 19th and early 20th centuries.

During World War I, the use of aromatic essences in civilian and military hospitals became widespread. One physician in France, Dr. Moncière, used essential oils extensively for their antibacterial and wound-healing properties and developed several kinds of aromatic ointments.

René-Maurice Gattefossé, Ph.D., a French cosmetic chemist, is widely regarded as the father of aromatherapy. He and a group of scientists began studying essential oils in 1907.

In his 1937 book, *Aromatherapy*, Dr. Gattefossé told the real story of his now-famous use of lavender on a serious burn. The tale has assumed mythic proportions in essential oil literature. While the event did *not* start him on the road to essential oil research (he was already studying the oils), his own words about this accident are even more powerful than what has been told over the years.

Dr. Gattefossé was literally aflame—covered in burning substances—following a laboratory explosion in July, 1910. After he extinguished the flames

by rolling on a grassy lawn, he wrote that "both my hands were covered with rapidly developing gas gangrene." Dr. Gattefossé said that, "just one rinse with lavender essence stopped 'the gasification of the tissue.' This treatment was followed by profuse sweating and healing began the next day."

Robert B. Tisserand, editor of *The International Journal of Aromatherapy,* searched for Dr. Gattefossé's book for 20 years. A copy was located and Tisserand edited the 1995 reprint. Tisserand noted that Dr. Gattefossé's burns "must have been severe to lead to gas gangrene, a very serious infection."

Dr. Gattefossé shared his studies with his colleague and friend, Jean Valnet, a medical doctor practicing in Paris. Exhausting his supply of antibiotics as a physician in Tonkin, China, during World War II, Dr. Valnet began using therapeutic-grade essential oils on patients suffering battlefield injuries. To his surprise, they exerted a powerful effect in combating and counteracting infection. He was able to save the lives of many soldiers who might otherwise have died.

Two of Dr. Valnet's students, Dr. Paul Belaiche and Dr. Jean Claude Lapraz, expanded his work. They clinically investigated the antiviral, antibacterial, antifungal, and antiseptic properties in essential oils.

Through the work of these doctors and chemists the worth of essential oils is again known to the public.

CHAPTER 2

How Do Essential Oils Work?

Therapeutic-Grade Essential Oils

Essential oils are volatile liquids that are distilled from various parts of plants, including seeds, bark, leaves, stems, roots, flowers, and fruit. One of the factors that determines the purity of an oil is its chemical constituents. These constituents can be affected by a vast number of variables, including: the part(s) of the plant from which the oil was produced, soil condition, fertilizer (organic or chemical), geographical region, climate, altitude, harvest season and methods, and distillation process. For example, common thyme *(Thymus vulgaris)* produces several different chemotypes (biochemically unique variants within one species), depending on the conditions of its growth, climate, and altitude. One chemotype of thyme will yield an essential oil with high levels of thymol, depending on the time of year it is distilled. The later it is distilled in the growing season (ie., mid-summer or fall), the more thymol the oil will contain.

The key to producing a therapeutic-grade essential oil is to preserve as many of the delicate aromatic compounds within the essential oil as possible. Fragile aromatic chemicals are easily destroyed by high temperature and pressure as well as contact with chemically reactive metals, such as copper or aluminum. This is why all therapeutic-grade essential oils should be distilled in stainless steel cooking chambers at low pressure and low temperature.

The plant material should also be free of pesticides, herbicides, and other agrichemicals. These can react with the essential oil during distillation to produce toxic compounds.

As we begin to understand the power of essential oils in the realm of personal, holistic healthcare, we will appreciate the necessity for obtaining the purest essential oils possible. No matter how costly pure essential oils may be, there can be no substitutes.

Although chemists have successfully recreated the main constituents and fragrances of some essential oils in the laboratory, these synthetic oils lack therapeutic benefits and may even carry risks. Why? Because essential oils contain hundreds of different chemical compounds, some of which have never been identified but which lend important therapeutic properties to the oil. Also, some essential oils contain molecules and isomers that are impossible to manufacture in the laboratory.

Anyone venturing into the world of aromatherapy and essential oils must use the purest quality oils available. Inferior quality or adulterated oils most likely will not produce therapeutic results and could possibly be toxic. In Europe, a set of standards has been established that outlines the chemical profile and principal constituents that a quality essential oil should have. Known as AFNOR and ISO standards, these guidelines help buyers differentiate between a therapeutic-grade essential oil and a lower grade oil with a similar chemical makeup and fragrance. All of the therapeutic effects of the essential oils in this book are based on oils that have been graded according to the AFNOR standard.

Science and Application

Essential oils of the plants and human blood share several common properties: They fight infection, contain hormone-like compounds, and initiate regeneration. Working as the chemical defense mechanism of the plant, essential oils possess potent antibacterial, antifungal, and antiviral properties. They also ward off attacks by insects and animals. Both essential oils and human blood contain hormone-like chemicals. The ability of some essential oils to work as hormones helps them bring balance to many physiological systems of the human body. Oils like clary sage and fennel, for example, have an estrogenic action. Essential oils also play a role in initiating the regeneration process for the plant, the same way the blood does in the human body.

This similarity goes deeper. Essential oils have a chemical structure that is similar to that found in human cells and tissues. This makes essential oils compatible with human protein and enables them to be readily identified and accepted by the body.

Essential oils have a unique ability to penetrate cell membranes and diffuse throughout the blood and tissues. The unique, lipid-soluble structure of essential oils is very similar to the makeup of our cell membranes. The molecules of essential oils are also relatively small, giving them the ability to easily penetrate the cells. When topically applied to the feet or elsewhere, essential oils can travel throughout the body in a matter of minutes.

The ability of some essential oils to decrease the viscosity or thickness of the blood can enhance circulation and immune function. Adequate circulation is vital to good health, since it affects the function of every cell and organ, including the brain.

Research indicates that when essential oils are diffused, they can increase atmospheric oxygen and provide negative ions, which can inhibit bacterial growth. This suggests that essential oils could play an important role in air purification and neutralizing odors. Because of their ionizing action, essential oils have the ability to break down and render potentially harmful chemicals nontoxic.

In the human body, essential oils stimulate the secretion of antibodies, neurotransmitters, endorphins, hormones, and enzymes. Oils containing limonene have been shown to be antiviral. Other oils, like lavender, have been shown to promote the growth of hair and increase the rate of wound healing. They increase the uptake of oxygen and ATP (adenosine triphosphate), the fuel for individual cells.

European scientists have studied the ability of essential oils to work as natural chelators, binding with heavy metals and petrochemicals and ferrying them out of the body.

Today about 200 types of oils are distilled, with several thousand chemical constituents and aromatic molecules identified and registered. The quantity, quality, and type of these aromatic compounds will vary depending on climate, temperature, and distillation factors. Ninety-eight percent of essential oils produced today are used in the perfume and cosmetic industry. Only about 2 percent are produced for therapeutic and medicinal applications.

Because essential oils are composites of hundreds of different chemicals, they can exert many different effects on the body. For example, clove oil can be simultaneously antiseptic and anaesthetic when applied topically. It can also be antitumoral. Lavender oil has been used for burns, insect bites, headaches, PMS, insomnia, stress, and hair growth.

Moreover, because of their complexity, essential oils do not disturb the body's natural balance or homeostasis: if one constituent exerts too strong an effect, another constituent may block or counteract it. Synthetic chemicals, in contrast, usually have only one action and often disrupt the body's natural balance or homeostasis.

Using European AFNOR/ISO Standards to Identify Therapeutic-Grade Oils

One of the most reliable indicators of essential oil quality is the AFNOR or ISO certification. This standard is more stringent and differentiates true therapeutic-grade essential oils from similar Grade A essential oils with inferior chemistry.

The AFNOR standard (Association French Normalization Organization Regulation) was written by a botanical chemist, Hervi Casabianca, Ph.D., while working with different analytical laboratories throughout France. He recognized that the constituents within an essential oil had to occur in certain percentages in order for the oil to be considered therapeutic. He combined his studies with research conducted by other scientists and doctors. The Central Service Analysis Laboratory is certified by the French government for essential oil analysis.

As a result, many oils that are listed as therapeutic-grade, such as, frankincense or lavender, can be checked to see if they meet AFNOR standards. If some constituents are too high or too low, the oils cannot be AFNOR or ISO certified.

For example, the AFNOR standard for *Lavandula angustifolia* (true lavender) dictates that the level of linalool should range from 30 to 34 percent and linalyl acetate range between 26-30 percent. As long as the oil's marker compounds are within a specific parameter, it can be recognized as a therapeutic-grade essential oil.

As a general rule, if two or more marker compounds in an essential oil fall outside of their proper percentages, the oil may not be able to meet the AFNOR standard. It cannot be recognized as therapeutic-grade essential oil, even though it is still Grade A and of high quality.

What distinguishes a therapeutic-grade essential oil from a Grade A essential oil that is not therapeutic-grade or AFNOR-certified? A lavender oil produced in one region of France might have a slightly different chemistry than that grown in another region and as a result may not meet the standard. It may have excessive camphor levels (1.0 instead of 0.5), a condition that might be caused by distilling lavender that was too green. Or the levels of lavandulol may be too low due to certain weather conditions at the time of harvest.

By comparing the chemistry of lavender essential oil with the AFNOR standard, you may also distinguish true lavender from various species of lavandin (hybrid lavender). Usually lavandin has high camphor levels, almost no lavandulol, and is easily identified. However, Tasmania produces a lavandin that yields an essential oil with naturally low camphor levels that mimics the chemistry of true lavender. Only by analyzing the chemical fingerprint of this Tasmanian lavandin using high resolution gas chromatography and comparing it with the AFNOR standard for genuine lavender can this hybrid lavender be identified.

Currently, there is no agency responsible for certifying that an essential oil is therapeutic grade. The only indication for a therapeutic-grade oil is if it meets ISO or AFNOR standards. (ISO is the International Standards Organization which has set standards for therapeutic-grade essential oils adopted from AFNOR.) The oils used in the products discussed in this book have been and are constantly being analyzed and graded according to the AFNOR standards.

To our knowledge, Young Living is the only essential oil producer in North America that has been collaborating with government-certified analytical chemists in Europe to ensure that its essential oils meet AFNOR standards.

In the United States, few companies use the proper analytical equipment and methods to properly analyze essential oils. Most labs use equipment best-suited for synthetic chemicals—not for essential oil analysis. We know of only two firms in the U.S. that use the proper machinery and test standards—Flora Research and Young Living Essential Oils. Both of these companies have made serious efforts to adopt the European testing standards, widely regarded as the gold standard for testing essential oils. In addition to operating its analytical equipment on the same standard as the European-certified laboratories, Young Living is also in the process of expanding its analytical library of chemicals in order to perform more thorough chemical analysis.

Properly analyzing an essential oil by gas chromatography is a complex undertaking. The injection mixture, film thickness, column diameter and length, and oven temperature must fall within certain parameters.

The column length should be at least 50 or 60 meters. However, almost all labs in the United States use a 30-meter column that is not long enough to achieve separation of all the essential oil constituents. While 30-meter columns are adequate for analyzing synthetic chemicals and marker compounds in vitamins, minerals, and herbal extracts, they are far too short to properly analyze the complex mosaic of natural chemicals found in an essential oil.

A longer column also enables double-phased ramping to be conducted, which enables constituents that occur in small percentages to be identified by increasing the separation of compounds. Without a longer column, it would be extremely difficult to identify these molecules, especially if they are chemically similar to each other or the marker compound.

While gas chromatography (GC) is an excellent tool for dissecting the anatomy of an essential oil, it does have limitations. Dr. Brian Lawrence, one of the foremost experts on essential oil chemistry, has commented that it is very difficult to distinguish between natural and synthetic compounds using GC analysis. If synthetic linalyl acetate was added to pure lavender, a GC analysis cannot tell whether that compound is synthetic or natural, only that it is linalyl acetate.

This is why oils must be analyzed by a technician specially trained on the interpretation of a gas chromatograph chart. The analyst examines the entire chemical fingerprint of the oil to determine its purity and potency, measuring how various compounds in the oil occur in relation to each other. If some chemicals occur in higher quantities than others, these provide important clues to determine if the oil is adulterated or pure.

Adulteration of essential oils will become more and more common as the supply of top-quality essential oils dwindles and demand explodes. These adulterated essential oils will jeopardize the integrity of aromatherapy in the United States and may put many people at risk.

(See AFNOR/ISO Standard charts in Appendix A. These charts show the standards of constituents—maximum or minimum—of therapeutic-grade essential oils).

Adulterated Oils and Their Dangers

Today most of the lavender oil sold in America is a hybrid called lavandin, grown and distilled in China, Russia, France, and Tasmania. It is brought into France, cut with synthetic linolyl acetate to improve the fragrance; propylene glycol, DEP, or DOP (solvents that have no smell and increase the volume), are then added and it is sold in the United States as lavender oil. Oftentimes lavandin is heated to evaporate the camphor and then is adulterated with synthetic linolyl acetate so that it appears as lavender. Most consumers don't know the difference, and are happy to buy and sell it for $5 to $7 per half ounce in health food stores, beauty salons, grocery and department stores, and through mail order. This is one of the reasons it is important to know about the integrity of the company that you are buying the essential from or the vendor who is selling it to you.

Frankincense is another example of a commonly adulterated oil. The frankincense resin that is sold in Somalia costs between $30,000 and $35,000 per ton. The essential oil requires 12 hours to be steam distilled from the resin and is very expensive. Frankincense oil that sells for $25 per ounce or less is invariably distilled with alcohol or other solvents. When these cut, synthetic, and adulterated oils cause rashes, burns, or other irritations, people wonder why they do not get the benefit they expected and conclude that essential oils do not have much value.

Statistics show that one company—Proctor & Gamble—uses twice as much essential oil as is produced in the entire world. From where are these "essential oils" coming?

In France, production of true lavender oil (*Lavandula angustifolia*) dropped from 87 tons in

1967 to only 12 tons in 1998. During this same period the demand for lavender oil grew over 100 times. So where did essential oil marketers obtain enough lavender to meet demand? They used a combination of synthetic and adulterated oils. There are huge chemical companies on the east coast of the U.S. that specialize in the duplication of every essential oil that exists. For every kilogram of pure essential oil that is produced, there are between 10 and 100 kilograms of synthetic oil created.

Adulterated and mislabeled essential oils present dangers for consumers. One woman who had heard of the ability of lavender oil to heal burns used lavender oil from a local health food store when she spilled boiling water on her arm. When the pain intensified and the burn worsened, she later complained that lavender oil was worthless for healing burns. When her "lavender" oil was later analyzed, it turned out to be lavandin, a hybrid lavender that is chemically very different from pure *Lavandula angustifolia*. Lavandin contains high levels of camphor (12-18 percent) and will burn the skin. In contrast, true lavender contains virtually no camphor and has burn-healing agents not found in lavandin.

Adulterated oils that are cut with synthetic extenders can be very detrimental, causing rashes, burning, and skin irritations. Petrochemical solvents, such dipropylene glycol and diethylphthalate, can all cause allergic reactions, besides being devoid of any therapeutic effects.

Some people assume that because an essential oil is 100 percent pure it will not burn their skin. This is not true. Pure essential oils may cause skin irritation if applied undiluted. If you apply straight oregano oil to the skin, it may cause severe reddening and burning. Citrus and spice oils, like orange and cinnamon, may also produce rashes. Even the terpenes in conifer oils, like pine, may cause skin irritation on sensitive people.

Some writers have claimed that a few compounds when isolated from the essential oil and tested in the lab can exert toxic effects. Even some nature-identical essential oils (a structured essential oil that has been chemically duplicated from 5 to 15 synthetic compounds) can produce unwanted side effects or toxicities. However, even though isolated compounds may be toxic, pure essential oils, in most cases, are not. This is because natural essential oils contain up to hundreds of different compounds, some of which balance and counteract each other, acting as buffers and balancers for the compounds that can be toxic.

Many tourists in Egypt are eager to buy local essential oils, especially lotus oil. Venders convince the tourists that the oils are 100 percent pure, even going so far as to touch a lighted match to the neck of the oil container to show that the oil is not diluted with alcohol or other petrochemical solvents. However, this test provides no reliable indicator of purity. Many synthetic marker compounds can be added to an essential oil that are not flammable. Or, flammable solvents can be added to a vegetable oil base that will have a hard time catching fire. Even more confusing is the fact that some natural essential oils high in terpenes can be flammable.

Fact or Fiction: Myths and Misinformation

Much current information available on essential oils should be regarded with caution. Many aromatherapy books are merely compilations of two or three other books. The content is similar, only phrased and worded differently. Because the information has been copied from sources that have never been documented, the same misinformation repeatedly resurfaces.

Many aromatherapy books claim that essential oils, like clary sage, fennel, sage, and bergamot, can trigger an abortion. In fact several years ago a rumor circulated about a laboratory research project in which the uterus of a rat was turned inside out and a cold drop of clary sage oil was applied to the exposed uterine wall. When this caused a contraction of the muscle, clary sage was labeled as abortion causing. One must ask, what would have happened if cold water had been dropped on the exposed uterus? Would the uterine wall have contracted using water also? Following this reasoning, water could be labeled as abortion-causing as well.

The truth is, that to our knowledge, there has never been a single documented case that any of these essential oils have caused an abortion. Sclareol is not an estrogen, although it can mimic estrogen if there is an estrogen deficiency. If there is not an estrogen deficiency, sclareol will not create more estrogen in the body. As a rule, essential oils bring balance to the human body.

The belief that pure essential oils will not leave a stain when poured on a tissue is unfounded. Any essential oil high in waxes will leave stains. Oils like frankincense, cedarwood, ylang ylang, or German chamomile will also leave a noticeable residue. However, an essential oil spiked with synthetic dilutents or solvent may or may not leave a stain.

The Powerful Influence of Aromas on Both Mind and Body

The fragrance of an essential oil can directly affect everything from your emotional state to your lifespan.

When a fragrance is inhaled, the odor molecules travel up the nose where they are trapped by olfactory membranes well protected by the lining inside the nose. Each odor molecule fits like a little puzzle piece into specific receptor cells lining a membrane known as the olfactory epithelium. Each one of these hundreds of millions of nerve cells is replaced every 28 days. When stimulated by odor molecules, this lining of nerve cells triggers electrical impulses to the olfactory bulb, which then transmits the impulses to the gustatory center (where the sensation of taste is perceived), the amygdala (where emotional memories are stored), and other parts of the limbic system of the brain. Because the limbic system is directly connected to those parts of the brain that control heart rate, blood pressure, breathing, memory, stress levels, and hormone balance, essential oils can have some very profound physiological and psychological effects.

The sense of smell is the only one of the five senses directly linked to the limbic lobe of the brain, the emotional control center. Anxiety, depression, fear, anger, and joy all emanate from this region. This is why the scent of a special fragrance can evoke memories and emotions before we are even consciously aware of it. Where smells are concerned, we react first and think later. In contrast, all other senses (touch, taste, hearing, and sight) are routed through the thalamus, which acts as the switchboard for the brain, passing stimuli onto the cerebral cortex and other parts of the brain.

The limbic lobe (a group of brain structures that includes the hippocampus and amygdala that is located below the cerebral cortex) can also directly activate the hypothalamus. The hypothalamus is one of the most important parts of the brain, acting as our hormonal control center. It releases chemical messengers that can affect everything from our sex drive to energy levels. The production of growth hormones, sex hormones, thyroid hormones, and neurotransmitters, like serotonin, are all governed by the hypothalamus. This is why the hypothalamus is referred to as the "master gland."

Essential oils—through their fragrance and unique molecular structure—can directly stimulate both the limbic lobe and the hypothalamus. In this way, essential oils can exert a profound effect on body and mind. Not only can inhalation of essential oils be used to combat stress and emotional trauma, but they can also stimulate the production of hormones from the hypothalamus that can result in increased thyroid hormone (our energy hormone) and growth hormone (our youth and longevity hormone).

Essential oils may also be used to reduce appetite and produce dramatic reductions in weight because of their ability to stimulate the ventromedial nucleus of the hypothalamus, a section of the brain that governs our feeling of satiety or fullness following meals. In one large clinical study, Alan Hirsch, M.D., used fragrances, including peppermint, to trigger significant weight losses in a large group of patients who had previously been unsuccessful in any type of weight-management program. During the course of the six-month study involving over 3,000 people, the average weight loss exceeded five pounds a month. According to Dr. Hirsch, some patients actually had to be dropped from the study to avoid becoming underweight.

Another double-blind, randomized study by Hirsch documents the ability of aroma to enhance libido and sexual arousal. When 31 male volunteers were subjected to the aromas of 30 different essential oils, each one exhibited a marked increase in arousal, based on measurements of brachial penile index and the measurement of both penile and brachial blood pressures. Among the scents that produced the most sexual excitement was a combination of lavender and pumpkin. This study shows that fragrances enhance sexual desire through their stimulation of the amygdala, which is the emotional center of the brain.

In 1989, Dr. Joseph Ledoux, of the New York Medical University discovered that the amygdala plays a major role in storing and releasing emotional trauma and that aroma may exert a profound effect in triggering a response from this gland.

In studies conducted at Vienna and Berlin Universities, researchers found that sesquiterpenes in the essential oils of sandalwood and frankincense can increase levels of oxygen in the brain by up to 28% (Nasel, 1992). Such an increase in brain oxygen may lead to a heightened level of activity in the hypothalamus and limbic systems of the brain, which can have dramatic effects not only on emotions, learning, and attitude, but also on many physical processes of the body, such as immune function, hormone balance, and energy levels. High levels of sesquiterpenes also occur in melissa, myrrh, and clove oil.

People who have undergone nose surgery or suffer olfactory impairment may find it difficult or impossible to detect a complete odor. The same is true of people who use makeup, perfume, cologne, hair sprays, hair coloring, perms, or other products with synthetic odors. These people may not derive the full physiological and emotional benefits of essential oils and their fragrances.

Proper stimulation of the olfactory nerves may present a powerful and entirely new form of therapy that may be used as an adjunct against many forms of illness. Essential oils, through inhalation, may occupy a key position in this relatively unexplored frontier in medicine.

Chemical Sensitivities and Allergies

Occasionally, individuals beginning to use essential oils will suffer rashes or allergic reactions. This may be due to using an undiluted spice, conifer, or citrus oil, or it may be caused by an interaction of the oil with residues of synthetic, petroleum-based personal care products that have leached into the skin.

When using essential oils on a daily basis, it is imperative to avoid personal care products containing ammonium or hydrocarbon-based chemicals. These include quaternary compounds, such as quarternarium 1-29 and polyquarternarium 1-14. These compounds are found ubiquitously in a variety of hand creams, mouthwashes, shampoos, antiperspirants, after-shave lotions, and hair-care products. In small concentrations they can be toxic and present the possibility of reacting with essential oils and producing chemical byproducts of unknown toxicity. These chemicals can be fatal when ingested, especially benzalkonium chloride, which is used in many personal care products.

Other compounds that present concerns are sodium lauryl sulfate, propylene glycol, and the aluminum salts found in many deodorants.

Of particular concern are the potentially-hazardous preservatives and synthetic fragrances that abound in virtually all modern personal-care products. Some of these include methylene chloride, methyl isobutyl ketone, and methyl ethyl ketone. These are not only toxic, in their own right, but can react with some compounds in natural essential oils. The result can be a severe case of dermatitis or even septicemia (blood poisoning).

A classic case of a synthetic fragrance causing widespread damage occurred in the 1970s. AETT (acetylethyltetramethyltetralin) appeared in numerous brands of personal care products throughout the United States. Even after a series of animal studies revealed that it caused significant brain and spinal cord damage, the FDA refused to ban the chemical. Finally, the cosmetic industry voluntarily withdrew it after allowing it to be distributed for years. How many other toxins masquerading as preservatives or fragrances are currently being used in personal care products?

Even worse, many chemicals are easily absorbed through the skin due to its permeability. One study found that 13 percent of BHT (butylated hydroxytoluene) and 49 percent of DDT (a carcinogenic pesticide) are absorbed into the skin (Steinman 1997). Once absorbed, they can become trapped in the fatty subdermal layers where they can leach into the blood stream. Sometimes these chemicals can remain trapped in fatty tissues underneath the skin for months or even years, where they harbor the potential of reacting with essential oils that may be topically applied later on. The user may mistakenly assume that the threat of an interaction between oils and synthetic cosmetics used months before is small. However, a case of dermatitis is an ever-present possibility.

CHAPTER 3

The Chemistry of Essential Oils

Essential Oil Constituents

Eugenol—An aromatic molecule found in several essential oils including clove. It has been used as an antiseptic for many years.

OH

OCH3

CH2

Unlike synthetic chemicals, essential oil chemicals are diverse in their effects. No two oils are alike. Some constituents, such as aldehydes found in lavender and chamomile, are antimicrobial and calming. Eugenol, found in cinnamon and clove, is antiseptic and stimulating. Ketones, found in lavender, hyssop, and patchouly, stimulate cell regeneration and liquefy mucous. Phenols, found in oregano and thyme oil, are highly antimicrobial. Sesquiterpenes, predominant in sandalwood and frankincense, are soothing to inflamed tissue and produce profound effects on emotions and hormonal balance.

The complex chemistry of essential oils makes them ideal for killing and preventing the spread of bacteria, since microorganisms have a hard time mutating in the presence of so many different antiseptic compounds. In 1985, Dr. Jean C. Lapraz stated that no microbe could survive in the presence of the essential oils of cinnamon or oregano. This is significant as we face life-threatening, drug-resistant viruses and bacteria.

The essential oils of ravensara, melissa, oregano, mountain savory, clove, cumin, cistus, Idaho tansy, hyssop, and frankincense are highly antibacterial and contain immune supportive properties that have been documented by many researchers, such as Daniel Pénoël, M.D. and Pierre Franchomme, Ph.D. These oils are found in varying amounts in the blends of ImmuPower, Thieves, and Exodus II.

Key Chemical Constituents in Essential Oils and their Effects

Constituent	Representative Oil	Property	Effect
Ketones	Sage	neurotoxic	mucolytic
Aldehydes	Lemongrass	irritant	calming
Esters	Lavender	soothing	balancing
Ethers	Tarragon	soothing	balancing
Alcohols	Ravensara	energizing	toning
Phenols	Savory	hepatotoxic	stimulant
Terpenes	Pine	skin irritant	stimulant

Understanding Essential Oil Chemistry

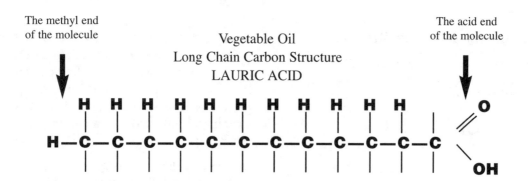

The methyl end of the molecule

The acid end of the molecule

Vegetable Oil
Long Chain Carbon Structure
LAURIC ACID

Basic Chemical Structure

The aromatic constituents of essential oils (i.e., terpenes, monoterpenes, phenols, aldehydes, etc.) are constructed from long chains of carbon and hydrogen atoms, which have a predominantly ring-like chemical structure. Links of carbon atoms form the backbone of these chains, with oxygen, hydrogen, nitrogen, sulfur, and other carbon atoms attached at various points of the chain.

Essential oils are chemically different from fatty oils (also known as fatty acids). In contrast to the simple linear carbon-hydrogen structure of fatty oils, essential oils have a far more complex aromatic-ring structure and contain sulfur and nitrogen atoms that fatty oils do not have.

The terpenoids found in many essential oils are actually constructed out of the same basic building block—a five-carbon molecule known as isoprene.

When two isoprene units link together, they create a monoterpene; when three join, they create a sesquiterpene; and so on. Some of largest molecules found in essential oils are triterpenoids, which consist of 30 carbon atoms or six isoprene units linked together. Carotenoids, which consist of 40 carbons or eight isoprene units, only occur in essential oils in tiny quantities because they are too heavy to be extracted via steam distillation.

Different molecules in an essential oil can exert different effects. For example, German chamomile (*Matricaria recutita*) contains azulene, a dark blue compound that has powerful anti-inflammatory compounds. German chamomile also contains bisobolol, a compound studied for its sedative and mood-balancing properties. There are other compounds in German chamomile that perform different functions, like speeding the regeneration of tissue.

Chemotypes

A single species of plant can have several different chemotypes based on chemical composition. This means that basil (*Ocimum basilicum*) grown in one area might produce an essential oil with a completely different chemistry than that from a basil grown in another location. The plant's growing environment, such as soil pH and mineral content, can dramatically affect the plant's chemistry as well. Following are the different chemotypes of basil:

Ocimum basilicum Linalol Fenchol CT (Germany)
• antiseptic

Ocimum basilicum Methyl Chavicol CT (Reunion, Comoro, or Egypt)
• anti-inflammatory

Ocimum basilicum Eugenol CT (Madagascar)
• anti-inflammatory, pain-relieving

Another species of plant that occurs in a variety of different chemotypes is rosemary (*Rosmarinus officinalis*).

Rosmarinus officinalis CT Camphor is high in camphor. Camphor serves best as a general stimulant and works synergistically with other oils, such as black pepper, and can be a powerful energy stimulant.

Rosmarinus officinalis CT Cineol is rich in 1,8 cineol, which is used in other countries for pulmonary congestion and to help with the elimination of toxins from the liver and kidneys.

Rosmarinus officinalis CT Verbenon is high in verbenon and is the most gentle of the rosemary chemotypes. It offers powerful regenerative properties and has outstanding benefits for skin care.

Thyme (*Thymus vulgaris*) also has several different chemotypes. Some of these are:

Thymus vulgaris CT Carvacrol is germicidal and anti-inflammatory.

Thymus vulgaris CT Linalool is anti-infectious.

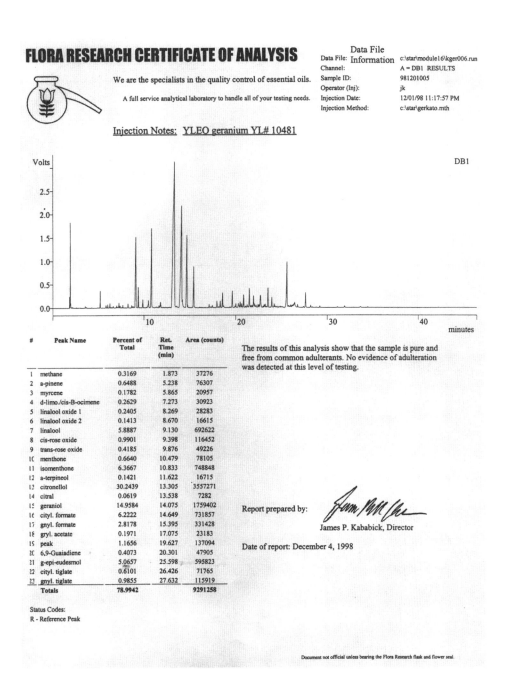

FLORA RESEARCH CERTIFICATE OF ANALYSIS

We are the specialists in the quality control of essential oils.

A full service analytical laboratory to handle all of your testing needs.

Injection Notes: YLEO geranium YL# 10481

Data File Information

Data File:	c:\star\module16\kger006.run
Channel:	A = DB1 RESULTS
Sample ID:	981201005
Operator (Inj):	jk
Injection Date:	12/01/98 11:17:57 PM
Injection Method:	c:\star\gerkato.mth

DB1

#	Peak Name	Percent of Total	Ret. Time (min)	Area (counts)
1	methane	0.3169	1.873	37276
2	a-pinene	0.6488	5.238	76307
3	myrcene	0.1782	5.865	20957
4	d-limo./cis-B-ocimene	0.2629	7.273	30923
5	linalool oxide 1	0.2405	8.269	28283
6	linalool oxide 2	0.1413	8.670	16615
7	linalool	5.8887	9.130	692622
8	cis-rose oxide	0.9901	9.398	116452
9	trans-rose oxide	0.4185	9.876	49226
10	menthone	0.6640	10.479	78105
11	isomenthone	6.3667	10.833	748848
12	a-terpineol	0.1421	11.622	16715
13	citronellol	30.2439	13.305	3557271
14	citral	0.0619	13.538	7282
15	geraniol	14.9584	14.075	1759402
16	cityl. formate	6.2222	14.649	731857
17	gnyl. formate	2.8178	15.395	331428
18	gryl. acetate	0.1971	17.075	23183
19	peak	1.1656	19.627	137094
20	6,9-Guaiadiene	0.4073	20.301	47905
21	g-epi-eudesmol	5.0657	25.598	595823
22	cityl. tiglate	0.6101	26.426	71765
23	gnyl. tiglate	0.9855	27.632	115919
	Totals	**78.9942**		**9291258**

Status Codes:
R - Reference Peak

The results of this analysis show that the sample is pure and free from common adulterants. No evidence of adulteration was detected at this level of testing.

Report prepared by:

James P. Kababick, Director

Date of report: December 4, 1998

Document not official unless bearing the Flora Research flask and flower seal.

17

CHAPTER 4

How to Safely Use Essential Oils

There are a few guidelines to follow when using essential oils, especially if you are unfamiliar with the oils and their benefits. Many guidelines are listed below and will be elaborated on throughout the chapter. However, no list of "do's and don'ts" could ever replace common sense. It is foolish to dive headlong into a pond when you don't know the depth of the water. The same is true when using these oils. Start gradually, and find what works best for you and your family.

Guidelines for Safe Use

1. Always keep a bottle of a pure vegetable oil handy when using essential oils. Vegetable oils dilute essential oils if they cause discomfort or skin irritation.

2. Keep bottles of essential oils tightly closed and store in a cool location away from light. If stored properly, essential oils will maintain their potency for many years.

3. Keep essential oils out of reach of children. Treat them as you would any product for therapeutic use.

4. Essential oils rich in menthol (such as peppermint) should not be used on the throat or neck area of children under 30 months of age.

5. Angelica, bergamot, grapefruit, lemon, orange, tangerine, and other citrus oils are photosensitive and may cause a rash or dark pigmentation on skin exposed to direct sunlight or UV rays within 3 to 4 days after application.

6. Keep essential oils away from eye area and never put directly into ears. Do not handle contact lenses or rub eyes with essential oils on your fingers. Oils with high phenol content—oregano, cinnamon, thyme, clove, lemongrass, and bergamot—may damage contacts and irritate eyes.

7. Pregnant women should consult a health care professional when starting any type of health program.

8. Epileptics and those with high blood pressure should consult their health care professional before using essential oils. Use caution with hyssop, fennel, basil, birch, nutmeg, rosemary, peppermint, sage, tarragon, and Idaho tansy oils.

9. People with high blood pressure should avoid using sage and rosemary.

10. People with allergies should test a small amount of oil on a small area of sensitive skin, such as the inside of the arm, before applying the oil on other areas.

The bottom of the feet is one of the safest, most effective places to use essential oils.

11. Before taking GRAS (Generally Regarded As Safe—see Appendix E) essential oils internally, dilute one drop of essential oil in one teaspoon of an oil-soluble liquid like honey, olive oil, or soy or rice milk. Never consume more than a few frops of diluted essential oil per day without the advice of a physician.

12. Do not add undiluted essential oils directly to bath water. Using Bath Gel Base for all oils applied to your bath is an excellent way to disperse the oils into the bath water.

When essential oils are put directly into bath water without a dispersing agent, they can harm the skin because essential oils are soluble with the lipid membranes of cells. The oils have an unmatched ability to disperse within minutes throughout the body when absorbed by the skin. This is similar to how nicotine and hormone skin patches rely on transdermal absorption to deliver drugs into the bloodstream.

13. Keep essential oils away from open flames, sparks, or electricity. Essential oils, including orange, fir, pine, and peppermint are potentially flammable.

Before You Start...

Always skin test an essential oil before using it. Each person's body is different, so apply oils to a small area first. Apply one oil or blend at a time. When layering oils that are new to you, allow enough time (3 to 5 minutes) for the body to respond before applying a second oil.

Exercise caution when applying essential oils to skin that has been exposed to cosmetics, personal care products, soaps, and cleansers containing synthetic chemicals. Some of them—especially petroleum-based chemicals—can penetrate and remain in the skin and fatty tissues for days or even weeks after use. Essential oils may react with such chemicals and cause skin irritation, nausea, headaches or other uncomfortable effects.

Essential oils can also react with toxins built up in the body from chemicals in food, water and work environment. If you experience a reaction to essential oils, it may be wise to temporarily discontinue their use and start an internal cleansing program before resuming regular use of essential oils. In addition, double your water intake while using essential oils.

You may also want to try the following alternative to a detoxification program to determine the cause of the problem:

- Dilute the oils—1 to 3 drops of oil to 1/2 tsp. massage oil, V-6 Mixing Oil, or any pure vegetable oil, such as jojoba or olive. More dilution may be needed, as necessary.

- Reduce the number of oils used at any time.

- Use single oils or oil blends, one at a time.

- Reduce the amount of oil used.

- Reduce the frequency of application.

- Drink more purified or distilled water.

- Ask your health care professional to monitor detoxification.

- Skin-test the diluted essential oil on a small patch of skin. If any redness or irritation results, cleanse skin thoroughly and reapply.

- If skin irritation or other uncomfortable side effects persist, discontinue using the oil(s).

You may also want to avoid using products that contain the following ingredients to eliminate potential problems:

- Cosmetics, deodorants, and skin care products containing aluminum, petrochemicals, or other synthetic ingredients.

- Perms, hair colors or dyes, hair sprays or gels containing synthetic chemicals. Avoid shampoos, toothpastes, mouth wash, and soaps containing synthetic chemicals such as sodium laurel sulfate, propylene glycol, or lead acetate.

- Garden sprays, paints, detergents, and cleansers containing toxic chemicals and solvents.

You can use essential oils anywhere on the body except on the eyes and ears. Caution: Essential oils may sting if applied in or around the eyes. Some oils may be painful on mucous membranes unless diluted properly. Immediate dilution is strongly recommended if skin becomes painfully irritated or if oil accidentally gets into eyes. Flushing the area with a vegetable oil should minimize discomfort almost immediately. DO NOT flush with water! Essential oils are oil soluble, not water soluble. Water will only spread the oils over a larger surface, possibly exacerbating the problem.

Keep all essential oils out of reach of children and only apply to children under skilled supervision. If a child or infant swallows an essential oil:

- Administer a mixture of milk, cream, yogurt, or another safe, oil-soluble liquid.

- Call a Poison Control Center or seek immediate emergency medical attention if necessary.

Topical Application

Many oils are safe to apply directly to the skin. Lavender is safe to use on children without dilution. However, you must be sure it is not lavandin that is labeled as lavender or is a genetically-engineered lavender. When applying most other essential oils on children, dilute them with a carrier oil. For dilution, add fifteen to thirty drops of essential oil to one ounce of a quality carrier oil as mentioned previously.

Carrier oils extend essential oils and provide more efficient use. When massaging, the carrier oil helps lubricate the skin. Some excellent carrier oils include cold-pressed grapeseed, olive, wheat germ, jojoba, and sweet almond oils, or a blend of any of these.

When starting an essential oil application, always apply the oil first to the bottom of the feet. This allows the body to become acclimated to the oil, minimizing the chance of a reaction. The Vita Flex foot charts (see pg. 41) identify areas for best application. Start by applying 3 to 6 drops of a single or blended oil, spreading it over the bottom of each foot.

When applying essential oils to yourself, use 1 to 2 drops of oil on two to three locations twice a day. Increase to four times a day if needed. Rub the oil and allow it to absorb for two to three minutes before applying another oil or getting dressed to avoid staining clothing.

As a general rule, when applying oils to yourself or another person for the first time, do not apply more than 2 singles or blends at one time.

When mixing carrier oil with essential oils, it is best to use containers made of glass or earthenware, rather than plastic. Plastic particles can leach into the oil and then into the skin once it is applied.

Massage

Start by applying 2 drops of a single oil or blend on location and massaging in. If working on a large area, such as the back, mix 1-3 drops of the selected essential oil into one teaspoon of pure carrier oil (such as V-6 Mixing Oil or Massage Oil Base).

Please keep in mind that many massage oils, such as olive, jojoba, or wheat germ oil may stain some fabrics.

Acupuncture

Licensed doctors can dramatically increase the effectiveness of acupuncture by using essential oils. To start, place several drops of essential oil into the palm of your hand. Dip the needle tip into the oil before inserting the needle. You can pre-mix several oils in your hand if you wish to use more than one oil.

Acupressure

When performing acupressure treatment, apply 1 to 3 drops of essential oil to the acupressure point with a finger. Using an auricular probe with a slender point to dispense oil can enhance the application. Start by pressing firmly and releasing. Avoid applying pressure to any particular pressure point too long. You may continue along the acupressure points and meridians or use the reflexology or Vita Flex points as well. Once you have completed small point stimulation, massage the general area with the oil.

Hot Packs

For deeper penetration of an essential oil, use hot packs. Start by dipping a cloth in comfortably hot water. Wring the cloth out and place it on location. After allowing it to cool, wrap it loosely with another dry towel or blanket to seal in the heat. Use this technique 1-3 times daily as needed.

Cold Packs

Apply essential oils on location, followed by cold water or ice packs when treating inflamed or swollen tissues. Frozen packages of peas or corn make excellent ice packs that will mold to the contours of the body part and will not leak. Keep the cold pack on until the swelling diminishes. For neurological problems, always use cold packs, never hot.

Layering

This technique consists of applying multiple oils one at a time. For example, place marjoram over a sore muscle, massage into the tissue gently until the area is dry, then apply the next oil, such as peppermint, until the oil is absorbed and skin is dry. Then layer on the third oil, such as basil.

Creating a Compress

- Rub 1-3 drops on location, diluted or neat, depending on the oil used and the skin sensitivity at that location.

- Cover with a hot, damp towel.

- Cover the moist towel with a dry towel for 10-60 minutes, depending on the need.

As the oil penetrates the skin, you may experience a warming or even a burning sensation, especially in areas where the greatest benefits occur. If burning becomes uncomfortable, apply a massage oil, V-6 Mixing Oil, or any pure vegetable oil to the location.

A second type of application is very mild and is even suitable for infants, children, or those with sensitive skin.

- Place 5 to 15 drops of essential oil into a basin filled with warm water.

- Vigorously agitate the water and let it stand for 1 minute.

- Water temperature should be approximately 100°F (38°C), unless the patient suffers neurological conditions; in this case, use cool water.

- Place a dry face cloth on top of the water to soak up oils that have floated to the surface.

- Wring out the water and apply the cloth on the location. To seal in warmth, cover with a thick towel for no more than 1 hour.

Bath

Adding essential oils to bath water is challenging because oil does not mix with water. For even dispersion, drop in the oils while running the bath, or add 2 to 3 drops of oil to a cup of Epsom salts or bath gel base and pass this mixture under the faucet. Either method will help the oils disperse evenly and prevent stronger oils from stinging sensitive areas.

You can also use premixed bath gels containing essential oils as a liquid soap in the shower or bath. Lather down with the bath gel, let it soak in, and then rinse. To maximize benefits, leave them on the skin or scalp for several minutes to allow the essential oils to penetrate. You can create your own aromatic bath gels by placing 5 to 15 drops of essential oil in 1/2 ounce of unscented bath gel base.

Shower

Essential oils may be added to bath or Epsom salts and used in the shower. The RainSpa shower head contains a special attached receptacle that may be loaded with essential oil salts. This allows essential oils to not only make contact with the skin but also diffuses the fragrance of the oils into the air. The shower head receptacle can hold approximately 1/4 to 1/2 cup of bath salts.

Start by adding several drops of essential oil to 1/4 cup of bath salt and filling the shower head receptacle. This should provide enough material for about 2 to 3 showers. The RainSpa shower head has a bypass feature that allows the user to switch from bath salt water to regular tap water.

How to Enhance the Benefits of Topical Application

The longer essential oils stay in contact with the skin, the more likely they are to be absorbed. Rose Ointment or AromaSilk Satin Body Lotion may be layered on top of the essential oils to reduce evaporation of the oils and enhance penetration. It also helps seal and protect cuts and wounds.

Other Uses

Inhalation

Direct

- Place 2 or more drops into the palm of the left hand, and rub clockwise with the right hand.

- Cup hands together over the nose and mouth and inhale deeply.

- Add several drops of an essential oil to a bowl of hot (not boiling) water.

- Inhale the vapors that rise from the bowl.

- To increase the intensity of the oil vapors inhaled, place a towel over the head and bowl.

- Apply oils to a cotton ball, tissue, or handkerchief (do not use synthetic fibers or fabric).

- Inhale directly.

Indirect or Subtle Inhalation (wearing as a perfume or cologne)

- Rub 2 or more drops of oil on your chest, neck, upper sternum, wrists, or under nose and ears.

- Breathe in the fragrance throughout the day.

Diffusing

Diffused oils alter the structure of molecules that create odors, rather than just masking them. They also increase oxygen availability and produce negative ions. Many essential oils, such as lemon, Purification, Citrus Fresh, and Thieves, are highly antibacterial and are extremely effective for eliminating and destroying airborne germs and bacteria.

A cold-air diffuser is designed to atomize a microfine mist of essential oils into the air, where they can remain suspended for up to several hours. Unlike aroma lamps or candles, it disperses oils without the heating or burning, which can render the oil therapeutically less beneficial and even create toxic compounds. Research shows (Chao, 1997) that cold air diffusing certain oils may:

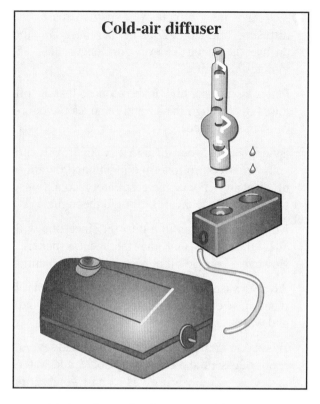

Cold-air diffuser

- Reduce bacteria, fungus, mold, and unpleasant odors.

- Relax the mind and body, relieve tension, and clear the mind.

- Help with weight management.

- Improve concentration, alertness, and mental clarity.

- Stimulate neurotransmitters.

- Stimulate secretion of endorphins.

- Stimulate growth hormone production and receptivity.

- Digest petrochemicals on the receptor sites.

- Improve the secretion of IgA antibodies that fight candida.

- Improve digestive function.

- Improve hormonal balance.

- Relieve headaches.

- Dispel odors.

23

Start by diffusing oils for 15-30 minutes a day. As you become accustomed to the oils and recognize their effects, you may increase the diffusing time to 1-2 hours per day. Do not diffuse the blend Thieves for longer than 15 minutes at a time.

Place the diffuser high in the room so that the oil mist falls through the air and removes the odor-causing substances.

By connecting your diffuser to a timer, you can gain better control over the length and duration of diffusing. For some respiratory conditions, you may diffuse the oils through the night.

Do not mix blends in a diffuser since this will alter the smell and the therapeutic benefit. However, a single oil may be added to a blend.

Always wash diffuser before using a different oil blend. Use ethyl (grain) alcohol or natural soap and water.

If you don't have a diffuser, you may add several drops of essential oil to a spray bottle, add water, and shake. You can use this to mist your entire house, work place, or car.

To freshen air, use the following blend:

- 20 drops lavender
- 10 drops lemon
- 6 drops bergamot
- 5 drops lime
- 5 drops grapefruit

Diffuse or put in 1/2 oz. of distilled water in a spray bottle; shake well.

OTHER EASY WAYS TO DIFFUSE OILS

- Add essential oils to cedar chips to make your own potpourri.

- Put scented cedar chips in closets or drawers to deodorize them.

- Place any conifer essential oil onto each log in the fireplace. As they burn, they will disperse a lovely smell. This method has little therapeutic benefit.

- Put essential oil on cotton balls and put in car or home air vents

- Place a bowl of water with a few drops of oil on a wood stove.

- Dampen a cloth, apply essential oils to it, and place it near the intake duct of your heating and cooling system.

Humidifier and Vaporizer

Essential oils like peppermint, lemon, and frankincense make ideal additions to humidifiers or vaporizers.

Vaginal Retention Implant

For systemic conditions, such as candida, a vaginal implant is one of the best ways to absorb essential oils into the body.

- Place 10-20 drops of essential oil into a tablespoon of carrier oil.

- Use a small syringe to implant the mixture into the vagina and retain it overnight.

- To use a capsule, place oils in the capsule and implant immediately after the oils are added.

- A pad or tampon may need to be used to aid in the retention of the essential oil solution.

Rectal Implant and Retention Enema

Enemas and rectal implants are the most efficient ways to deliver essential oils to the urinary tract and reproductive organs. Always use sterile applicator.

- Mix 20-35 drops of essential oil in a teaspoon of carrier oil.

- Place mixture in a small syringe and inject into the rectum.

- Retain mixture through the night (or longer for best results).

- Clean and disinfect applicator after each use.

Water Distillers and Filters

You can apply oils like peppermint, lemon, clove, and cinnamon to the post-filter side of your water purifier. This will help purify the water.

Dishwashing Soap

To add fragrance or improve the antiseptic action of your soap, add several drops of essential oils such as lavender, lemon, bergamot, and orange.

Cleaning and Disinfecting

A few drops of oil may be added to the dishwasher to help disinfect and purify. Some popular oils are lemon and peppermint, although any antibacterial oil would work well.

Painting

When painting, add a 5 ml. bottle of your favorite essential oil, such as White Angelica, Abundance, or Sacred Mountain, to 1 gallon of paint. Mix well. The oil will counteract the unpleasant smell of paint. Because essential oils are not fatty oils, they will leave no oil spots on the walls.

Laundry

Essential oils may be used to enhance the cleanliness and fragrance of your laundry. As unpleasant as it seems, dust mites live in your bedding, feeding from the dead skin cells you constantly shed. Recent research has shown that eucalyptus oil kills dust mites. To achieve effective dust mite control, add 25 drops of eucalyptus to each load, or approximately 1/2 ounce to a bottle of liquid laundry detergent.

Instead of using toxic and irritating softening agents in the dryer, place a washcloth dampened with 10 drops of lavender, lemon, melaleuca, bergamot, or other oils . While the oils will not reduce static cling, they will impart a distinctive fragrance to the clothes.

In addition, because clothing (like everything else) has a frequency, consider moving toward natural fabrics instead of synthetics. Cotton, linen, silk, and wool possess energy frequencies harmonious to the human body.

Surface Cleansers: Counters, Furniture, etc.

Instead of purchasing standard household cleaners for surfaces, you can create your own natural, safe version by filling a plastic spray bottle with water and a squirt of dishwashing soap. Add 3 to 5 drops each of lavender, lemon, and pine essential oils. Shake the spray bottle well, and your homemade cleaner is ready to spray. This simple solution is extremely economical, yet it cleans and disinfects as well as any commercial cleaner.

Please keep in mind that some of the oils used directly may stain some surfaces, such as linoleum.

Additional antibacterial and antiviral oils that are excellent for cleaning include cinnamon, clove, eucalyptus, thyme, spruce, lemongrass, and grapefruit.

Floors and Carpet

By combining essential oils with common household products, you can create your own nontoxic aromatic floor and carpet cleaners.

To clean hard floors, add 1/4 cup of white vinegar to a bucket of water. Then add 5-10 drops of lemon, pine, spruce, melaleuca, Purification, or another suitable oil. If the floor is especially dirty, add several drops of dishwashing soap. This will clean even the dirtiest floor.

To make a carpet freshener, add sixteen to twenty drops of essential oils to a cup of baking soda or borax powder. Mix well and place in a covered container overnight so that the oil can be absorbed. Sprinkle over your carpet the next day and then vacuum the powder up.

You may also saturate a disposable cloth or tissue with several drops of essential oil and place it into the collecting bag of your vacuum. This will diffuse a pleasant odor as you clean. If your vacuum collects dirt into water, simply add a few drops into the water reservoir before cleaning. This refreshes both the carpet and the room.

Insecticide and Repellent: Dust Mites, Fleas, Ticks, Ants, Spiders, etc.

Many of us use synthetic chemicals to deal with insects. Essential oils and oil blends, such as lavender, lemon, peppermint, lemongrass, cypress, eucalyptus globulus, cinnamon, thyme, basil, Thieves, Purification, and citronella, effectively repel many types of insects including mites, lice, and fleas. Peppermint placed on entryways prevents ants from entering.

If you need moth repellents for your linens and woolens, avoid toxic commercial mothballs made of naphthalene. Natural essential oils, like citronella, lavender, lemongrass, Canadian red cedar, or rosemary, can just as effectively repel moths and other insects. You can make a sachet by placing several drops of essential oil on a cotton ball. Wrap and tie this in a small handkerchief or square of cotton. Hang this cloth in storage areas or add it to your chest of linens. Refresh as often as necessary.

You can put this sachet in your bureau drawers to keep your clothes freshly scented. Lavender and rose are classic scents. For children's sleepwear, Roman chamomile is especially fragrant and relaxing. To scent stationery, stretch out a scented cotton ball and place in an envelope.

Hot Tubs and Saunas

Hot tubs, jacuzzis, and saunas act as reservoirs for germs, especially if used frequently. Lavender, cinnamon, clove, eucalyptus, thyme, lemon, or grapefruit can be used to disinfect and fragrance the water. Use 3 drops per person. For saunas, add several drops of rosemary, thyme, pine, or lavender to a spray bottle with water and then spray down the surfaces. Scented water can also be used to splash on hot sauna stones.

Deodorizing: Kitchens, Bathrooms, etc.

The kitchen and bathroom are often a source of odors and bacteria. Use the following mixtures to freshen, deodorize, and disinfect the air, work areas, cupboards, bathroom fixtures, sinks, tiles, woodwork, carpets, etc. These blends are safe for the family and the environment.

Since the oils separate easily from water, always shake well and keep on shaking the bottle as you use these mixtures. They will deodorize and clean the air, instead of covering the odors.

Single oils:

• Rosemary with lemon, eucalyptus, and lavender.

Blends:

• Lavender with Purification.

Mix:
• 2 drops rosemary
• 4 drops lemon
• 3 drops eucalyptus
• 4 drops lavender with 1 quart water.

Shake well and put in a spray bottle.

Mix:
• 3 to 4 drops lavender
• 5 to 6 drops Purification with 1 quart water.

Shake well and put in a spray bottle.

Cooking

Many essential oils make excellent food flavorings. They are so concentrated that only 1-2 drops of an essential oil is equivalent to a full bottle of dried herbs.

As a general rule, spice oils impart a far stronger flavor than citrus oils do. For stronger spice oils (such as oregano, nutmeg, cinnamon, marjoram, thyme, or basil), you may choose to dip a toothpick into the oils and stir food with toothpick; therefore, better controlling the amount of essential oil that is put into the food.

Oils that can be used as spices: Basil, cinnamon, clove, fennel, ginger, lemon, lavender, marjoram, mountain savory, nutmeg, oregano, peppermint, rosemary, sage, spearmint, tarragon, and thyme.

For a recipe that serves four to six people, add 1 to 2 drops of an oil and stir in after cooking and just before serving, so the oil does not evaporate.

Cooking uses:

- Salad dressings or salad oil: Lemon, lavender, rosemary, clove, or peppermint in V-6 Mixing Oil.

- Cakes, frosting, puddings, fruit pies: Lavender, lemon, clove, or peppermint.

- Pie Crusts: V-6 Mixing Oil has been reported to produce very flaky crusts.

- Herbal teas: Lavender, lemon, peppermint, and melissa.

- Cool refreshing drink: Lemon or peppermint added to a pitcher of cold water.

- Flavored honey: warm until it becomes a thin liquid, then stir in your favorite oil, such as cinnamon, chamomile, or lemon.

Internal and Oral Use as a Dietary Supplement

All essential oils that are Generally Regarded As Safe (GRAS) or certified as Food Additives (FA) by the FDA may be safely taken internally as dietary supplement. In fact, some oils (valerian, lemon, grapefruit, orange, and tangerine) are more effective when taken orally.

Essential oils should be diluted in vegetable oil, honey, soy milk, or rice milk prior to ingestion. More or less dilution may be required, depending on how strong the oil is. More potent oils, like cinnamon, oregano, lemongrass, and thyme, will require far more dilution than relatively mild oils, like lavender or lemon (which may not need any dilution at all). As a general rule, dilute 1 drop of essential oil in 1 teaspoon of honey or in 4 ounces of a beverage like soy milk or rice milk.

Usually no more than 2 or 3 drops should be ingested at one time (during any four to eight hour period). Because essential oils are so concentrated, 1 to 2 drops are often sufficient to achieve significant benefits.

Essential oils should not be given as dietary supplements to children under six years of age. Parents should exercise caution before orally administering essential oils to any child, and oils should always be diluted prior to ingestion.

Essential oils are extremely concentrated, so they should be kept out of reach of infants and children. If a large quantity of oil is ingested at one time (more than 5 drops), please contact your health care physician or Poison Control Center immediately.

Producing Therapeutic-Grade Essential Oils

Organic Herb Farming

The key to producing oils that are of genuine therapeutic quality starts with the proper cultivation of the herbs in the field.

- Plants should be grown on virgin land uncontaminated by chemical fertilizers, pesticides, fungicides, or herbicides. They should also be grown away from factories and heavily-populated cities, if possible.

- Because robust, healthy plants produce higher quality essential oils, the soil should be nourished with enzymes, minerals, and organic bio-solids. The mineral content of the soil is crucial to the proper development of the plant, and soils that lack minerals result in plants that produce inferior oils.

- Land should be watered with reservoir or water-shed water. Mountain stream water is best because of its purity and high mineral content. Municipally-treated water or secondary run-off water from residential and commercial areas can introduce undesirable chemicals and residues into the plant and the essential oil.

- Different varieties of plants produce different qualities of oils. Only those cultivars that produce the highest quality essential oil should be selected.

- The timing of the harvest is one of the most important factors in the production of therapeutic-grade oils. If the plant is harvested at the wrong time of the season or even at the incorrect time of day, a substandard essential oil can be produced. In some instances, changing harvest time by even a few hours can make a huge difference. For example, German chamomile harvested in the morning will produce an oil with far more azulene (a powerful anti-inflammatory compound) than chamomile harvested in the late afternoon. Other factors that should be taken into consideration during the harvest include the amount of dew on the leaves, the percentage of plant in bloom, and weather conditions during the two weeks prior to harvest.

- To prevent herbs from drying out prior to being distilled, distillers should be located as close to the field as possible. Transporting herbs to distillers hundreds or thousands of miles away heightens the risk of exposure to pollutants, dust, and petrochemical residues.

Steam Distillation

Essential oils can be extracted from the plant by a variety of methods, including solvent extraction, carbon-dioxide extraction, and steam distillation. Steam distillation is one of the most common and has several advantages over other methods.

Steam distillation involves creating steam and sending it into a cooking chamber that holds the raw plant material. As the steam rises, it ruptures the oil membranes in the plant and releases the essential oil. The steam then carries the oil to the condenser, where the oil-water mixture reliquefies. It is then sent to a separator where the oil is separated from the water. The run-off water is called "floral water."

Distillation

Distillation can determine or destroy the value of the oil. The operator of the distiller must have a full understanding of the value of essential oils in order to produce quality oils. If the pressure or temperature is too high, it may change the molecular structure of the fragrance molecule, altering the chemical constituents. For example, the distilling process for lavender should not exceed three pounds of pressure, and temperatures should not exceed 245° F.

However, there are many variants of steam distillation. Subtle differences in distillation equipment and processing conditions can translate into huge differences in essential oil quality. The size of cooking chamber, the type of condenser and separator, and the degree of temperature and pressure can all have a huge impact on the oil. In many respects the way essential oils are steam distilled can enhance or destroy them. Distillation is more than a science; it is an art. If the pressure or temperature is too high, or if the cooking chambers are constructed from reactive metals, the oil may not be therapeutic grade, even though it still may technically be "Grade A."

Vertical steam distillation gives us the greatest potential for protecting the therapeutic benefits and quality of essential oils. In ancient distillation, low pressure (5 pounds or lower) and low temperature were extremely important to produce the therapeutic benefits. Marcel Espieu, president of the Lavender Growers Association in Southern France has long maintained that the best oil quality can only be produced when the pressure is zero pounds during distillation.

Temperature also has a distinct effect. At certain temperatures, the oil fragrance, as well as the chemical constituents, may be altered. High pressures and high temperatures seem to cause a harshness in the oil. Even the oil pH and the electrical polarity are greatly affected.

For example, cypress requires a minimum of 24 hours of distillation at 265° F and 5 pounds of pressure to extract most of the therapeutically-active constituents. If distillation time is cut by only two hours, 18 to 20 constituents will be missing from the oil. However, most cypress is distilled for only 2 hours and 15 minutes. The short distillation times allow the producer to cut costs and produce a cheaper oil, since money is saved on fuel to generate the steam. It also causes less wear and tear on equipment.

In France, lavender produced commercially is often distilled for only 15 to 20 minutes at 155 lbs. of pressure with a steam temperature approaching 350 degrees F. Although this oil costs less and is easily marketed, it is of poor quality. It retains few, if any, of the therapeutic properties of high-grade lavender distilled at zero pounds of pressure for two hours.

In many large commercial operations, distillers introduce chemicals into the steam distillation process to increase the volume of oil produced. Chemical trucks can now pump solvents directly into the boiler water. This expands oil production by as much as 18 percent. These chemicals inevitably leach into the distilling water and mix with the

Pressure/Temperature Chart for Distilling Some Therapeutic-Grade Essential Oils

Essential Oil	Starting Material	Oil Production	Optical Rotation	Pressure in lbs.	Distilling Temp.	Distilling Time
Cypress	2000 lb	1 lb	24	0	220	24 hrs.
Pine	1000 lb	1 lb	2	0	180	8 hrs.
Myrtle	500 kl	1 kl	22	1-2	200	7-9 hrs.
Palmarosa	600 kl	1 kl	6	2	200	4 hrs.
Lemongrass	650 kl	17.5 kl	0	5	230	2.75 hrs.
Citronella	150 lb	1 lb	0	5	225	4.5 hrs.
Rosewood	500 kl	1 kl	-4	30	287	3 hrs.
Cinnamon	1300 lb	5 oz	0	5	225-235	9-24 hrs.
Clove	450 kl	5 lit	0	10	229	18 hrs.
Eucalyptus	250 lb	1 lb	5	5	225	3-18 hrs.
Melaleuca	1000 lb	10-15 lb	3	3	218	2-3 hrs.
Geranium	500 lb	6 lb	-8	1.2	200	1-3 hrs.

essential oil, fracturing the molecular structure of the oil and altering both its fragrance and therapeutic value. These chemicals remain in the oil after it is sold because it is almost impossible to completely separate them from the oil.

Other ways that essential oil producers can increase the quantity of oil extracted is through redistillation. This refers to the repeated distillation of the plant material to maximize the volume of oil by using second, third, and fourth stages of steam distillation, with each distillation generating successively weaker and less potent essential oils. Such essential oils are also degraded due to prolonged exposure to water used in the redistillation; this water can hydrolize or oxidize the oil and begin to chemically break down the constituents responsible for its aroma and therapeutic properties.

Combining Traditional Steam Distillation with Modern Technology

Few people appreciate how chemically complex essential oils are. They are rich tapestries of literally hundreds of chemical components, some of which—even in small quantities—contribute important therapeutic benefits. The key to preserving as many as possible of these delicate aromatic constituents is to steam distill plant material in small batches using low pressure and low heat. This is the traditional method of distillation that has been used for centuries in Europe but is being abandoned in favor of high-volume pressure cookers designed to operate at over 400° F and over 50 pounds of pressure.

Even more important, the cooking chamber where the plants are distilled should be constructed of a non-reactive metal, like stainless steel, to reduce the possibility of the essential oil being chemically altered by more reactive metals such as steel or copper.

No solvents or synthetic chemicals should be used or added to the water used to generate steam because they might jeopardize the integrity of the essential oil. Even the addition of chemicals to water used in the closed-loop heat-exchange systems of the condenser can be dangerous, since there is no guarantee that they can be completely isolated from the essential oil. It is unfortunate that many essential oils distilled commercially are

---

Different Types of Oil Production

Expressed oils are pressed from the rind of fruits, such as grapefruit, lemon, orange, and tangerine. Rich in terpene alcohols, expressed oils are not technically "essential oils," even though they are highly regarded for their therapeutic properties. Expressed oils should only be obtained from organically grown crops, since pesticide residues can become highly concentrated in the oil.

Steam distillation is the oldest and most traditional method of extraction. Plant material is inserted into a cooking chamber, and steam is passed through it. After the steam is collected and condensed, it is run through a separator to collect the oil.

Solvent-extraction involves the use of oil-soluble solvents, such as hexane, dimethylenechloride, and acetone. Because there can be no guarantee that solvent residues will not be found in the finished product, none of Young Living's essential oils are processed using solvent extraction.

Absolutes are technically not "essential oils" but are "essences." They are obtained from the grain alcohol extraction of a concrete, which is the solid waxy residue that is derived from the extraction of plant materials, usually flower petals. This method of extraction is used primarily for botanicals where the fragrance and therapeutic parts of the plant can only be unlocked using solvents. Jasmine and neroli are extracted this way.

---

processed using boiler water laden with chemicals and descaling agents.

Absolutely no pesticides, herbicides, fungicides, or agricultural chemicals of any kind should be used in the cultivation of herbs earmarked for distillation. These chemicals—even in minute quantities—can react with the essential oil and degrade its purity and quality and render it less therapeutically effective. During distillation, pesticide residue leaches into plant material.

Essential Oil Production

Producing pure essential oils is very costly. It often requires several hundred or even thousands of pounds of raw plant material to produce a single pound of essential oil. For example, it takes three tons of melissa to produce one pound of oil. Its extremely low yield explains why it sells for $9,000 to $15,000 a kilo. It takes 5,000 pounds of rose petals to produce one pound of rose oil. It is not difficult to understand why these oils are so expensive.

The vast majority of oils are produced for the perfume industry, which is only interested in their aromatic qualities. High pressure, high temperatures, and the use of chemical solvents are used in this distillation process to produce greater quantities of oil at a faster rate. To many people, these oils smell exquisite but lack true therapeutic properties. Many of the important chemical constituents necessary to produce therapeutic results are either flashed off with the high heat or are not released from the plant material.

The Benefits of Therapeutic-Grade Essential Oils

1. Essential oils are so small in molecular size that they can quickly penetrate the tissues of the skin.

2. Essential oils are lipid soluble and are capable of penetrating cell membranes, even if the membranes have hardened because of an oxygen deficiency. According to Jean Valnet, M.D., essential oils can affect every cell of the body within 20 minutes and are then metabolized like other nutrients.

3. Essential oils contain oxygen molecules which help to transport nutrients to starving human cells. Because a nutritional deficiency is an oxygen deficiency, disease begins when cells lack the oxygen for proper nutrient assimilation. By providing the needed oxygen, essential oils also work to stimulate the immune system.

4. Essential oils are very powerful antioxidants that create an unfriendly environment for damaging free radicals. They may prevent mutations, fungus, and oxidation in cells, and work as free-radical scavengers.

5. Essential oils are antibacterial, anticancerous, antifungal, anti-infectious, antimicrobial, antitumoral, antiparasitic, antiviral, and antiseptic. Some essential oils have been shown to destroy all tested bacteria and viruses while simultaneously restoring physiological balance to the body.

6. Essential oils may detoxify the cells and blood in the body.

7. Essential oils containing sesquiterpenes have the ability to pass the blood-brain barrier.

8. Essential oils are aromatic and when diffused may provide air purification by:

   A. Removing metallic particles and toxins from the air;

   B. Increasing ozone and negative ions in the area, which inhibit bacterial growth;

   C. Eliminating odors from mold, cigarettes, and animals; and

   D. Filling the air with a fresh, aromatic scent.

9. Essential oils promote emotional, physical, and spiritual well being.

10. Essential oils have a bio-electrical frequency that is several times greater than the frequency of herbs, food, and even the human body.

CHAPTER 6

Single Oils

This section describes over 80 single essential oils, including botanical information, therapeutic and traditional uses, and chemical constituents of each oil. Extraction method, safety data, and application instructions are also provided.

How to be Sure Your Essential Oils are Therapeutic Grade

There are many ways to be sure if your essential oils are of the highest quality therapeutic grade. For a better idea of the quality of your oils, answer the following questions about your essential oil and supplier:

Are the fragrances subtle, rich, organic, and delicate? Do they "feel" natural? Do the fragrances of your oils vary from batch to batch as an indication that they are pure and painstakingly distilled in small batches rather than industrially processed on a large scale?

Does your supplier send each batch of essential oils it receives through up to five different chemical analyses before it is released?

Are these tests performed by independent labs?

Does your supplier grow and distill its own organically grown herbs?

Are the distillation facilities part of the farm where the herbs are grown so they are freshly distilled, or do the herbs wait for days to be processed; thereby losing their potency?

Does your supplier use low pressure and low temperature to distill essential oils and preserve all of their fragile chemical constituents? Are the distillation cookers fabricated from costly stainless steel alloys to reduce the likelihood of the oils chemically reacting with metal?

Does your supplier have representatives traveling worldwide to personally inspect the fields and distilleries where the herbs are grown and distilled?

Do they scrutinize the facilities to check that no synthetic chemicals are being used in any of these processes?

How many years has your supplier been doing all of this?

Young Living Essential Oils has taken all of these questions into consideration. Responsible consumers should ask these questions of the providers of their essential oils.

How to Maximize the Shelf Life of Your Essential Oils

The highest quality essential oils are bottled in dark glass. The reason for this is two-fold: glass is more stable than plastic and does not "breathe" the same way plastic does. Also, the darkness of the glass protects the oil from light that may chemically alter or degrade it over time.

After using an essential oil, keep the lid tightly sealed. Bottles that are improperly sealed can result in the loss of some of the lighter, lower-molecular-weight parts of the oil, especially the monoterpenes and sesquiterpenes. In addition, over time, oxygen in the air may react with and oxidize the essential oil.

Store essential oils away from light, especially sunlight. While the amber glass of the oil bottles does afford some protection against visible light, the darker the storage conditions the longer your oil will last.

Store essential oils in a cool location. Excessive heat can derange the molecular structure of the oil the same way ultraviolet light can. This can lead to changes in the fragrance of the essential oil.

Angelica (*Angelica archangelica*)

Botanical Family: Apiaceae or Umbelliferae (parsley)

Plant Origin: France, Belgium

Extraction Method: Steam distilled from root.

Chemical Constituents: Monoterpenes (73%): phellandrene, α– and β-pinenes, limonene (13%); Esters; Terpene alkaloids; Coumarins: bergoptene.

Action: Angelica is anticoagulant and sedating to the nervous system. It reduces inflammation of the intestinal wall. Emotionally, it is calming, assisting in the release of pent-up negative feelings.

Found In: Awaken, Forgiveness, Grounding, Harmony, Passion, and Surrender.

Traditional Uses: Known as the "holy spirit root" or the "oil of angels" by the Europeans, angelica had healing powers so strong that it was believed to be of divine origin. From the time of Paracelsus, it was credited with the ability to protect from the plague. The stems were chewed during the plague of 1660 to prevent infection. When burned, the seeds and roots were thought to purify the air.

Indications: Angelica may help with bruises, colic, coughs, respiratory infections, indigestion, menopause, premenstrual tension, loss of appetite, and rheumatic conditions.

Application: Apply to Vita Flex points of shoulders, on bottom of feet or diffuse.

Fragrant Influence: Angelica brings memories back to the point of origin before trauma or anger was experienced, helping us to release and let go of negative feelings. It is soothing and calming.

Safety Data: If pregnant or under a doctor's care, consult your physician. Avoid if diabetic. Avoid direct sunlight after use.

Companion Oils: Patchouly, vetiver, clary sage, and most citrus oils.

Frequency: Physical and emotional: approximately 85 MHz.

NOTE: Because angelica contains bergopten, it may be photo-sensitizing and should not be applied to skin that will be exposed to direct sunlight or ultraviolet light within 72 hours.

Basil (*Ocimum basilicum*)

Botanical Family: Lamiaceae or Labiatae (mint

Plant Origin: Egypt, India, Utah, France

Extraction Method: Steam distilled from leaves, stems, and flowers.

Chemical Constituents: Methyl chavicol (70-75%), 12-14% linalol; Terpene alcohols: linalol, citronnellol; Terpene esters: fenchyle acetate, linalyl acetate: Phenols: eugenol: Phenols methyl-ethers (90%): methyl chavicol (85-88%), methyl eugenol: Ketones: camphor; Oxides: 1,8 cineol.

Action: Powerful antispasmodic, anti-infectious, antiviral, anti-inflammatory, decongestant (veins, arteries of the lungs, prostate), and antibacterial.

Found In: Aroma Siez, Clarity, and M-Grain

Traditional Uses: Used extensively in traditional Asian Indian medicine, basil's name is derived from "basileum," the Greek name for king. In the 16th century, the powdered leaves were inhaled to treat migraines and chest infections. The Hindu people put basil sprigs on the chests of the dead to protect them from evil spirits. Italian women wore basil to attract possible suitors.

Indications: Migraines, mental fatigue, and scanty menstrual periods.

Other Uses: Basil is relaxing to both striated and smooth muscles, soothing for insect bites, and stimulating to the sense of smell. It may help bronchitis and chest infections.

Application: Apply basil to tip of nose, on temples, and on location of stings and bites. For mental fatigue, inhale first, then apply to crown of head, forehead, heart, and navel. May be added to food or water as a dietary supplement.

Fragrant Influence: Helps with mental fatigue.

Safety Data: If pregnant or under a doctor's care, consult your physician. Do not use if epileptic. Skin test for sensitivity.

Companion Oils: Bergamot, birch, cypress, geranium, lavender, lemongrass, and marjoram.

Frequency: Low (Physical); approximately 52 MHz.

Selected Research:

Fyfe L., et al. "Inhibition of *Listeria monocytogenes* and *Salmonella enteriditis* by combinations of plant oils and derivatives of benzoic acid: the development of synergistic antimicrobial combinations." *Int J Antimicrob Agents*. 1997;9(3):195-9.

Wan J, et al. "The effect of essential oils of basil on the growth of *Aeromonas hydrophila* and *Pseudomonas fluorescens*." *J Appl Microbiol*. 1998;84(2):152-8.

Lachowicz KJ, et al. "The synergistic preservative effects of the essential oils of sweet basil (*Ocimum basilicum* L.) against acid-tolerant food microflora." *Lett Appl Microbiol*. 1998;26(3):209-14.

Bergamot *(Citrus bergamia)*

Botanical Family: Rutaceae (citrus)

Plant Origin: Italy, Ivory Coast

Extraction Method: Pressed from the rind Rectified and void of terpenes. Produced by solvent extraction or vacuum distilled.

Chemical Constituents: Monoterpenes, α-pinene, Aldehydes: citrals (45%); Furocoumarins.

Action: Calming, antiseptic, anti-infectious, anti-inflammatory, hormonal support, antibacterial.

Found In: Awaken, Clarity, Dream Catcher, Forgiveness, Gentle Baby, Harmony, Joy, and White Angelica.

Traditional Uses: It is believed that Christopher Columbus brought bergamot to Bergamo in Northern Italy from the Canary Islands. A mainstay in traditional Italian medicine, bergamot has been used in the Middle East for hundreds of years for skin conditions associated with an oily complexion. Bergamot is responsible for the distinctive flavor of the renowned Earl Grey Tea, and was used in the first genuine eau de cologne.

Indications: Stress, loss of appetite, indigestion, agitation, depression, infection, inflammation, intestinal parasites, rheumatism, insomnia, vaginal candida, and as an insect repellent.

Other Uses: Bergamot may help bronchitis, cold sores, oily complexion, anxiety, nervous tension, coughs, urinary tract infections, respiratory infection, sore throat, thrush, and tonsillitis. Jean Valnet, M.D., recommends it as an antidepressant and to regulate appetite.

Application: Diffuse, apply to forehead, on temples, and on location of stings and bites. Apply where you would a deodorant. May be added to food or water as a dietary supplement.

Fragrant Influence: It may help to relieve anxiety, stress, and tension, and has many constituents contributing refreshing, mood-lifting qualities.

Safety Data: If pregnant or under a doctor's care, consult your physician. *Citrus bergamia* is *very* photo-sensitizing and should NOT be applied to skin that will be exposed to direct sunlight or ultraviolet light within 72 hours.

Birch *(Betula alleghaniensis)*

Botanical Family: Betulaceae

Plant Origin: Canada, Scandinavia

Extraction Method: Steam distilled from wood.

Chemical Constituents: Esters: methyl salicylate (89%)

Action: Analgesic, antispasmodic, anti-inflammatory, liver stimulant, and supports bone function.

Found In: PanAway and Raven

Traditional Uses: The American Indians and early European settlers flavored their tea with birch bark. Birch's main constituent, methyl salicylate, is also found in willow trees and is similar to the salicylic acid used in aspirin.

Indications: Arthritis, rheumatism, inflammation, muscular pain, tendonitis, hypertension, and for cramps. Contains an active principle similar to cortisone and is beneficial for bone, muscle, and joint discomfort.

Other Uses: Birch oil may be beneficial for cystitis, acne, bladder infection, gout, gall-stones, edema, eczema, osteoporosis, skin diseases, ulcers, and urinary tract disorders.

Application: Birch oil is safest to apply after diluting with massage oil or V-6 Mixing Oil. It also may be applied neat to the bottom of the feet. For baths, add 3 to 5 drops to bath water with 1/2 oz. of Bath Gel Base.

Fragrant Influence: It stimulates and increases awareness in all levels of the sensory system.

Safety Data: If pregnant or under a doctor's care, consult your physician. Do not use if epileptic. Skin test for allergies.

Companion Oils: Basil, cypress, geranium, juniper, lavender, lemongrass, marjoram, peppermint, and Roman chamomile.

Cajeput *(Melaleuca leucadendra)*

Botanical Family: Myrtaceae (myrtle)

Chemical Constituents: Cineol (45-70%); Aldehydes: benzoic, butyric, valeric; Monoterpenes: pinene; Terpene Alcohols: terpineol.

Action: Antimicrobial, analgesic (mild), antispasmodic, antineuralgic, antiseptic (pulmonary, urinary, and intestinal), insecticidal, and as an expectorant.

Traditional Uses: In Malaysia and other Indonesian islands, cajeput was used for respiratory infections, headaches, rheumatism, toothache, skin conditions, throat infections, and sore muscles. Cajeput derives its name from the Malaysian word for white tree.

Indications: Cajeput may help with arthritis, acne, respiratory infections, asthma, bronchitis, urinary complaints, coughs, cystitis, stiff joints, toothache, hay fever, bursitis, headaches, insect bites, intestinal problems, laryngitis, dysentery, psoriasis, rheumatism, sinusitis, oily skin, sore throat, and viral infections.

Application: Diffuse or rub on bottom of feet.

Safety Data: If pregnant or under a doctor's care, consult your physician. Use with caution. Do not use synthetic cajeput, as it could cause further blistering and skin eruption. Skin test for sensitivity.

Companion Oils: Birch, eucalyptus, juniper, and peppermint.

Canadian Red Cedar *(Thuja plicata)*

Botanical Family: Cupressaceae (Cypress)

Plant Origin: Canada

Extraction Method: Steam distilled from bark and sawdust.

Chemical Constituents: Thujle acid methyl ester, Terpinen-4-ol, Sesquiterpene: β−caryophylline; Monoterpene ester: Linalyl acetate.

Action: Antifungal, antibacterial, hair follicle stimulator, antiparasitic, and insect repellent.

Traditional Uses: It was used traditionally by the Native American Indians to help them enter a higher spiritual realm. They used it to stimulate the scalp and as an antimicrobial and antiseptic agent.

Application: Diffuse. Apply on crown of head or on location.

Safety Data: If pregnant or under a doctor's care, consult your physician.

Cardamom *(Elettaria cardamomum)*

Botanical Family: Zingiberaceae (ginger)

Chemical Constituents: Monoterpenes: sabinene, mycene, limonene; monoterpenols; linalol, terpinene; Esters (40%); linalyle acetate (3.4%), terpenal acetate (30-45%); Terpene oxides (45%): 1.9 ceneole (40-45%).

Action: Antispasmodic (neuro muscular), antibacterial, expectorant, anti-infectious, and combats worms.

Found In: Clarity

Traditional Uses: Cardamom has been used for paralysis, rheumatism, cardiac disorders, epilepsy, spasms, pulmonary disease, digestive, intestinal, and urinary complaints.

Indications: Cardamom may help with indigestion, loss of appetite, coughs, debility, halitosis, mental fatigue, headaches, heartburn, nausea, and sciatica. It may also alleviate menstrual problems and irregularities.

Application: Diffuse, rub on bottom of feet, stomach, solar plexus, and thighs.

Fragrant Influence: Uplifting, refreshing, and invigorating.

Safety Data: If pregnant or under a doctor's care, consult your physician.

Companion Oils: Bergamot, cedarwood, cinnamon, cistus, clove, neroli, orange, rose, and ylang ylang.

Cassia *(Cinnamomum cassia)*

Botanical Family: Lauraceae (laurel)

Plant Origin: China

Extraction Method: Steam distilled from bark.

Chemical Constituents: t-cinnamaldehyde, Benzaldehyde, t-cinamyl acetate, t-cinnamic alcohol.

Action: Antibacterial, antiviral, and antifungal.

Found In: Exodus II

Safety Data: If pregnant or under a doctor's care, consult your physician.

NOTE: While its aroma is similar to cinnamon, cassia is chemically and physically quite different.

Cedarwood *(Cedrus atlantica)*

Botanical Family: Pinaceae (pine)

Plant Origin: Morocco, USA. *Cedrus atlantica* is the species most closely related to the biblical Cedars of Lebanon.

Extraction Method: Steam distilled from bark.

Chemical Constituents: Sesquiterpenes (50%): Sesquiterpenols (30%); Sesquiterpenones (20%).

Action: Mildly antiseptic, cedarwood may be effective against hair loss (alopecia areata), tuberculosis, bronchitis, gonorrhea, and skin disorders such as acne and psoriasis. It can reduce hardening of artery walls. It is high in sesquiterpenes which can stimulate the limbic region of the brain (the center of our emotions). It also may help stimulate the pineal gland, which releases melatonin, an antioxidant hormone associated with deep sleep.

Found In: Brain Power, Grounding, Inspiration, Into The Future, Passion, Sacred Mountain, and SARA.

Traditional Uses: Throughout antiquity, cedarwood has been used in medicines and cosmetics. The Egyptians used it for embalming the dead. It was used as both a traditional medicine and incense in Tibet. It is recognized for its calming, purifying properties and is used to benefit the skin and underlying tissues.

Indications: Bronchitis, anger/hysteria, hair loss, arteriosclerosis, diuretic, tuberculosis, calming, nervous tension, and urinary infections.

Other Uses: Cedarwood may help with acne, anxiety, arthritis, congestion, coughs, cystitis, dandruff, psoriasis, purification, respiratory system, sinusitis, skin diseases, and fluid retention. It may help open the pineal gland. It also helps to reduce skin oilness.

Application: Diffuse or apply topically on location.

Safety Data: If pregnant or under a doctor's care, consult your physician.

Companion Oils: Bergamot, cypress, eucalyptus, juniper, and rosemary.

Bible References: (see additional Bible references in Appendix D)

Leviticus 14:4— "Then shall the priest command to take for him that is to be cleansed two birds alive [and] clean, and cedar wood, and scarlet, and hyssop."

Leviticus 14:6— "As for the living bird, he shall take it, and the cedar wood, and the scarlet, and the hyssop, and shall dip them and the living bird in the blood of the bird [that was] killed over the running water."

Leviticus 14:49— "And he shall take to cleanse the house two birds, and cedar wood, and scarlet, and hyssop."

Selected Research:

Hay IC, et al. "Randomized trial of aromatherapy. Successful treatment for alopecia areata." *Arch Dermatol.* 1998;134(11):1349-52.

Chamomile (German) *(Matricaria recutita)*

Botanical Family: Asteraceae or Compositae (daisy)

Plant Origin: Utah, Egypt, Hungary

Extraction Method: Steam distilled from flowers.

Chemical Constituents: Sesquiterpenes: chamazulene; Sesquiterpenols: α bisabolol, farnesol; Sesquiterpene oxides; Sesquiterpenes lactones; Coumarins; Ethers.

Action: Sedating, calming, anti-inflammatory, antispasmodic, decongestant. It supports digestive, liver and gallbladder function, reduces scarring, and relieves allergies.

Found In: EndoFlex and Surrender.

Traditional Uses: German chamomile has been highly esteemed for over 3,000 years and has been used for many types of skin conditions and stress-related complaints.

Indications: Insomnia, nervous tension, stress, bursitis, tendonitis, inflammation, carpal tunnel syndrome, headaches, acne, liver and gallbladder disease, parasites, and ulcers.

Other Uses: German chamomile is a cleanser of the blood, helps increase liver function and secretion, and supports the pancreas. German chamomile promotes the regeneration of skin and can be used for abscesses, burns, rashes, cuts, dermatitis, teething pains, acne, eczema, chronic gastritis, infected nails, cystitis, inflamed joints, menopausal problems, sores, skin disorders, stress-related complaints, toothaches, ulcers, and wounds.

Application: Diffuse, add to food or water as a dietary supplement, or apply topically on location. Among the gentlest oils used in aromatherapy, the chamomiles are suitable for use on children.

Fragrant Influence: Dispels anger, stabilizes emotions, and helps release emotions linked to the past. It may also be used to soothe and clear the mind.

Safety Data: If pregnant or under a doctor's care, consult your physician.

Companion Oils: Birch, fir, geranium, helichrysum, hyssop, lavender, lemongrass, marjoram, melaleuca, sandalwood, spearmint, and spruce.

Frequency: Emotional; approximately 105 MHz.

Chamomile (Roman) *(Chamaemelum nobile)*

Botanical Family: Asteraceae or Compositae (daisy)

Plant Origin: Utah, Egypt

Extraction Method: Steam distilled from flowers.

Chemical Constituents: Alcohols terpenes; Esters (75-80%); acetates, isobutyrate d'isobutyle; Terpene ketones; pinocarvone (13%); Lactones sesquiterpenes.

Action: Calming for preanesthesia and tension, antispasmodic, anti-inflammatory, antiparasitic, and skin regeneration.

Found In: Awaken, Clarity, Forgiveness, Gentle Baby, Harmony, Joy, JuvaFlex, Motivation, M-Grain, and Surrender

Traditional Uses: Roman chamomile is used extensively in Europe for the skin. For centuries, mothers have used chamomile to calm crying children, ease earaches, reduce fevers, soothe stomachaches and indigestion, and relieve toothaches and teething pain.

Indications: It may help calm and relieve restlessness and tension. Its anti-infectious properties benefit cuts, scrapes, and bruises.

Other Uses: Roman chamomile neutralizes allergies and increases the ability of the skin to regenerate. It is a cleanser of the blood and also helps the liver discharge poisons. This oil may help with allergies, bruises, cuts, depression, insomnia, muscle tension, nerves (calming and promoting nerve health), restless legs, and skin conditions, such as acne, dermatitis, eczema, rashes, and sensitive skin. It can effectively minimize irritability and nervousness in hyperactive children.

Application: Diffuse, apply topically on bottom of feet, ankles, wrists or on location. Add to food or water as a dietary supplement. Among the gentlest oils used in aromatherapy, all of the chamomiles are suitable for use on children.

Fragrant Influence: Because it is calming and relaxing, it can combat depression, insomnia, and stress. It minimizes anxiety, irritability, and nervousness. It may also dispel anger, stabilize the emotions, and help to release emotions that are linked to the past.

Safety Data: If pregnant or under a doctor's care, consult your physician. Test for skin sensitivity.

Companion Oils: Clary sage, geranium, lavender, or rose.

Cinnamon Bark (*Cinnamomum verum*)

Botanical Family: Lauraceae (laurel)

Plant Origin: Sri Lanka, Madagascar, India

Extraction Method: Steam distilled from bark.

Chemical Constituents: Esters; Phenols; Aldehydes arom.: cinnamaldehyde (63-76%), hydroxycinnamald; Coumarins.

Action: Highly antimicrobial, anti-infectious, antibacterial for large spectrum of infection, antiviral, antifungal (candida), general tonic, sexual stimulant, increases blood flow when previously restricted, and light anticoagulant.

Found In: Abundance, Christmas Spirit, Exodus II, Gathering, Magnify Your Purpose, and Thieves.

Traditional Uses: Cinnamon bark is one of the most antimicrobial essential oils. It has been produced in Sri Lanka for over 2,000 years. Research has found that pathogenic microorganisms cannot live in the presence of cinnamon oil (Yousef, 1980).

Indications: Sexual stimulant, tropical infection, typhoid, and vaginitis.

Other Uses: This oil may be beneficial for circulation, infections, coughs, exhaustion, respiratory infections, digestion, rheumatism, and warts. This oil also fights viral and infectious diseases.

Application: Diffuse, apply topically on bottom of feet, ankles, and wrists. May be added to food or water as a dietary supplement.

Fragrant Influence: Thought to attract wealth.

Safety Data: If pregnant or under a doctor's care, consult your physician. Repeated use can result in extreme contact sensitization. Skin test for sensitivity. Diffuse with caution; cinnamon may irritate the nasal membranes if it is inhaled directly from the diffuser.

Companion Oils: All citrus oils, frankincense, cypress, juniper, geranium, lavender, rosemary, and all spice oils.

Bible Reference: (see additional Bible references in Appendix D)

Exodus 30:23 — "Take thou also unto thee principal spices, of pure myrrh five hundred [shekels], and of sweet cinnamon half so much, [even] two hundred and fifty [shekels], and of sweet calamus two hundred and fifty [shekels]…"

Proverbs 7:17 — "I have perfumed my bed with myrrh, aloes, and cinnamon."

Song of Solomon 4:14 — "Spikenard and saffron; calamus and cinnamon, with all trees of frankincense; myrrh and aloes, with all the chief spices:"

Selected Research:

Tantaoui-Elaraki A, et al. "Inhibition of growth and aflatoxin production in *Aspergillus parasiticus* by essential oils of selected plant materials." *J Environ Pathol Toxicol Oncol.* 1994;13(1):67-72.

Cistus (Cistus ladanifer)

Botanical Family: Cistaceae

Plant Origin: France, Spain

Extraction Method: Steam distilled from branches.

Chemical Constituents: Monoterpenes; α pinene (50%), camphene (4%); Aldehydes; Centones.

Action: Anti-infectious, antiviral, antibacterial, powerful antihemorraging agent, helps reduce inflammation, neurotonic for the sympathetic nervous system.

Found In: ImmuPower

Traditional Uses: Cistus is also known as "rock rose" and has been studied for its effects on the regeneration of cells.

Indications: Bronchitis, respiratory infections, coughs, rhinitis, urinary infections, wounds, and wrinkles.

Other Uses: Cistus may strengthen and support the immune system (due to phenol action).

Application: Diffuse or apply topically mixed with massage oil.

Fragrant Influence: Calming to the nerves, elevates the emotions.

Safety Data: If pregnant or under a doctor's care, consult your physician.

Companion Oils: Bergamot, clary sage, cypress, juniper, lavender, lavandin, patchouly, pine, sandalwood, and vetiver.

Citronella (Cymbopogon nardus)

Botanical Family: Poaceae or Gramineae (grasses)

Plant Origin: Sri Lanka, Philippines, Egypt

Extraction Method: Steam distilled from leaves.

Chemical Constituents: Terpene alcohols (35%): geraniol (18%), borneol (6%), citronnellol (8%); Aldehydes (5-15%): citronnellal (5%); Esters (9%); Phenols (9%): methyl isoeugenol (7%).

Action: Antibacterial, insect-repellent, antifungal, anti-inflammatory, antiseptic, antispasmodic, deodorant, and insecticidal.

Found In: Purification

Traditional Uses: Various cultures have used this oil to treat intestinal parasites, digestive and menstrual problems, and as a stimulant.

Indications: Citronella oil may alleviate headaches, respiratory infections, neuralgia, fatigue, oily skin, and headaches.

Other Uses: This oil can be used as an antiseptic to sanitize and deodorize surfaces. It makes an excellent insect repellent when combined with cedarwood.

Application: Diffuse or apply topically on bottom of feet or on location diluted with massage oil.

Fragrant Influence: Insecticidal and soothing to the tissues.

Safety Data: If pregnant or under a doctor's care, consult your physician. Repeated use can result in extreme contact sensitization. Skin test for sensitivity.

Companion Oils: Bergamot, cedarwood, geranium, lemon, orange, and pine.

Clary Sage (Salvia sclarea)

Botanical Family: Lamiaceae or Labiatae (mint)

Plant Origin: Utah, France

Extraction Method: Steam distilled from flowering plant.

Chemical Constituents: Contains over 250 constituents: Monoterpenes: α and β-pinenes, camphene, myrcene, limonene; Sesquiterpenes; Monoterpenols (15%): linalol (6-16%), terpinene; Sesquiterpenols; Diterpenols: sclareol; Terpene esters (75%): linalyle acetate (62-75%); Ethers; oxides: 1,8 cineol, linalol oxide; Ketones; Aldehydes; Coumarins.

Clary sage distilled in Utah contains 5-7% sclareol.

Action: Antidiabetic, helps reduce high cholesterol, estrogen-like, supports hormones, anti-infectious, antifungal, antispasmodic, relaxing, antibacterial, may help with epilepsy, menopause, and PMS.

Found In: Dragon Time, Into the Future, and Passion

Traditional Uses: The name "clary" sage came from the nickname "clear eyes," given in the Middle Ages, for its ability to cure eye conditions.

Indications: Treats bronchitis, cholesterol, hemorrhoids, hormonal imbalance, insomnia, intestinal cramps, menstrual cramps, PMS, premenopause, and weak digestion.

Other Uses: This oil may be used for menstrual problems, depression, headaches, dandruff, insect bites, insomnia, kidney disorders, dry skin, throat reaction, ulcers, circulatory problems, and whooping cough.

Application: Diffuse, apply topically on bottom of feet, ankles, and wrists. May be added to food or water as a dietary supplement.

Fragrant Influence: Enhances one's ability to dream and is very calming and stress-relieving.

Safety Data: If pregnant or under a doctor's care, consult your physician. Use caution with infants and children.

Companion Oils: Bergamot, cedarwood, citrus oils, cypress, geranium, juniper, lavender, and sandalwood.

Clove *(Syzygium aromaticum)*

Botanical Family: Myrtaceae (myrtle)

Plant Origin: Madagascar, Spice Islands

Extraction Method: Steam distilled from bud and stem.

Chemical Constituents: Eugenol Acetate, β–Caryophyllene, α-Humelene

Action: Highly antimicrobial, antiseptic, analgesic, bactericidal, antioxidant, hemostatic (blood thinning), anti-inflammatory.

Found In: Abundance, En-R-Gee, ImmuPower, Melrose, PanAway, and Thieves

Traditional Uses: The people on the island if Ternate were free from epidemics until the sixteenth century, when Dutch conquerors destroyed the clove trees that flourished on the islands. Many of the islanders died from the epidemics that followed. Eugenol, clove's principal constituent, is used in the dental industry for the numbing of gums. Courmont et al. demonstrated that a solution of .05% eugenol from clove oil was sufficient to kill the tuberculosis bacillus (Gattefossé 1990).

Indications: Infectious diseases, intestinal parasites, tuberculosis, respiratory infections, pain, toothache, scabies, and wounds (infected).

Other Uses: According to Jean Valnet, M.D., clove oil can prevent contagious disease and may treat arthritis, bronchitis, cholera, cystitis, dental infection, amoebic dysentery, diarrhea, tuberculosis, acne, fatigue, thyroid dysfunction, halitosis, headaches, hypertension, insect bites, nausea, neuritis, dermatitis, rheumatism, sinusitis, skin cancer, chronic skin disease, bacterial colitis, sores (speeds healing of mouth and skin sores), viral hepatitis, warts, and lymphoma.

Application: Diffuse, apply topically diluted with massage oil, add one to two drops in four ounces of water and use as a gargle. May be applied neat on palms of hands, bottom of feet, and on gums and teeth. May be added to food or water as a dietary supplement. For oral hygiene, rub directly on the gums surrounding an infected tooth. To break tobacco addiction, place a drop on tongue with finger. For tickling cough, put a drop on back of tongue.

Fragrant Influence: It may influence healing, serve as a mental stimulant, encourage sleep, stimulate dreams, and create a sense of protection and courage.

Safety Data: If pregnant or under a doctor's care, consult your physician. Repeated use can result in contact sensitization. Skin test for sensitivity. Clove essential oil can act as a blood thinner and should be avoided if taking a prescription blood thinner such as Warfarin or Coumarin.

Companion Oils: Basil, bergamot, cinnamon bark, clary sage, clove, grapefruit, lavender, lemon, nutmeg, orange, peppermint, rose, rosemary, and ylang ylang.

Selected Research:

Nishijima H, et al. "Mechanisms mediating the vasorelaxing action of eugenol, a pungent oil, on rabbit arterial tissue." *Jpn J Pharmacol.* 1999 Mar;79(3):327-34.

Jayashree T, et al. "Antiaflatoxigenic activity of eugenol is due to inhibition of lipid peroxidation." *Lett Appl Microbiol.* 1999; 28(3):179-83.

Wie MB, et al. "Eugenol protects neuronal cells from excitotoxic and oxidative injury in primary cortical cultures." *Neurosci Lett.* 1997: 4;225(2):93-6.

Coriander *(Coriandrum sativum)*

Botanical Family: Apiaceae or Umbelliferae (parsley)

Plant Origin: Russia, India

Extraction Method: Steam distilled seeds.

Chemical Constituents: Monoterpenes: Phellandrene; Aldehydes (85-95%); octanal, decanal, undecanal.

Action: Anti-inflammatory, sedative.

Traditional Uses: The seeds were found in the ancient Egyptian tomb of Ramses II. This oil has been researched at Cairo University for its effects in lowering glucose and insulin levels and supporting pancreatic function. It has been studied for its effects in strengthening the pancreas.

Indications: It also has soothing, calming properties.

Other Uses: Coriander may help with arthritis, diarrhea, respiratory infections, indigestion, digestive spasms, poor circulation, rheumatism, gout, infections (general), measles, headaches, nausea, muscular aches and pains, neuralgia, skin conditions (acne, psoriasis and dermatitis), and stress. It may also help during convalescence and after a difficult childbirth. Because of its estrogen content, coriander may regulate and help control pain-related to menstruation.

Application: Apply topically. May be added to food or water as a dietary supplement or flavoring.

Fragrant Influence: Soothing and calming.

Safety Data: If pregnant or under a doctor's care, consult your physician. Use sparingly, as coriander can be stupefying in large doses.

Companion Oils: Bergamot, cinnamon, citronella, clary sage, cypress, ginger, jasmine, neroli, petitgrain, pine, sandalwood, and other spice oils.

Cumin *(Cuminum Cyminum)*

Botanical Family: Apiaceae or Umbelliferae (parsley)

Plant Origin: Egypt

Extraction Method: Steam distilled from seeds.

Chemical Constituents: Monoterpenes (30-60%): pinene (13-22%), paracymene (3-9%), terpinene (12-32%); Coumarins.

Action: Antiviral, helps appetite and digestion, and acts as a liver regulator.

Found In: ImmuPower, ParaFree, and Protec

Traditional Uses: The Hebrews used cumin as an antiseptic for circumcision.

Indications: Immune stimulant, antiviral. This oil may help with poor circulation, indigestion, digestive spasms, headaches, and migraines. It may also help with wound healing and scars.

Other Uses: *Nigella damascena* is more rare and expensive than the commonly used white cumin found in supermarkets. It is antiseptic, calming, and a powerful support to the immune system.

Application: Diffuse or apply topically. Dilution may be required. Skin test for sensitivity before using without carrier oil.

Fragrant Influence: Stimulates appetite.

Safety Data: If pregnant or under a doctor's care, consult your physician. Avoid direct sunlight for up to 12 hours after use.

Companion Oils: Cinnamon, frankincense, jasmine, myrrh, patchouly, rose, sandalwood, and ylang ylang.

Cypress *(Cupressus sempervirens)*

Botanical Family: Cupressaceae (cypress)

Plant Origin: France, Spain

Extraction Method: Steam distilled from branches.

Chemical Constituents: Monoterpenes: α-pinene; Sesquiterpenes; Sesquiterpenols; Diterpenols.

Action: Improves circulation and supports the nerves and intestines. Anti-infectious, antibacterial, antimicrobial, and strengthens blood capillaries. Acts as an insect repellent.

Found In: Aroma Life, Aroma Siez, and R.C.

Traditional Uses: Cypress is one of the oils most used for the circulatory system.

Indications: Arthritis, bronchitis, circulation, cramps, hemorrhoids, insomnia, intestinal parasites, menopausal problems, menstrual pain, pancreas insufficiencies, pulmonary infections, rheumatism, spasms, tuberculosis, throat problems, varicose veins, and fluid retention. Jean Valnet, M.D. suggests that it may be helpful for some cancers.

Other Uses: This oil may be beneficial for asthma, strengthening blood capillary walls, reducing cellulite, circulatory system, strengthening connective tissue, coughs, edema, improving energy, gallbladder, bleeding gums, hemorrhaging, laryngitis, liver disorders, muscular cramps, nervous tension, nose bleeds, and ovarian cysts. It is outstanding when used in skin care, lessening scar tissue.

Application: Use topically with a massaging action toward the center of the body. Apply where you would wear a deodorant.

Fragrant Influence: Cypress influences, strengthens, and helps ease the feeling of loss. It creates a feeling of security, grounding, and it helps heal emotional trauma.

Safety Data: If pregnant or under a doctor's care, consult your physician.

Companion Oils: Bergamot, clary sage, juniper, lavender, lemon, orange, and sandalwood.

Bible Reference:

Isaiah 44:14—"He heweth him down cedars, and taketh the cypress and the oak, which he strengtheneth for himself among the trees of the forest: he planteth an ash, and the rain doth nourish [it]."

Davana *(Artemisia pallens)*

Botanical Family: Asteraceae or Compositae (daisy)

Chemical Constituents: Davanone

Action: Anti-infectious

Found In: Trauma Life

Indications: Stimulates the endocrine system, improves hormonal balance, and soothes rough, dry, and chapped skin.

Application: Diffuse or apply topically.

Safety Data: If pregnant or under a doctor's care, consult your physician.

Dill *(Anethum graveolens)*

Botanical Family: Apiaceae or Umbelliferae (parsley)

Plant Origin: Austria, Hungary

Extraction Method: Steam distilled from whole plant.

Chemical Constituents: Carvone, limonene, phellandrene (depending on extraction method), eugenol, pinene, and others.

Action: Antispasmodic, antibacterial, expectorant, and stimulant.

Traditional Uses: The dill plant is mentioned in the Papyrus of Ebers from Egypt (1550 BC). Roman gladiators rubbed their skin with dill before each match. It is used in European hospitals.

Indications: Dill has been researched at Cairo University for its effects in glucose and insulin levels and supporting pancreatic function.

Other Uses: This oil may help bronchial, indigestion, constipation, headaches, indigestion, liver deficiencies, lower glucose levels, nervousness, normalize insulin levels, promote milk flow in nursing mothers, and support pancreatic function.

Application: Apply topically on abdomen and bottom of feet. May be added to food or water as a dietary supplement.

Fragrant Influence: Dill calms the autonomic nervous system and, when diffused with Roman chamomile, may help calm fidgety children.

Safety Data: If pregnant or under a doctor's care, consult your physician.

Companion Oils: Nutmeg and citrus oils.

Elemi *(Canarium luzonicum)*

Botanical Family: Burseraceae (frankincense)

Plant Origin: Philippines

Extraction Method: Steam distilled from the gum of the tree.

Chemical Constituents: Monoterpenes; Sesquiterpenes; Alcohols sesquiterpenes: elemol.

Action: Antiseptic and antimicrobial .

Traditional Uses: Elemi has been used in Europe for hundreds of years in salves for skin and is included in celebrated healing ointments, such as *baum paralytique*. Used by a 17th century physician, J. J. Wecker, on the battle wounds of soldiers, elemi belongs to the same botanical family as frankincense (*Boswellia carteri*) and myrrh (*Commiphora myrrha*). The Egyptians used elemi for

embalming, and subsequent cultures used it for skin care.

Indications: Stimulates glands, helps reduce scarring, calms stomach, and fights against amoebic dysentery.

Other Uses: It is widely regarded today for soothing sore muscles, protecting and rejuvenating the skin, reducing wrinkles, and stimulating nerves. Its fragrance is very conducive toward meditation.

Application: Apply topically or diffuse. May be added to food or water as a dietary supplement. It is one of the gentlest oils in aromatherapy, and suitable for use on children.

Safety Data: If pregnant or under a doctor's care, consult physician.

Eucalyptus citriodora

Botanical Family: Myrtaceae (myrtle)

Plant Origin: China

Extraction Method: Steam distilled from leaves.

Chemical Constituents: Monoterpene alcohols: citronnellol (15-20%), trans-pinocarveol, geraniol; Terpene Esters; Terpene aldehydes: citronnellal (40-80%).

Action: Analgesic, antiseptic, antiviral, antibacterial, antifungal, deodorant, expectorant, and insecticidal.

Found In: R.C.

Traditional Uses: *Eucalyptus citriodora* has been used to perfume linen closets, and as an insect repellent, especially for cockroaches and silverfish.

Indications: Asthma, athlete's foot and other fungal infections, respiratory infections, cuts, dandruff, fevers, herpes, infectious skin conditions, laryngitis, scabs, shingles, sore throat, sores, and wounds.

Application: Diffuse or rub on bottom of feet or on location.

Safety Data: If pregnant or under a doctor's care, consult your physician. Do not take internally.

Eucalyptus dives

Botanical Family: Myrtaceae (myrtle)

Plant Origin: Australia, Brazil

Extraction Method: Steam distilled from leaves.

Chemical Constituents: Phellandrene, eucalyptol.

Action: This species has a different, more specific antibacterial action than other eucalyptus oils.

Application: Apply topically or diffuse. May be added to food or water as a dietary supplement. Avoid direct inhalation.

Safety Data: If pregnant or under a doctor's care, consult your physician.

Eucalyptus globulus

Botanical Family: Myrtaceae (myrtle)

Plant Origin: Australia, Brazil

Extraction Method: Steam distilled from leaves.

Chemical Constituents: Monoterpenes: α-pinenes (10-12%); Sesquiterpenes: Sesquiterpenols; Terpene oxides: 1,8 cineole (70-75%).

Action: Expectorant, mucolytic, antimicrobial, antibacterial, antifungal (candida), antiviral, and antiseptic.

Found In: R.C.

Traditional Uses: For centuries, Australian Aborigines used the leaves as a disinfectant to cover wounds. Shown by laboratory tests to be a powerful antimicrobial agent, *E. globulus* contains a high percentage of eucalyptol (a key ingredient in many antiseptic mouth rinses). Often used for the respiratory system, eucalyptus has been investigated for its powerful insect repellant effects (Trigg, 1996). Eucalyptus trees have been planted throughout parts of North Africa to successfully block the spread of malaria. According to Jean Valnet, M.D., a solution of 2% eucalyptus oil sprayed in the air will kill 70% of airborne staph bacteria. Some doctors still use solutions of eucalyptus oil in surgical dressings.

Indications: Asthma, candida, coughs, diabetes, herpes, hypoglycemia, lungs, measles, headaches, respiratory infections, sinusitis, shingles, and tuberculosis.

Other Uses: This oil may be used for aches/pains, acne, allergies, arthritis, bronchitis, burns, decongestant, respiratory infections, cystitis, endometriosis, increasing energy, gonorrhea, inflammation of the ear, eye, and sinus, malaria, rheumatism, respiratory infections, skin and throat infection/sores, ulcers, vaginitis, and wounds.

Application: Apply topically, diffuse, or use in a humidifier. May be added to food or water as a dietary supplement.

Fragrant Influence: It promotes health, well-being, purification, and healing.

Safety Data: If pregnant or under a doctor's care, consult your physician. Do not take internally.

Companion Oils: Geranium, juniper, lavender, lemon, lemongrass, melissa, pine, sandalwood, and thyme.

Selected Research:

Tovey ER, et al. "A simple washing procedure with eucalyptus oil for controlling house dust mites and their allergens in clothing and bedding." *J Allergy Clin Immunol*. 1997; 100(4):464-6.

Weyers W, et al. "Skin absorption of volatile oils. Pharmacokinetics." *Pharm Unserer Zeit*. 1989;18(3):82-6.

Zanker KS, et al. "Evaluation of surfactant-like effects of commonly used remedies for colds." *Respiration*. 1980;39(3):150-7.

Eucalyptus polybractea

Botanical Family: Myrtaceae (myrtle)

Plant Origin: Australia

Extraction Method: Steam distilled from leaves.

Chemical Constituents: Terpene oxides: 1,8 cineole (10%), Paracymene (30%), Sesquiterpenols.

Action: Anti-infectious, antiviral, antibacterial, anti-inflammatory, expectorant, mucolytic, and insect repellent.

Indications: Acne and cystitis.

Application: Diffuse or apply topically.

Safety Data: If pregnant or under a doctor's care, consult your physician.

Eucalyptus radiata

Botanical Family: Myrtaceae (myrtle)

Plant Origin: Australia

Extraction Method: Steam distilled from leaves.

Chemical Constituents: Monoterpenes (8%); α-pinene; Monoterpenols (20%): linalol, borneal, geraniol, α-terpinol (14%); Monoterpenals: Terpene oxides: 1,8 cineol (62-72%).

Action: Anti-infectious, antibacterial, antiviral, expectorant, and anti-inflammatory.

Found In: R.C., Raven, and Thieves

Traditional Uses: An antimicrobial oil studied for its action against viruses. This oil is used extensively for respiratory infections.

Indications: Conjunctivitis, vaginitis, acne, sinusitis, and bronchitis.

Other Uses: This oil, when combined with bergamot, has been used effectively on herpes simplex. It may also help with acne, bronchitis, ear (inflammation), endometriosis, nasal and sinus congestion, sinusitis, and vaginitis.

Application: Diffuse or rub on bottom of feet or on location.

Safety Data: If pregnant or under a doctor's care, consult your physician.

Fennel *(Foeniculum vulgare)*

Botanical Family: Apiaceae or Umbelliferae (parsley)

Plant Origin: Australia, Spain

Extraction Method: Steam distilled from the crushed seeds.

Chemical Constituents: Monoterpenes; α-pinene, limonene; Monoterpenols: fenchol; Phenols: methyl chavicol; Aldehydes; Ketones, camphor, Oxides: 1.9 cineol; Coumarins and furocoumarins.

Action: Stimulates estrogen production, facilitates birthing, increases lactation, promotes digestion, reduces indigestion, supports the heart and respiratory system, expels worms, stimulating to the circulatory and respiratory systems. It is antiseptic, antispasmodic, and analgesic.

Found In: Di-Tone, Dragon Time, JuvaFlex, and Mister.

Traditional Uses: Fennel was believed to ward off evil spirits and to protect against spells cast by witches during medieval times. Sprigs were hung over doors to fend off evil spirits. For hundreds of years, fennel seeds have been used as a digestive aid to balance menstrual cycles. Recently it has been used in mouthwashes and toothpastes.

Indications: Cystitis, sluggish digestion, fluid retention, gout, intestinal parasites, intestinal spasms, nausea, menopause and pre-menopause problems.

Other Uses: Fennel oil may be used for indigestion, stimulating the cardiovascular system, constipation, digestion, balancing hormones, supporting pancreatic function, PMS, and stimulating the respiratory system. It may break up fluids and toxins, and cleanse the tissues.

Application: Apply topically mixed with massage oil. Add to food or water as a dietary supplement or flavoring.

Safety Data: If pregnant or under a doctor's care, consult your physician. Use caution if epileptic.

Companion Oils: Basil, geranium, lavender, lemon, rosemary, and sandalwood.

Selected Reference:

Fyfe L, et al. "Inhibition of *Listeria monocytogenes* and *Salmonella enteriditis* by combinations of plant oils and derivatives of benzoic acid: the development of synergistic antimicrobial combinations." *Int J Antimicrob Agents.* 1997;9(3):195-9.

Fir *(Abies alba)*

Botanical Family: Pinaceae (pine)

Plant Origin: Balkans

Extraction Method: Steam distilled from needles.

Chemical Constituents: Monoterpenes (90-95%): alpina-Pinenes (24%), camphene (21%), limonene (34%).

Action: Antiseptic, anticatarrahal, and stimulant.

Found In: En-R-Gee, Grounding, Into The Future, and Sacred Mountain.

Traditional Uses: Fir is used today as the traditional Christmas tree. Though highly regarded for its fragrant scent, the fir tree has been prized through the ages for its medicinal virtues in regards to respiratory conditions and muscular and rheumatic pain. It has been researched for its ability to kill airborne germs and bacteria.

Indications: Bronchitis, respiratory congestion, and fatigue.

Other Uses: It may be beneficial for discomfort from respiratory infections, fighting airborne bacteria, treating arthritis, asthma, bronchial obstructions, coughs, rheumatism, sinusitis, and urinary tract infections.

Application: Diffuse or apply topically.

Fragrant Influence: Grounding, stimulating to the mind, and relaxing to the body.

Safety Data: If pregnant or under a doctor's care, consult your physician. Skin test for sensitivity.

Companion Oils: Blue chamomile, cedarwood, frankincense, lavender, lemon, myrtle, and rosewood.

Bible References: (see additional Bible references in Appendix D)

2 Samuel 6:5 — "And David and all the house of Israel played before the Lord on all manner of [instruments made of] fir wood, even on harps, and on psalteries, and on timbrels, and on cornets, and on cymbals."

1 Kings 5:8 — "And Hiram sent to Solomon, saying, I have considered the things which thou sentest to me for: [and] I will do all thy desire concerning timber of cedar, and concerning timber of fir."

1 Kings 5:10 — "So Hiram gave Solomon cedar trees and fir trees [according to] all his desire."

Fleabane *(Conyza canadensis)*

Botanical Family: Asteraceae or Compositae (daisy)

Plant Origin: Canada

Extraction Method: Steam distilled from stems, leaves, and flowers.

Chemical Constituents: Monoterpenes; Sesquiterpenes: Terpene alcohols, Esters: lactones.

Action: Stimulates liver and pancreas, anti-rheumatic, antispasmodic, hormone-like, cardiovascular dilator. Daniel Penoël, M.D., used it to treat children with retarded puberty.

Found In: Ultra Young

Safety Data: If pregnant or under a doctor's care, consult your physician.

Note: This oil is still under study.

Frankincense (*Boswellia carteri*)

Botanical Family: Burseraceae (Frankincense)

Plant Origin: Somalia

Extraction Method: Steam distilled from gum/resin.

Chemical Constituents: Monoterpenes (40%); α pinene (43%), limonese; Sesquiterpenes; Alcohols terpenes: borneol.

Action: Expectorant, antitumoral, immuno-stimulant, and antidepressant.

Found In: Abundance, Acceptance, Brain Power, Exodus II, Forgiveness, Gathering, Harmony, Humility, ImmuPower, Inspiration, Into The Future, 3 Wise Men, Trauma Life, and Valor.

Traditional Uses: Also known as "olibanum," or "Oil from Lebanon" the name frankincense is derived from the Medieval French word for "real incense." Frankincense is considered the "holy anointing oil" in the Middle East and has been used in religious ceremonies for thousands of years. It was well known during the time of Christ for its anointing and healing powers and was one of the gifts given to Christ at His birth. "Used to treat every conceivable ill known to man," frankincense was valued more than gold during ancient times, and only those with great wealth and abundance possessed it. Researchers today have discovered that frankincense is high in sesquiterpenes, which helps stimulate the limbic system of the brain (the center of emotions) as well as the hypothalamus, pineal and pituitary glands. The hypothalamus is the master gland of the human body, controlling the release of many hormones including thyroid and growth hormone. Frankincense is now being researched and used therapeutically in European hospitals and is being investigated for its ability to improve human growth hormone production.

Indications: Asthma, depression, and ulcers. High in sesquiterpenes, it is stimulating and elevating to the mind and helps in overcoming stress and despair, as well as supporting the immune system.

Other Uses: This oil may help with allergies, bites (insect and snake), bronchitis, cancer, respiratory infections, diphtheria, headaches, hemorrhaging, herpes, high blood pressure, inflammation, stress, tonsillitis, typhoid, and warts. It contains sesquiterpenes, enabling it to go beyond the blood brain barrier. It increases the activity of leukocytes in defense of the body against infection.

Application: Diffuse or apply topically. May be added to food or water as a dietary supplement.

Fragrant Influence: It increases spiritual awareness and promotes meditation. Frankincense may also help improve attitude and uplift spirits, which may help to strengthen the immune system.

Safety Data: If pregnant or under a doctor's care, consult physician.

Companion Oils: All oils.

Bible Reference: There are over 52 references to frankincense (considering that "incense" is translated from the Hebrew/Greek "frankincense" and is referring to the same oil). (See additional Bible references in Appendix D)

Exodus 30:34—"And the Lord said unto Moses, Take unto thee sweet spices, stacte, and onycha, and galbanum; [these] sweet spices with pure frankincense: of each shall there be a like [weight]:"

Leviticus 2:1—"And when any will offer a meat offering unto the Lord, his offering shall be [of] fine flour; and he shall pour oil upon it, and put frankincense thereon:"

Leviticus 2:2—"And he shall bring it to Aaron's sons the priests: and he shall take thereout his handful of the flour thereof, and of the oil thereof, with all the frankincense thereof; and the priest shall burn the memorial of it upon the altar, [to be] an offering made by fire, of a sweet savour unto the Lord:"

Selected Research:

Michie, C.A., et al. "Frankincense and myrrh as remedies in children." *J R Soc Med.* 1991;84(10):602-5.

Wang, L.G., et al. "Determination of DNA topoisomerase II activity from L1210 cells--a target for screening antitumor agents." Chung Kuo Yao Li Hsueh Pao. 1991;12(2):108-14.

Galbanum *(Ferula gummosa)*

Botanical Family: Apiaceae or Umbelliferae (parsley)

Plant Origin: Iran

Extraction Method: Steam distilled from resin derived from stems and branches.

Chemical Constituents: Monoterpenes (65-85%), α-pinene (45-50%), camphene, limonene, myrcene, carvone; Sesquiterpenols; Esters; Coumarins.

Action: Anti-infectious, stimulant, supporting to the kidneys and menstruation, analgesic, and light antispasmodic.

Found In: Exodus II and Gathering.

Traditional Uses: Mentioned in Egyptian papyri and the Old Testament (Exodus 30:34) it was esteemed for its medicinal and spiritual properties. Dioscorides, an ancient Roman historian, records that galbanum was used for its antispasmodic, diuretic, and pain-relieving properties.

Indications: Recognized for its antimicrobial and body supporting properties.

Other Uses: Galbanum may also help with abscesses, acne, asthma, bronchitis, chronic coughs, cramps, cuts, indigestion, inflammation, muscular aches and pains, nervous tension, poor circulation, rheumatism, scar tissue, stress, wrinkles, and wounds. Although galbanum has a low frequency, when combined with other oils, such as frankincense or sandalwood, the frequency rises dramatically.

Application: Apply topically. May be added to food or water as a dietary supplement.

Fragrant Influence: Harmonic and balancing. It may help increase spiritual awareness and meditation.

Safety Data: If pregnant or under a doctor's care, consult physician.

Companion Oils: All oils.

Bible Reference:

Exodus 30:34—"And the Lord said unto Moses, Take unto thee sweet spices, stacte, and onycha, and galbanum; [these] sweet spices with pure frankincense: of each shall there be a like [weight]:"

Geranium *(Pelargonium graveolens)*

Botanical Family: Geraniaceae

Plant Origin: Egypt, India

Extraction Method: Steam distilled from the leaves.

Chemical Constituents: Monoterpenes; Sesquiterpenes; Monoterpene alcohols (60-68%): linalol, citronnellol (33%), geraniol (25%), nerol, menthol, Sesquiterpene alcohols; Terpene esters (20-33%); Oxides: 1,8 cineole: Aldehydes: neral, geranial (9.8%); Ketones.

Action: Antispasmodic, antitumoral, adrenal cortex stimulant, anti-inflammatory, astringent, hemostatic (stops bleeding) anti-infectious, antibacterial, antifungal, revitalizes skin tissue, and dilates bile ducts for liver detoxification. Geranium balances the sebum, which is the fatty secretion in the sebaceous glands of the skin that keep the skin supple. Helps cleanse oily skin and restores and enlivens pale skin.

Found In: Acceptance, Awaken, Clarity, EndoFlex, Envision, Forgiveness, Gathering, Gentle Baby, Harmony, Humility, Joy, JuvaFlex, Release, SARA, Trauma Life, and White Angelica.

Traditional Uses: Geranium has been used for centuries for skin care.

Indications: Skin conditions (dermatitis, eczema, psoriasis, vitiligo), herpes, shingles, bleeding, tumor growths, and hormone imbalances.

Other Uses: This oil may be used for acne, burns, circulatory problems (improves blood flow), depression, gingivitis, liver problems, sterility, digestion, eczema, insomnia, menstrual problems, neuralgia (severe pain along the nerve), regenerating tissue and nerves, pancreas imbalances, ringworm, shingles, sore throats, and wounds. Jean Valnet, M.D., recommends it for liver disorders and hepatitis.

Application: Diffuse and apply topically. May be added to food or water as a dietary supplement. Apply where you would use a deodorant.

Fragrant Influence: It may help to release negative memories. It may also help ease nervous tension and stress, balance the emotions, lift the spirit, and foster peace, well-being, and hope.

Safety Data: If pregnant or under a doctor's care, consult physician.

Companion Oils: All oils.

Selected Research:

Lis-Balchin, M., et al. "Antimicrobial activity of Pelargonium essential oils added to a quiche filling as a model food system." *Lett Appl Microbiol.* 1998;27(4):207-10.

Lis-Balchin, M., et al. "Comparative antibacterial effects of novel Pelargonium essential oils and solvent extracts." *Lett Appl Microbiol.* 1998;27(3):135-41.

Fang, H.J., et al. "Studies on the chemical components and anti-tumour action of the volatile oils from Pelargonium graveoleus." *Yao Hsueh Hsueh Pao.* 1989;24(5):366-71.

Ginger *(Zingiber officinale)*

Botanical Family: Zingiberaceae (ginger)

Plant Origin: China

Extraction Method: Steam distilled from root.

Chemical Constituents: Monoterpenes: α pinene, camphene, β-pinene, myrcene, limonene; Sesquiterpenes: zingiberene (30%); Hydrocarbons: Monoterpene alcohols: Sesquiterpene alcohols; Aldehydes; Ketones.

Action: Digestive tonic, sexual tonic, reduces pain, and expectorant.

Found In: Abundance, Di-Tone, Magnify Your Purpose, and Passion.

Traditional Uses: Ginger is used to combat the effects of motion sickness and has been studied for its gentle, simulating effects. Women in the West African country of Senegal weave belts of ginger root to restore their mates' sexual potency.

Indications: Arthritis, rheumatism, indigestion, digestive disorders, and motion sickness.

Other Uses: Ginger may be used for alcoholism, loss of appetite, arthritis, chills, respiratory infections, congestion, coughs, digestive disorders, infectious diseases, muscular aches/pains, nausea, rheumatism, sinusitis, sore throats, and sprains.

Application: Diffuse and apply topically. May be added to food or water as a dietary supplement or flavoring.

Fragrant Influence: Gentle, stimulating, endowing physical energy, and courage.

Safety Data: If pregnant or under a doctor's care, consult your physician. Repeated use can possibly result in contact sensitization. Avoid direct sunlight after use.

Companion Oils: All spice oils, all citrus oils, eucalyptus, frankincense, geranium, myrtle, rosemary, and spearmint.

Grapefruit *(Citrus x paradisi)*

Botanical Family: Rutaceae (citrus)

Plant Origin: California. (Grapefruit is a hybrid between *Citrus maxima* and *Citrus sinensis*.)

Extraction Method: Cold press from rind.

Chemical Constituents: Monoterpenes: limonene (96-98%); Aldehydes; Coumarins and furocoumarins.

Action: Antiseptic, disinfecting, detoxifying, and diuretic. Like many cold-pressed citrus oils, it has unique fat-dissolving characteristics. It is exceptionally cleansing for oily skin. Psychologically, it is antidepressant and emotionally uplifting.

Found In: Citrus Fresh

Indications: Helps with acne, cellulite, digestion, and fluid retention.

Other Uses: Grapefruit oil may help with depression, drug withdrawal, eating disorders, fatigue, jet lag, liver disorders, migraine headaches, pre-menstrual tension, and stress. It may also have a cleansing effect on the kidneys, the lymphatic system, and the vascular system.

Application: Diffuse and apply topically. Add to food or water as a dietary supplement or flavoring. Grapefruit is not photosensitizing unlike other oils with furocoumarins.

Fragrant Influence: Refreshing and uplifting.

Safety Data: If pregnant or under a doctor's care, consult physician.

Companion Oils: Basil, bergamot, cedarwood, chamomile, cypress, frankincense, geranium, juniper, lavender, peppermint, rosemary, rosewood, and ylang ylang.

Helichrysum *(Helichrysum italicum)*

Botanical Family: Asteraceae or Compositae (daisy)

Plant Origin: Yugoslavia, Corsica

Extraction Method: Steam distilled from flower.

Chemical Constituents: Sesquiterpenes; Monoterpenols: nerol; Terpene esters; neryle acetate (75%); Ketones.

Action: Anticoagulant, anesthetic, dissolves hematomas (blood clots), mucolytic, expectorant, antispasmodic, stimulates liver, reduces scar tissue and skin discoloration. It balances blood pressure, chelates chemicals and toxins.

Found In: Aroma Life, Brain Power, Forgiveness, JuvaFlex, M-Grain, PanAway, Passion, and Trauma Life.

Traditional Uses: Helichrysum has been studied by European researchers for regenerating tissue and nerves and improving circulation and skin conditions.

Indications: Hematoma (swelling or blood-filled tumor), bleeding, arteriosclerosis, atherosclerosis, hypertension, congestive heart failure, cardiac arrhythmias, thrombosis, embolisms, liver disorders, phlebitis, sciatica, sinus infection, and skin conditions (eczema, dermatitis, psoriasis).

Other Uses: This oil may help blood circulation, hearing loss, pain (acute), respiratory conditions, scar tissue, and varicose veins. It may regenerate tissue, detoxify and stimulate the liver cell function.

Application: Diffuse. Apply topically around outside of ear, temple, forehead, back of neck, or on location.

Fragrant Influence: It is uplifting to the subconscious.

Safety Data: If pregnant or under a doctor's care, consult physician.

Hyssop *(Hyssopus officinalis)*

Botanical Family: Lamiaceae or Labiatae (mint)

Plant Origin: France, Hungary

Extraction Method: Steam distilled from stems/leaves.

Chemical Constituents: Monoterpenes (25-30%); β–pinenes; Sesquiterpenes (12%); Sesquiterpenols (5-10%); Phenols methylethers, methyl chavicol; Monoterpenones (45-58%); α and β– thujones, camphor, isopinocamphone (31-32%); pinocamphone (53%).

Action: Anticatarrhal, mucolytic, decongestant, expectorant, cleansing, purifying, and helps reduce fats in the tissue. Hyssop raises low blood pressure, regulates menstrual flow, and increases perspiration.

Found In: Exodus II, Harmony, ImmuPower, Relieve It, and White Angelica.

Traditional Uses: While there is some uncertainty that *Hyssopus officinalis* is the same species of plant as the hyssop referred to in the Bible, there is no question that *H.*

officinalis has been used medicinally for almost a millennium for its antiseptic, disinfecting, and anti-infectious properties. It has also been used for opening the respiratory system.

Indications: Anxiety, arthritis, asthma, bruises, respiratory infections, coughs, cuts, dermatitis, indigestion, fatigue, nervous tension, parasites (expelling worms), rheumatism, sore throats, viral infections, and wounds.

Application: Diffuse and apply topically. May be added to food or water as a dietary supplement.

Fragrant Influence: Stimulates creativity and meditation.

Safety Data: If pregnant or under a doctor's care, consult your physician. Do not use if epileptic.

Companion Oils: All citrus oils, clary sage, fennel, geranium, myrtle, and sage.

Bible References: (see additional Bible references in Appendix D)

Exodus 12:22 — "And ye shall take a bunch of hyssop, and dip [it] in the blood that [is] in the bason, and strike the lintel and the two side posts with the blood that [is] in the bason; and none of you shall go out at the door of his house until the morning."

Leviticus 14:4 — "Then shall the priest command to take for him that is to be cleansed two birds alive [and] clean, and cedar wood, and scarlet, and hyssop:"

Leviticus 14:6 — "As for the living bird, he shall take it, and the cedar wood, and the scarlet, and the hyssop, and shall dip them and the living bird in the blood of the bird [that was] killed over the running water:"

Idaho Tansy (*Tanacetum vulgare*)

Botanical Family: Asteraceae or Compositae (daisy)

Plant Origin: Idaho, Washington

Extraction Method: Steam distilled from leaves.

Chemical Constituents: Thujone, Camphor, Sabinene, Camphene.

Action: Insect repellent, analgesic, antitumoral, hemostat, and immune stimulant.

Found In: ImmuPower and Into The Future.

Traditional Uses: This antimicrobial oil has been used extensively as an insect repellent. According to E. Joseph Montagna's P.D.R. on herbal formulas, it may help numerous skin conditions and tone the entire system.

Indications: May help respiratory infections, stomach conditions, arthritis, irritable bowel syndrome, aneurysm, bruises, diarrhea, freckles, and gout.

Application: Diffuse or apply topically.

Safety Data: If pregnant or under a doctor's care, consult your physician.

Companion Oils: Birch, clary sage, elemi, hyssop, myrtle, pine, valerian, and vetiver.

Jasmine (*Jasminum officinale*)

Botanical Family: Oleaceae (olive)

Plant Origin: India

Extraction Method: Absolute extraction from flower. Jasmine is actually an "essence" not an essential oil. The flowers must be picked at night to maximize fragrance.

Chemical Constituents: Benzyl Acetate, Benzyl Benzoate, Methyl Anthranilate, Linalol, Phytol, Methyl Palmitate.

Action: Beneficial for skin, uplifting, antidepressant, and stimulating.

Found In: Awaken, Clarity, Dragon Time, Forgiveness, Gentle Baby, Harmony, Inner Child, Into The Future, Joy, Passion, and Sensation.

Traditional Uses: Jasmine has been nicknamed as the "queen of the night" and "moonlight of the grove." For centuries, women have treasured jasmine for its beautiful, seductive fragrance.

Indications: Beneficial for dry, greasy, irritated, or sensitive skin. Helps anxiety, stress, and depression.

Other Uses: This oil may help with eczema (when caused by emotions), frigidity, labor pains, laryngitis, lethargy (abnormal drowsiness), menstrual pain and problems, and stress. It is ideal for skin care (dry, greasy, irritated, and sensitive).

Application: Diffuse and apply topically. May be added to food or water as a dietary supplement.

Fragrant Influence: Uplifting and stimulating in times of hopelessness and nervous exhaustion. It helps to reduce anxiety, apathy, depression, dilemmas that deal with relationships, indifference, and listlessness. When worn as a cologne, it increases excitability.

Safety Data: If pregnant or under a doctor's care, consult physician.

Companion Oils: Bergamot, frankincense, geranium, helichrysum, lemongrass, mandarin, melissa, orange, palmarosa, rose, rosewood, sandalwood, and spearmint.

Note: One pound of jasmine oil requires about 1,000 pounds of jasmine or 3.6 million fresh unpacked blossoms. The blossoms must be collected before sunrise, or much of the fragrance will have evaporated. The quality of the blossoms may also be compromised if they are crushed. A single pound of pure jasmine oil may cost between $1,200 to $4,500. In contrast, synthetic jasmine oils can be obtained for $3.50 per pound, but they obviously do not possess the same therapeutic qualities as pure jasmine oil. The properties mentioned above are based on pure jasmine oil, not synthetic oil.

Juniper (*Juniperus osteosperma* and/or *J. scopulorum*)

Botanical Family: Cupressaceae (cypress)

Plant Origin: Utah

Extraction Method: Steam distilled from berries and twigs.

Chemical Constituents: Monoterpenes: α pinene (34-46%), sabinene (9-28%), myrcene (6-8%); Sesquiterpenes; Terpene alcohols; Aldehydes; Ketones mono and sesquiterpenes: camphor, pinocamphone.

Action: Antiseptic, astringent, digestive stimulant, purifying, and detoxifying. Juniper increases circulation through kidneys and promotes excretion of uric acid and toxins.

Found In: Di-Tone, Dream Catcher, En-R-Gee, Grounding, Hope, and Into the Future.

Traditional Uses: Bundles of juniper berries were hung over doorways to ward off witches during medieval times. It has been used for centuries as a diuretic. Until recently, French hospital wards burned sprigs of juniper and rosemary to protect from infection.

Indications: It may help acne, dermatitis, eczema, depression, fatigue, liver problems, sore muscles, rheumatism, ulcers, urinary infections, fluid retention, and wounds.

Other Uses: Juniper oil may work as a detoxifier and a cleanser, as well as being beneficial for the skin. It may possibly assist with nerve regeneration.

Application: Diffuse and apply topically. May be added to food or water as a dietary supplement.

Fragrant Influence: Juniper evokes feelings of health, love, and peace and may help to elevate one's spiritual awareness.

Safety Data: If pregnant or under a doctor's care, consult physician.

Companion Oils: Bergamot, all citrus oils, cypress, geranium, lavender, melaleuca, Melrose, and rosemary.

Bible Reference:

Job 30:45—"Who cut up mallows by the bushes, and juniper roots [for] their meat."

Selected Research:

Takacsova M, et al. "Study of the antioxidative effects of thyme, sage, juniper and oregano." *Nahrung.* 1995;39(3):241-3.

Laurus nobilis (Bay laurel)

Botanical Family: Lauraceae

Plant Origin: France

Extraction Method: Steam distilled from leaves.

Chemical Constituents: Monoterpenes: α pinene, β–pinene, sabinene; Sesquiterpenes; Monoterpenols: linalol (8-16%); Terpene Esters; Phenols: eugenol (3%); Oxides: 1,8 cineol (35-45%); Lactones sesquiterpenes.

Action: Antiseptic, antimicrobial, expectorant, mucolytic, anti-infectious, antibacterial (staph, strep, *E. coli*), candida, and anticoagulant.

Traditional Uses: Both the leaves and the black berries were also used to alleviate indigestion, and loss of appetite. During the Middle Ages, it was used for angina pectoris, asthma, gout, migraine, palpitations, and liver and spleen complaints.

Indications: Nerve regeneration, arthritis (rheumatoid), and oral infections.

Other Uses: Laurel may help with loss of appetite, asthmatic conditions, chronic bronchitis, hair loss (after an infection), lice, scabies, and viral infections.

Application: Diffuse or apply topically on the abdomen or on location. Add to food or water as a dietary supplement or flavoring.

Fragrant Influence: Laurel has been used as a fragrance component in cosmetics and perfumes.

Safety Data: If pregnant or under a doctor's care, consult your physician. Use in moderation.

Lavandin (*Lavandula* x *hybrida*)

Botanical Family: Lamiaceae or Labiatae (mint)

Chemical Constituents: Lynalyl acetate (30-32%), linalol, cineol, camphene (8-12%), pinene, and others.

Action: Antibacterial, antifungal, and strong antiseptic. (See lavender for additional properties.)

Found In: Purification, Release.

Traditional Uses: Also known as *Lavandula* x *intermedia*, lavandin is a hybrid plant developed by crossing true lavender with spike lavender or aspic (*Lavandula latifolia*). It has been used to sterilize the animal cages in veterinary clinics and hospitals throughout Europe.

Indications: There is not a long history of the therapeutic use of lavandin.

Other Uses: Lavandin is best used as an antiseptic. Its greater penetrating qualities make it well suited to help with respiratory, circulatory, and muscular conditions.

Application: Diffuse or apply topically.

Fragrant Influence: It has the same calming effects as lavender.

Safety Data: If pregnant or under a doctor's care, consult your physician. **DO NOT USE FOR BURNS.**

Companion Oils: Bergamot, cinnamon, citronella, clove, cypress, clary sage, geranium, lime, patchouly, pine, rosemary, and thyme.

Lavender (*Lavandula angustifolia*)

Botanical Family: Lamiaceae or Labiatae (mint)

Plant Origin: Utah, Idaho, France

Extraction Method: Steam distilled from flowering top.

Chemical Constituents: Monoterpene; α pinene, β–pinene, camphene; Sesquiterpenes; Non terpene alcohols (45%), geraniol, borneol, lavandulol; Esters: linalyl acetate (30-34%); lavanduyle, Oxides: 1,8 cineole; Ketones; Sesquiterpenones; Aldehydes; Lactones: Coumarins.

Action: Antiseptic, analgesic, antitumoral, anticonvulsant, sedative, anti-inflammatory. Lavender is beneficial for cleansing cuts and wounds and is ideal for skin care, since it prevents the build up of excess sebum, a skin oil that bacteria feed on. Lavender has also been clinically evaluated for its relaxing effects.

Found In: Aroma Siez, Brain Power, Dragon Time, Envision, Forgiveness, Gathering, Gentle Baby, Harmony, Mister, Motivation, M-Grain, R.C., SARA, Surrender, and Trauma Life.

Traditional Uses: The French scientist René Gatefossé was the first to discover lavender's ability to promote tissue regeneration and speed wound healing when he severely burned his arm in a laboratory accident. Today, lavender is one of the few essential oils to still be listed in the British Pharmacopoeia.

Indications: Burns (cell renewal), sunburns (including lips), dandruff, hair loss, allergies, convulsions, herpes, headaches, indigestion, insomnia, high blood pressure, menopausal conditions, nausea, phlebitis, tumors, premenstrual conditions, scarring (minimizes), skin conditions (acne, dermatitis, eczema, psoriasis, and rashes) and stretch marks. It may be used to cleanse cuts, bruises, and skin irritations.

Other Uses: Lavender is a universal oil with many different applications. It may help arthritis, asthma, bronchitis, convulsions, depression, earaches, heart palpitations, high blood pressure, hives (urticaria), insect bites, laryngitis, nervous tension, respiratory infections, rheumatism, and throat infections.

Application: Diffuse or apply topically. Has a wide range of uses. Apply where you would use a deodorant. Safe for use on small children. May also be added to food or water as a dietary supplement.

Fragrant Influence: Calming, relaxing, and balancing, both physically and emotionally.

Safety Data: If pregnant or under a doctor's care, consult physician.

Companion Oils: Most oils, especially citrus oils, chamomile, clary sage, and geranium.

Selected Research:

Larrondo JV, et al. "Antimicrobial activity of essences from labiates." *Microbios*. 1995; 82(332):171-2.

Guillemain J, et al. "Neurodepressive effects of the essential oil of *Lavandula angustifolia* Mill." *Ann Pharm Fr*. 1989;47(6):337-43.

Kim HM, et al. "Lavender oil inhibits immediate-type allergic reaction in mice and rats." *J Pharm Pharmacol*. 1999;51(2):221-6.

Lemon *(Citrus limon)*

Botanical Family: Rutaceae (citrus)

Plant Origin: California, Italy

Extraction Method: Cold pressed from rind. It takes 3,000 lemons to produce a kilo of oil.

Chemical Constituents: Monoterpenes: limonene (54-72%); Sesquiterpenes; Aldehydes; Coumarins and furocoumarins, contains flavonoids, carotenoids, steroids.

Action: Anti-infectious, disinfectant, antibacterial (spores), antiseptic, antiviral. Lemon improves microcirculation, promotes white blood cell formation, and improves immune function.

Found In: Awaken, Citrus Fresh, Clarity, Forgiveness, Gentle Baby, Harmony, Joy, Raven, Surrender, and Thieves.

Traditional Uses: Lemon has antiseptic-like properties and contains compounds that have been studied for their effects on immune function. According Jean Valnet, M.D., the vaporized essence of lemon can kill meningococcus bacteria in 15 minutes, typhoid bacilli in one hour, *Staphylococcus aureus* in two hours, and *Pneumococcus* bacteria within three hours. Even a 0.2% solution of lemon oil can kill diphtheria bacteria in 20 minutes and inactivate tuberculosis bacteria. Lemon oil has been widely used in skin care to cleanse skin and reduce wrinkles.

Indications: Anemia, asthma, herpes, warts, shingles, bleeding, malaria, parasites, rheumatism, throat infection, ureter infections, and varicose veins.

Other Uses: Lemon oil may be beneficial for anxiety, blood pressure, digestive problems, respiratory infections, and sore throats. It helps promote leukocyte formation, improves memory, strengthens nails, cleans the skin, and promotes a sense of well-being. It may also help brighten a pale, dull complexion by removing the dead skin cells. It serves as an effective insect repellent and works well in removing gum, wood stain, oil, and grease spots.

Application: Diffuse or add a few drops to a spray bottle to deodorize and sterilize the air. Add 2 drops to water for purification or combine with peppermint (*Mentha piperita*) to provide a refreshing lift. Add to food or water as a dietary supplement or flavoring.

Fragrant Influence: It promotes clarity of thought and purpose, as well as health, healing, physical energy, and purification. Its fragrance is invigorating, enhancing, and warming.

Safety Data: If pregnant or under a doctor's care, consult your physician. Lemon oil is very photosensitizing, so avoid applying it to skin that will be exposed to direct sunlight or UV light.

Companion Oils: Chamomile, eucalyptus, fennel, frankincense, geranium, juniper, peppermint, sandalwood, and ylang ylang.

Lemongrass *(Cymbopogon flexuosus)*

Botanical Family: Poaceae or Gramineae (grasses)

Plant Origin: India, Guatemala

Extraction Method: Steam distilled from leaves.

Chemical Constituents: Alcohol monoterpenes; α terpenol, borneol, geraniol; Alcohol sesquiterpenes: farnesol (12.8%); Monoterpene aldehydes (60-85%): citrals (75%), neral (27.7%), geranial (46.6%); Monoterpene aldehydes.

Action: Support digestion, tones and helps regenerate connective tissues and ligaments, dilates blood vessels, strengthens vascular walls, promotes lymph flow, and is anti-inflammatory and sedative.

Found In: Di-Tone, En-R-Gee, Inner Child, and Purification.

Traditional Uses: Lemongrass is used for purification and digestion. Research was published in *Phytotherapy Research* on topically applied lemongrass for its powerful antifungal properties.

Indications: Bladder infection, digestive disturbances, parasites, torn ligaments, edema, fluid retention, kidney disorders, and varicose veins.

Other Uses: Lemongrass oil may help improve circulation, digestion, eyesight, as well as combat headaches, infections, respiratory problems, sore throats, and fluid retention. It aids in tissue regeneration.

Application: Diffuse or apply topically.

Fragrant Influence: Promotes psychic awareness and purification.

Safety Data: If pregnant or under a doctor's care, consult your physician. Skin test for sensitivity/ irritation.

Companion Oils: Basil, cedarwood, eucalyptus, geranium, lavender, melaleuca, and rosemary.

Selected Research:

Pattnaik S, et al. "Antibacterial and antifungal activity of ten essential oils in vitro." *Microbios*. 1996;86(349):237-46.

Lorenzetti BB, et al. "Myrcene mimics the peripheral analgesic activity of lemongrass tea." *J Ethnopharmacol*. 1991;34(1):43-8.

Elson CE, et al. "Impact of lemongrass oil, an essential oil, on serum cholesterol." *Lipids*. 1989;24(8):677-9.

Mandarin *(Citrus reticulata)*

Botanical Family: Rutaceae (citrus)

Plant Origin: Madagascar, Italy, China

Extraction Method: Cold press from rind.

Chemical Constituents: Monoterpenes; limonene (65-94%); Esters; Aldehydes; Coumarins and furocoumarins. Contains flavonoids, carotenoids, and steroids.

Action: Light antispasmodic, digestive tonic (digestoid), antiseptic, antifungal, and stimulates gallbladder.

Found In: Citrus Fresh, Joy, and Awaken

Traditional Uses: This fruit was traditionally given to Imperial Chinese officials named the Mandarins.

Other Uses: This oil may help acne, digestive problems, fluid retention, insomnia, intestinal problems, skin problems (congested and oily skin, scars, spots, tones the skin), stretch marks (when combined with either jasmine, lavender, sandalwood, and/or frankincense), nervous tension, and restlessness. Recommended for children and pregnant women because it is very gentle.

Application: Diffuse or apply topically.

Fragrant Influence: It is appeasing, gentle, and promotes happiness.

Safety Data: If pregnant or under a doctor's care, consult your physician. Avoid direct sunlight after use.

Companion Oils: Cinnamon, clove, lavender, neroli, nutmeg, and other citrus oils and spice oils.

Marjoram (*Origanum majorana*)

Botanical Family: Lamiaceae or Labiatae (mint)

Plant Origin: France

Extraction Method: Steam distilled from leaves.

Chemical Constituents: Monoterpenes (40%): α and β–pinenes, myrcene; Sesquiterpenes; Monoterpenols (50%): linalol; Terpene esters: terpenyle acetates, geranyle acetates.

Action: Anti-infectious, antibacterial, dilates blood vessels, regulates blood pressure, soothes muscles, promotes intestinal peristalsis, tones the parasympathetic nervous system, and supports respiratory system.

Found In: Aroma Life, Aroma Siez, Dragon Time, M-Grain, and R.C.

Traditional Uses: Marjoram was known as the "herb of happiness" to the Romans and "joy of the mountains" to the Greeks. It was believed to increase longevity.

Indications: Aches, arthritis, asthma, bronchitis, indigestion, constipation, cramps, insomnia, migraine headaches, neuralgia, rheumatism, and sprains.

Other Uses: Marjoram may be relaxing and calming to the muscles that constrict and sometimes contribute to headaches. It may help anxiety, nervous tension, bruises, burns, sores, cuts, circulatory disorders, respiratory infections, fungal and viral infections, menstrual problems, ringworm, shingles, shock, sores, spasms, sunburns, and fluid retention.

Application: Diffuse or apply topically. Massage to calm stressed muscles. Add to food or water as a dietary supplement or flavoring.

Fragrant Influence: Assists in calming the nerves.

Safety Data: If pregnant or under a doctor's care, consult physician.

Companion Oils: Bergamot, cedarwood, chamomile, cypress, lavender, nutmeg, orange, rosemary, rosewood, and ylang ylang.

Melaleuca alternifolia

Botanical Family: Myrtaceae (myrtle)

Plant Origin: Australia

Extraction Method: Steam distilled from leaves.

Chemical Constituents: Monoterpenes: α pinene, β–pinene, myrcene; Sesquiterpenes; Monoterpene alcohols (45-50%); Terpene oxides.

Action: Anti-infectious, antibacterial (large spectrum action of gram positive and gram negative bacteria), antifungal, antiviral, antiparasitic, antiseptic, anti-inflammatory, immunostimulant, cardiotonic, decongestant of the veins, reduces phlebitis, neurotonic, analgesic, and protects against radiation.

Found In: Melrose, Purification

Traditional Uses: Highly regarded as an antimicrobial and antiseptic essential oil. It has high levels of terpinenol, which is the key active constituent.

Indications: Athlete's foot, fungal infections, bronchitis, respiratory infections, gum disease, rash, sore throat, sunburn, tonsillitis, and vaginal thrush.

Other Uses: This oil may help acne, burns, candida, cold sores, inflammation, viral infections, ingrown nails, warts, and wounds (promotes healing).

Application: Diffuse or apply topically. Safe for use on children and pets.

Fragrant Influence: Promotes cleansing and purity.

Safety Data: If pregnant or under a doctor's care, consult your physician. Repeated use can possibly result in contact sensitization.

Companion Oils: All citrus oils, cypress, eucalyptus, lavender, rosemary, and thyme.

Selected Research:

Syed TA, et al. "Treatment of toenail onychomycosis with 2% butenafine and 5% *Melaleuca alternifolia* (tea tree) oil in cream." *Trop Med Int Health*. 1999;4(4):284-7.

Hammer KA, et al. "In vitro susceptibilities of lactobacilli and organisms associated with bacterial vaginosis to *Melaleuca alternifolia* (tea tree) oil." Antimicrob Agents Chemother. 1999;43(1):196.

Concha JM, et al. 1998 William J. Stickel Bronze Award. "Antifungal activity of *Melaleuca alternifolia* (tea-tree) oil against various pathogenic organisms." *J Am Podiatr Med Assoc*. 1998;88(10):489-92.

Melaleuca ericifolia (formerly called Australian Rosalina)

Botanical Family: Myrtaceae (myrtle)

Plant Origin: Australia

Chemical Constituents: α-Pinene, 1,8 Cineol, Linalook, α-Terpineol, Limonene, para-Cymene.

Application: Diffuse or apply topically.

Safety Data: If pregnant or under a doctor's care, consult physician.

Note: This oil is still under study. It has been found beneficial for bronchitis, asthma, respiratory infection, cynitis, and sinus infection.

Melaleuca quinquenervia

Botanical Family: Myrtaceae (myrtle)

Plant Origin: Australia

Extraction Method: Steam distilled from leaves and limbs.

Chemical Constituents: Sesquiterpenes; Monoterpene alcohols: linalol; Sesquiterpene alcohols: (+)-trans- nerolidol (81-82%), farnesols; Terpene oxides: 1.9 cineol.

Action: Male hormone-like, anti-inflammatory, anti-infectious, antibacterial, antiviral, and antiparasitic (amoeba and parasites in the blood).

Found In: Melrose

Indications: Relieves mucous in the respiratory passages, urinary tract, and genital organs, digestive tonic, and reduces hypertension (high blood pressure).

Other Uses: This oil may help with the respiratory tract and respiratory allergies, infections, and hemorrhoids.

Application: Diffuse or apply topically.

Fragrant Influence: Sweet and delicate.

Safety Data: If pregnant or under a doctor's care, consult your physician. Repeated use can possibly result in contact sensitization.

Melissa *(Melissa officinalis)*

Botanical Family: Lamiaceae or Labiatae (mint)

Plant Origin: Utah, Idaho, France

Extraction Method: Steam distilled from leaves and flowers.

Chemical Constituents: Monoterpenols: linalol, nerol, geraniol, citronnellol, α terpineol; Sesquiterpenols; Terpene esters: geranial acetates, Terpene oxides: 1,8 cineole; Monoterpenals: citrals, neral (15%) geranial (15%); Coumarins.

Action: Calming, sedative, hypotensive (low blood pressure), fights against cholera, and anti-inflammatory.

Found In: Brain Power, Forgiveness, Hope, Humility, Passion, and White Angelica.

Traditional Uses: Melissa has powerful anti-microbial constituents. The nature of the plant is very gentle and delicate and helps to bring out those characteristics in an individual. Anciently, melissa was used for nervous disorders and many different ailments dealing with the heart or the emotions. It was also used to promote fertility. Melissa was the main ingredient in Carmelite water, distilled in France since 1611 by the Carmelite monks.

Indications: Dr. Dietrich Wabner, a professor at the Technical University of Munich, reported that a one-time application of true melissa oil led to complete remission of Herpes Simplex lesions.

Other Uses: Allergies, anxiety, asthma, bronchitis, chronic coughs, respiratory infections, cold-sore blisters, indigestion, depression, dysentery, eczema, fevers, hypertension, indigestion, insect bites, insomnia, menstrual problems, migraine, nausea, nervous tension, palpitations, throat infections, and vertigo.

Application: Diffuse or apply topically.

Fragrant Influence: Melissa brings out gentle characteristics within people. It is calming and uplifting and may help to balance the emotions. It may also help to remove emotional blocks and instill a positive outlook on life.

Safety Data: If pregnant or under a doctor's care, consult physician.

Companion Oils: Geranium, lavender, and other floral and citrus oils.

Selected Research:

Yamasaki K, et al. "Anti-HIV-1 activity of herbs in Labiatae." *Biol Pharm Bull.* 1998;21(8):829-33.

Larrondo JV, et al. "Antimicrobial activity of essences from labiates." *Microbios.* 1995;82(332):171-2.

Kucera LS, et al. "Antiviral activities of extracts of the lemon balm plant." *Ann NY Acad Sci.* 1965 Jul 30;130(1):474-82.

Mountain Savory *(Satureja montana)*

Botanical Family: Lamiaceae or Labiatae

Plant Origin: France

Extraction Method: Steam distilled from flowering plant.

Chemical Constituents: Monoterpenes: α thujene, α and β–pinenes, camphene, sabinene, myrcene, limonene; Sesquiterpenes; Monoterpenes: linalol; Terpene alcohols, Terpene esters; Phenols: thymol, carvacrol (25-50%), eugenol; Phenols methyl-ethers: methyl carvacrol; Terpene oxides: 1,8 cineol; Ketones, camphor.

Action: Strong anti-infectious, antibacterial, antifungal, antiviral, antiparasitic, immuno-stimulant, general tonic and stimulant.

Found In: ImmuPower, Surrender

Traditional Uses: Mountain savory has been used historically as a general tonic for the body.

Indications: Reduces acute pain and is a tonic for the nerves and circulatory systems.

Other Uses: Due to its high phenol content, mountain savory is a very strong antiseptic and has been used to hasten the formation of scar tissue, and to help with abscesses, burns, and cuts. It is also known to stimulate the adrenal gland. Recent research suggests that the extract may have anti-HIV activity.

Application: Diffuse or apply topically mixed with massage oil.

Fragrant Influence: It may produce strong psychological effects and may help revitalize and stimulate the nervous system. It is a powerful energizer and motivator.

Safety Data: If pregnant or under a doctor's care, consult your physician. Dilution is recommended when using topically. Always skin test for sensitivity.

Selected Research:

Yamasaki K, et al. "Anti-HIV-1 activity of herbs in Labiatae." *Biol Pharm Bull*. 1998; 21(8):829-33.

Panizzi L, et al. "Composition and antimicrobial properties of essential oils of four Mediterranean Lamiaceae." *J Ethnopharmacol*. 1993;39(3):167-70.

Myrrh *(Commiphora myrrha)*

Botanical Family: Burseraceae (Frankincense)

Plant Origin: Somalia

Extraction Method: Steam distilled from gum/resin.

Chemical Constituents: Hydrocarbons; Sesquiterpenes; Sesquiterpenes furanics; Sesquiterpenones furanics; Ketones; Aldehydes.

Action: Anti-infectious, antiviral, antiparasitic, hormone-like, anti-inflammatory, soothes skin conditions, antihyperthyroid, and supports immune system.

Found In: Abundance, Exodus II, Hope, Humility, 3 Wise Men, and White Angelica.

Traditional Uses: The Arabian people used myrrh for many skin conditions, such as chapped and cracked skin and wrinkles. It has one of the highest levels of sesquiterpenes, a class of compounds that has direct effects on the hypothalamus, pituitary, and amygdala, the seat of our emotions. Myrrh is widely used today in oral hygiene products.

Indications: Bronchitis, diarrhea, dysentery, hyperthyroidism, stretch marks, thrush, ulcers, vaginal thrush, and viral hepatitis.

Other Uses: This oil may help asthma, athlete's foot, candida, coughs, eczema, digestion, fungal infection, gingivitis, gum infections, hemorrhoids, mouth ulcers, ringworm, sore throats, skin conditions (chapped and cracked), wounds, and wrinkles.

Application: Apply topically on location or in a massage. May be added to food or water as a dietary supplement.

Fragrant Influence: Myrrh promotes spiritual awareness and is uplifting.

Safety Data: If pregnant or under a doctor's care, consult physician.

Companion Oils: Frankincense, lavender, patchouly, sandalwood, and all spice oils.

Bible References: (see additional Bible references in Appendix D)

Genesis 37:25—"And they sat down to eat bread: and they lifted up their eyes and looked, and, behold, a company of Ishmeelites came from Gilead with their camels bearing spicery and balm and myrrh, going to carry [it] down to Egypt."

Genesis 43:11—"And their father Israel said unto them, If [it must be] so now, do this; take of the best fruits in the land in your vessels, and carry down the man a present, a little balm, and a little honey, spices, and myrrh, nuts, and almonds:"

Exodus 30:23—"Take thou also unto thee principal spices, of pure myrrh five hundred [shekels], and of sweet cinnamon half so much, [even] two hundred and fifty [shekels], and of sweet calamus two hundred and fifty [shekels],"

Selected Research:

Al-Awadi FM, et al. "Studies on the activity of individual plants of an antidiabetic plant mixture." *Acta Diabetol Lat*. 1987;24(1):37-41.

Dolara P, et al. "Analgesic effects of myrrh." *Nature*. 1996 Jan 4;379(6560):29.

Michie CA, et al. "Frankincense and myrrh as remedies in children." *J R Soc Med*. 1991;84(10):602-5.

Myrtle *(Myrtus communis)*

Botanical Family: Myrtaceae (myrtle)

Plant Origin: Tunisia, Morocco

Extraction Method: Steam distilled from leaves.

Chemical Constituents: Monoterpenes: α pinene (24-25%), β–pinene; Sesquiterpenes; Monoterpene alcohols: linalol, geraniol; Terpene esters: linalyle acetate, geranyle, bornyle; Terpene oxides: 1,8 cineole (45%); Aldehydes: Lactones.

Action: Expectorant, anti-infectious, liver stimulant, prostate decongestant, light antispasmodic, hormone-like for the thyroid and ovary, and a tonic for the skin.

Found In: EndoFlex, Inspiration, Mister, Purification, and R.C.

Traditional Uses: Myrtle has been researched by Dr. Daniel Pénoël for normalizing hormonal imbalances of the thyroid and ovaries, as well as balancing the hypothyroid. It has also been researched for its soothing effects on the respiratory system.

Indications: Bronchitis, coughs, hypothyroidism, insomnia, thyroid hormone-like effects, prostate decongestant, respiratory tract ailments, sinus infection, tuberculosis, and ureter infections.

Other Uses: This oil may help anger, asthma, respiratory infections, cystitis, diarrhea, dysentery, dyspepsia (impaired digestion), flatulence (gas), hemorrhoids, hormonal imbalances, support immune system, infections, infectious diseases, pulmonary disorders, skin conditions (acne, blemishes, bruises, oily skin, psoriasis, etc.), and sinusitis. Useful on children for chest complaints and coughs.

Application: Apply topically, diffuse, or use in a humidifier. Suitable for use on children.

Fragrant Influence: Elevating and euphoric.

Safety Data: If pregnant or under a doctor's care, consult physician.

Companion Oils: Bergamot, lavender, lemon, lemongrass, melaleuca, rosewood, rosemary, spearmint, and thyme.

Bible Reference: (see additional Bible references in Appendix D)

Nehemiah 8:15—"And that they should publish and proclaim in all their cities, and in Jerusalem, saying, Go forth unto the mount, and fetch olive branches, and pine branches, and myrtle branches, and palm branches, and branches of thick trees, to make booths, as [it is] written."

Isaiah 41:19—"I will plant in the wilderness the cedar, the shittah tree, and the myrtle, and the oil tree; I will set in the desert the fir tree, [and] the pine, and the box tree together:"

Isaiah 55:13—"Instead of the thorn shall come up the fir tree, and instead of the brier shall come up the myrtle tree: and it shall be to the Lord for a name, for an everlasting sign [that] shall not be cut off."

Neroli *(Citrus aurantium)*

Botanical Family: Rutaceae (citrus)

Plant Origin: Morocco, Tunisia

Extraction Method: Absolute extraction from flowers of the orange tree.

Chemical Constituents: Monoterpenes (35%); α pinene, β–pinenes (17.75%), limonene (11.45%); Alcols arom. (40%); linalol (30-32%); Esters; Aldehydes; Ketones: jasmone.

Action: Anti-infectious, antibacterial, antiparasitic, digestive tonic, antidepressive, and hypotensive (lowers blood pressure).

Found In: Acceptance, Awaken, Humility, Inner Child, Passion, and Present Time.

Traditional Uses: Loved by the Egyptian people for its great attributes for healing the mind, body, and spirit.

Indications: Neroli may support the digestive system and fight bacteria, infections, parasites, and viruses. It may also help with anxiety, depression, digestive spasms, fear, headaches, heart arrhythmia, hysteria, insomnia, nervous nervous tension, palpitations, PMS, poor circulation, scars, shock, stress-related conditions, stretch marks, tachycardia, thread veins, and wrinkles.

Other Uses: In support of the skin, neroli works at the cellular level to help shed the old skin cells and stimulate new cell growth. It is particularly beneficial for mature and sensitive skin.

Application: Diffuse or apply topically.

Fragrant Influence: As a natural tranquilizer, neroli has some powerful psychological effects. It has been used successfully to treat depression, anxiety, and shock. It is calming and relaxing to body and spirit. It may also help to strengthen and stabilize the emotions and bring relief to seemingly hopeless situations. Neroli encourages confidence, courage, joy, peace, and sensuality. It brings everything into focus at the moment.

Safety Data: If pregnant or under a doctor's care, consult physician.

Companion Oils: Cedarwood, geranium, jasmine, lavender, lemon, rose, and sandalwood.

Nutmeg (Myristica fragrans)

Botanical Family: Myristicaceae

Plant Origin: Tunisia, Indonesia

Extraction Method: Steam distilled from fruits and seeds.

Chemical Constituents: Monoterpenes: α and β-pinenes 915-10%), myrcene (12%), sabinene (15%), limonene (4%); Monoterpenols: terpinene; Phenols.

Action: Antiseptic, antiparasitic, reduces pain, analgesic, promotes menstruation, and improves circulation.

Found In: EndoFlex, En-R-Gee, and Magnify Your Purpose.

Traditional Uses: It has been used historically to benefit circulation to muscles and joints, and relieve muscle pain. It also helps to support the nervous system, overcome fatigue, and support immune and nervous systems.

Indications: Appetite (loss of), chronic debility, digestion (helps with starchy foods and fats), gallstones, halitosis, and rheumatism.

Other Uses: This oil has adrenal cortex-like activity, which helps support the adrenal glands for increased energy. It may also help treat arthritis, bacterial infection, frigidity, gout, impotence, menstrual problems, nausea, severe nerve pain.

Application: Apply topically mixed with massage oil. Add to food or water as a dietary supplement or flavoring.

Safety Data: If pregnant or under a doctor's care, consult your physician. Do not use if epileptic. Dilute with massage oil or only apply a single undiluted drop at a time when applied topically.

Companion Oils: Cinnamon bark, clove, cypress, frankincense, lemon, melaleuca, melissa, orange, patchouly, and rosemary.

Orange (Citrus sinensis)

Botanical Family: Rutaceae (citrus)

Plant Origin: USA, South Africa, Italy, China

Extraction Method: Cold pressed from rind.

Chemical Constituents: Monoterpenes (90-92%); limonene (90%); Esters; Aldehydes; Coumarins and furocoumarins; contains flavonoids, β-carotene, steroids, and acids.

Action: Calming, sedative, anti-inflammatory, antitumoral, anticoagulant, and improves circulation.

Found In: Abundance, Christmas Spirit, Citrus Fresh, Envision, Harmony, Inner Child, Into The Future, Peace & Calming, and SARA.

Traditional Uses: Palpitation, scurvy, jaundice, bleeding, heartburn, relaxed throat, prolapse of the uterus and the anus, diarrhea, and blood in the feces.

Indications: Angina (false), cardiac spasm, insomnia, menopause, and tumor growth.

Other Uses: Orange oil may help appetite, bones (rickety), bronchitis, respiratory infections, indigestion (dilute for infants; helps them sleep), complexion (dull and oily), dermatitis, digestive system, lowers high cholesterol, mouth ulcers, muscle soreness, sedation, tissue repair, fluid retention, and wrinkles.

Application: Diffuse, apply topically on location, or add to food or water as a dietary supplement flavoring.

Fragrant Influence: Uplifting, works as an antidepressant.

Safety Data: If pregnant or under a doctor's care, consult your physician. Citrus oils should NOT be applied to skin that will be exposed to direct sunlight or UV light within 72 hours.

Companion Oils: Cinnamon bark, clove, cypress, frankincense, geranium, juniper, lavender, nutmeg, and rosewood.

Selected Research:

Reddy BS, et al. "Chemoprevention of colon carcinogenesis by dietary perillyl alcohol." *Cancer Res.* 1997;57(3):420-5.

Oregano *(Origanum compactum)*

Botanical Family: Lamiaceae or Labiatae (mint)

Plant Origin: Utah, Turkey, France

Extraction Method: Steam distilled from leaves and flowers.

Chemical Constituents: Monoterpenes (25%): α and β–pinenes, myrcene; Sesquiterpenes; Monoterpenols: linalol; Monoterpene phenols (60-72%): carvacrol, thymol: Phenols: methyl chavicol; Monoterpene ketones: camphor.

Action: Powerful anti-infectious agent (for respiratory, intestines, genital, nerves, blood, and lymphatics) with large-spectrum action against bacteria, mycobacteria, fungus, virus, and parasites. It is a general tonic and immune stimulant.

Found In: ImmuPower

Indications: Asthma, bronchitis (chronic), mental disease, pulmonary tuberculosis, rheumatism (chronic), and whooping cough.

Other Uses: This oil may help respiratory infections, digestion problems, balance metabolism, viral and bacterial pneumonia, respiratory system problems, and strengthen the vital centers.

Application: Apply topically neat to bottom of feet. Mix with massage oil if applying elsewhere on the skin. May be used undiluted in Raindrop Therapy. Add to food or water as a dietary supplement or flavoring.

Fragrant Influence: Creates a feeling of security.

Safety Data: If pregnant or under a doctor's care, consult your physician. Skin test for sensitivity.

Companion Oils: Basil, fennel, geranium, lemongrass, myrtle, pine, rosemary, and thyme.

Palmarosa *(Cymbopogon martinii)*

Botanical Family: Poaceae or Gramineae (grasses)

Plant Origin: India, Conoros

Extraction Method: Steam distilled from leaves.

Chemical Constituents: Monoterpenes; limonene; Alcohols: geraniol (35-65%); Monoterpenones; carvone.

Action: Antimicrobial, antibacterial, antifungal, antiviral, uterine tonic, and cardiotonic.

Found In: Awaken, Clarity, Forgiveness, Gentle Baby, Harmony, Joy.

Traditional Uses: Helps with skin problems. A relative of lemongrass, palmarosa is antimicrobial and supportive to the nerves and circulation.

Indications: This oil may be beneficial for candida, cardiovascular system, circulation, digestion, infection, nervous system, and rashes. It is valuable for all types of skin problems because it stimulates new cell growth, regulates oil production, moisturizes, and speeds healing.

Application: Apply topically.

Fragrant Influence: Creates a feeling of security. It also helps to reduce stress and tension and promotes recovery from nervous exhaustion.

Safety Data: If pregnant or under a doctor's care, consult physician.

Companion Oils: Basil, fennel, geranium, lemongrass, myrtle, pine, rosemary, and thyme.

Patchouly (Pogostemon cablin)

Botanical Family: Lamiaceae or Labiatae (mint)

Plant Origin: Indonesia, India

Extraction Method: Steam distilled from flowers.

Chemical Constituents: Monoterpenes; α and β−pinenes; Sesquiterpenes (40-45%); Sesquiterpenolnes: pathoulenone; Acids; Sesquiterpenes alkaloids.

Action: Tonic and stimulant, soothing to digestion, decongestant, anti-inflammatory, anti-infectious, antimicrobial, antiseptic, and soothes wrinkled or chapped skin.

Found In: Abundance, Di-Tone, Magnify Your Purpose, Passion, and Peace & Calming.

Traditional Uses: It is very beneficial for the skin and may help prevent wrinkles or chapped skin. It is a general tonic and stimulant and helps the digestive system. It is also antimicrobial, antiseptic, and helps relieve itching.

Indications: Allergies, dermatitis, eczema, hemorrhoids, and tissue regeneration.

Other Uses: This oil is a digester of toxic material in the body. It may also help acne, curb appetite, bites (insect and snake), cellulite, congestion, dandruff, depression, digestive system, relieve itching from hives, skin conditions (chapped and tightens loose skin), fluid retention, weeping wounds, weight reduction, and prevent wrinkles.

Application: Diffuse or apply topically.

Fragrant Influence: It is sedating, calming, and relaxing, allowing it to reduce anxiety. It may have some particular influence on sex, physical energy, and money.

Safety Data: If pregnant or under a doctor's care, consult physician.

Companion Oils: Bergamot, clary sage, frankincense, geranium, ginger, lavender, lemongrass, myrrh, pine, rosewood, and sandalwood.

Pepper (Black) (Piper nigrum)

Botanical Family: Piperaceae

Plant Origin: Madagascar, Egypt, India

Extraction Method: Steam distilled from berries.

Chemical Constituents: Monoterpene: α and β−pinenes; Sesquiterpenes (85-90%); Terpene alcohols; Ketones; Acetophenones: Aldehydes.

Action: May help with toothache, expectorant, stimulates digestive secretions, reduces pain, and dispels fever.

Found In: Dream Catcher, En-R-Gee, and Relieve It.

Traditional Uses: Pepper was used by the Egyptians in mummification as evidenced by the discovery of black pepper in the nostrils and abdomen of Ramses II. Indian monks ate several black pepper corns a day to maintain their incredible stamina and energy.

Other Uses: This oil may increase cellular oxygenation, support digestive glands, stimulate endocrine system, increase energy, and help rheumatoid arthritis. It may also help with loss of appetite, chills, cholera, respiratory infections, indigestion, constipation, coughs, diarrhea, dysentery, dysuria, flatulence (when combined with fennel), heartburn, influenza, nausea, neuralgia, poor circulation, poor muscle tone, quinsy, sprains, toothache, vertigo, viruses, and vomiting.

Application: Apply topically to bottom of feet. Dilute with massage oil when applying topically elsewhere. Add to food or water as a dietary supplement or flavoring.

Fragrant Influence: Comforting and stimulating.

Safety Data: If pregnant or under a doctor's care, consult your physician. Skin test for irritation.

Companion Oils: cumin, fennel, frankincense, lavender, marjoram, rosemary, sandalwood, and other spice oils.

Selected Research:

Unnikrishnan MC, et al. "Tumour reducing and anticarcinogenic activity of selected spices." *Cancer Lett.* 1990;51(1):85-9.

Peppermint (*Mentha piperita*)

Botanical Family: Lamiaceae or Labiatae (mint)

Plant Origin: North America

Extraction Method: Steam distilled from leaves, stems, and flower buds.

Chemical Constituents: Monoterpenes: α pinene, β–pinene, limonene: Monoterpenols: menthol (38-48%); Monoterpenones: menthone (20-30%); Terpene oxides: 1,8 cineol; Terpene esters: menthol acetate; Coumarins, Sulfurs: dimenthalsulfide.

Action: Anticarcinogenic, supports digestion, expels worms, decongestant, anti-infectious, antibacterial, antifungal, mucolytic, stimulant, hypertensive, cardiotonic, stimulates gallbladder, pain-relieving, expectorant, and anti-inflammatory for the intestinal and urinary tract. It can heighten or restore the sense of taste by stimulating the trigeminal nerve.

Found In: Aroma Siez, Clarity, Di-Tone, M-Grain, Mister, PanAway, R.C., Raven, and Relieve It.

Traditional Uses: Peppermint is one of the oldest and most highly regarded herbs for soothing digestion. Jean Valnet, M.D.,

studied peppermint's effect on the liver and respiratory systems. Other scientists have also researched peppermint's role in affecting impaired taste and smell when inhaled. Dr. Dember of the University of Cincinnati studied peppermint's ability to improve concentration and mental accuracy. Alan Hirsch, M.D., studied peppermint's ability to directly affect the brain's satiety center (the ventromedial nucleus of the hypothalamus) which triggers a sensation of fullness after meals.

Indications: Asthma, bronchitis, candida, diarrhea, digestive aid, reduces fever, halitosis, heartburn, hemorrhoids, hot flashes, indigestion, menstrual irregularity, headaches, motion sickness, nausea, tumor growth, respiratory infections, shock, itchy skin, throat infections, and varicose veins.

Other Uses: This oil may help arthritis, indigestion, depression, skin conditions (eczema, psoriasis, dermatitis), food poisoning, headaches, hives, hysteria, inflammation, morning sickness, nerve regeneration, rheumatism, elevate and open sensory system, toothaches, and tuberculosis.

Application: Diffuse. Massage on the stomach or add to water or tea. Apply to bottom of feet or rub on the temples to treat headaches. To improve concentration, alertness, and memory, place several drops on the tongue. Add to food as a flavoring and preservative.

Fragrant Influence: It is purifying and stimulating to the conscious mind.

Safety Data: If pregnant or under a doctor's care, consult your physician. Avoid contact with eyes, mucus membranes, or sensitive skin areas. Do not apply neat to a fresh wound or burn.

Selected Research:

Gobel H, et al. "Effect of peppermint and eucalyptus oil preparations on neurophysiological and experimental algesimetric headache parameters." *Cephalalgia.* 1994; 14(3):228-34.

Juergens UR, et al. "The anti-inflammatory activity of L-menthol compared to mint oil in human monocytes in vitro: a novel perspective for its therapeutic use in inflammatory diseases." *Eur J Med Res*. 1998; 3(12):539-45.

Samman MA, et al. "Mint prevents shamma-induced carcinogenesis in hamster cheek pouch." *Carcinogenesis*. 1998;19(10):1795-801.

Petitgrain *(Citrus aurantium)*

Botanical Family: Rutaceae (citrus)

Plant Origin: Italy

Extraction Method: Steam distilled from leaves and twigs.

Chemical Constituents: Monoterpenes (10%); myrcene; Terpene esters (50-70%), linalyle (45-55%).

Action: Antispasmodic, anti-inflammatory, anti-infectious, antibacterial.

Traditional Uses: Petitgrain derives its name from the extraction of the oil, which at one time was from the green unripe oranges when they were still about the size of a cherry.

Other Uses: This oil may help re-establish nerve equilibrium. It may also help with acne, fatigue, greasy hair, insomnia, and excessive perspiration.

Application: Diffuse or apply topically.

Fragrant Influence: Petitgrain is uplifting and helps to refresh the senses, clear confusion, reduce mental fatigue, and reduce depression. It may also stimulate the mind, support memory, and gladden the heart.

Safety Data: If pregnant or under a doctor's care, consult physician.

Companion Oils: Bergamot, cistus, clary sage, clove, geranium, jasmine, lavender, neroli, orange, palmarosa, and rosemary.

Pine *(Pinus sylvestris)*

Botanical Family: Pinaceae (pine)

Plant Origin: Austria, Russia, Canada

Extraction Method: Steam distilled from needles.

Chemical Constituents: Monoterpenes: α and β-pinenes, limonene (25-30%); Sesquiterpenes; Monoterpenols: borneol; Sesquiterpenols; Terpene esters: bornyle acetate.

Action: Hormone-like, antidiabetic, cortisone-like, sexual stimulant, hypertensive (high blood pressure), anti-infectious, antifungal, and antiseptic.

Found In: Grounding and R.C.

Traditional Uses: Pine was first investigated by Hippocrates, the father of Western medicine, for its benefits to the respiratory system. In 1990, Dr. Pénoël and Dr. Franchomme described pine oil's antiseptic properties in their medical textbook. Pine is used in massage for stressed muscles and joints. It shares many of the same properties as *Eucalyptus globulus*, and the action of both oils is enhanced when blended. Native Americans stuffed mattresses with pine needles to repel lice and fleas. It was used to treat lung infections and even added to baths to revitalize those suffering from mental or emotional fatigue.

Indications: Asthma, pulmonary infections, bronchitis, diabetes, severe infections, rheumatoid arthritis, and sinusitis.

Other Uses: This oil may help dilate the respiratory system, particularly the bronchial tract. It may also help with respiratory infections, coughs, cuts, cysts, fatigue, gout, lice, nervous exhaustion, scabies, skin parasites, sores, stress, and urinary infection. Pine oil may also help increase blood pressure and stimulate the adrenal glands and the circulatory system. Pine is a good recommendation for any first aid kit.

Application: Diffuse or apply topically. Dilute to avoid possible skin irritation. Put two drops in palms of hands, place over mouth and nose, and inhale. Add 2 to 4 drops to warm bathwater. Disperse with Bath Gel Base if desired.

Fragrant Influence: Pine helps soothe mental stress, relieve anxiety, freshen and deodorize a room, and revitalize the entire body.

Safety Data: If pregnant or under a doctor's care, consult your physician. Avoid oils adulterated with turpentine, a low-cost, but potentially hazardous filler.

Companion Oils: Cedarwood, eucalyptus, juniper, lavender, lemon, marjoram, melaleuca, and rosemary.

Bible Reference:

Nehemiah 8:15—"And that they should publish and proclaim in all their cities, and in Jerusalem, saying, Go forth unto the mount, and fetch olive branches, and pine branches, and myrtle branches, and palm branches, and branches of thick trees, to make booths, as [it is] written."

Isaiah 41:19—"I will plant in the wilderness the cedar, the shittah tree, and the myrtle, and the oil tree; I will set in the desert the fir tree, [and] the pine, and the box tree together:"

Isaiah 60:13—"The glory of Lebanon shall come unto thee, the fir tree, the pine tree, and the box together, to beautify the place of my sanctuary; and I will make the place of my feet glorious."

Ravensara (*Ravensara aromatica*)

Botanical Family: Lauraceae

Plant Origin: Madagascar

Extraction Method: Steam distilled from branches.

Chemical Constituents: Monoterpenes: α and β−pinene; Sesquiterpenes; Monoterpenols: Terpene esters: terpenyle acetate; Terpene oxides; 1,8 cineole.

Action: Anti-infectious, antiviral, antibacterial, expectorant, antimicrobial, and supports nerves and respiratory system.

Found In: ImmuPower and Raven.

Traditional Uses: Ravensara is referred to by the people of Madagascar as "the oil that heals." It is antimicrobial and supporting to the nerves and respiratory system.

Indications: Bronchitis, cholera, herpes, infectious mononucleosis, insomnia, muscle fatigue, rhinopharyngitis, shingles, sinusitis, viral hepatitis.

Other Uses: Ravensara may help asthma, cystitis, burns, cancer, respiratory infections, cuts, pneumonia, strengthen the respiratory system, scrapes, viral infections, and wounds.

Application: Diffuse or apply topically.

Safety Data: If pregnant or under a doctor's care, consult physician.

Rose (*Rosa damascena*)

Botanical Family: Rosaceae

Plant Origin: Bulgaria, Turkey

Extraction Method: Steam distilled from flower (a two-part process).

Chemical Constituents: Hydrocarbures; Monoterpenols: geraniol; Sesquiterpene alcohols: farnesol; Terpene esters; Phenols: eugenol, methyl eugenol; Oxides: rose oxides.

Action: Anti-inflammatory, prevents and reduces scarring, and balances and elevates mind.

Found In: Envision, Forgiveness, Gathering, Gentle Baby, Humility, Harmony, Joy, SARA, Trauma Life, and White Angelica.

Traditional Uses: Rose has been used for the skin for thousands of years. The Arab physician, Avicenna, was responsible for first distilling rose oil, eventually authoring an entire book on the healing attributes of the rose water derived from the distillation of rose. Throughout much of ancient history, the oil was produced by enfleurage, a process of pressing the petals along with a vegetable oil to extract the essence. Today, however, almost all rose oils are solvent extracted.

NOTE: The Bulgarian *Rosa damascena* (high in citronellol) is very different from Morrocan *Rosa centifolia* (high in phenyl ethanol). They have different colors, aromas, and therapeutic actions.

Other Uses: This oil may help asthma, chronic bronchitis, herpes simplex, impotence, scarring, sexual debilities, skin diseases, and wrinkles.

Application: Diffuse or apply topically.

Fragrant Influence: Its beautiful fragrance is intoxicating and aphrodisiac-like. It helps bring balance and harmony, allowing one to overcome insecurities. It is stimulating and elevating to the mind, creating a sense of well-being.

Safety Data: If pregnant or under a doctor's care, consult physician.

Selected Research:

Sysoev NP. "The effect of waxes from essential-oil plants on the dehydrogenase activity of the blood neutrophils in mucosal trauma of the mouth." *Stomatologiia* 1991;70(1):12-3.

Mahmood N, et al. "The anti-HIV activity and mechanisms of action of pure compounds isolated from Rosa damascena." *Biochem Biophys Res Commun.* 1996;229(1):73-9.

Rosemary Cineol *(Rosmarinus officinalis* 1,8 Cineol CT*)*

Botanical Family: Labiatae

Plant Origin: France, U.S.

Extraction Method: Steam distilled from leaves.

Chemical Constituents: Monoterpenes: α-pinene (12%), β-pinene, camphene (22%), myrcene (1.5%) α-and β-phellandrene, limonene (0.5 to 2%) α-and γ-terpinenes, paracymene (2%); Sesquiterpenes: β-caryophyllene (3%); Monoterpenols: linalol (0.5 to 1%), terpinen 1-ol-4, α-terpineol (1.5%), borneol (3.5%), isoborneol, cis and trans thujanol-4, p-cymene-8-ol; Terpene Esters: bornyl acetate (0.2%) α-fenchyl acetate; Terpene Oxides: 1,8 cineole (30%) caryophyllene oxide, humulene epoxides I and II; Non-terpene Ketones: 3-hexanone, methyl heptanone; Monoterpenones: camphor (30%), verbenone, carvone (0.4%).

Action: Antifungal, antibacterial, antiseptic, antiparasitic, general stimulant, enhances mental clarity, and supports nerves and endocrine gland balance.

Found In: Clarity, En-R-Gee, JuvaFlex, Melrose, Purification, and Thieves.

Traditional Use: Rosemary was part of the "Marseilles Vinegar" or "Four Thieves Vinegar" used by grave-robbing bandits to protect themselves during the 15th century plague. The name of the oil is derived from the latin words for dew of the sea (ros + marinus), According to folklore history, rosemary originally had white flowers; however they turned red after the Virgin Mary laid her cloak on the bush. Since the time of ancient Greece (about 1000 BC), rosemary was burnt as incense. Later cultures believed that it warded off devils, a practice that eventually became adopted by the sick who instead burned rosemary to protect against infection. Until recently, French hospitals continued to use rosemary this way in order to disinfect the air.

Indications: Rheumatism, arthritis, myalgia, hepatitis, liver conditions, menstrual disturbances, hypertension (weak doses), hypotension (strong doses), indigestion, bronchitis, respiratory and lung infections, hair loss (alopecia areata), asthma.

Other Uses: Improves concentration, stimulates the scalp.

Application: Diffuse, inhale, or apply topically on location. May also be added to food or water as a dietary supplement.

Fragrant Influence: Helps overcome mental fatigue and improves mental clarity and focus.

Safety Data: Epileptics should use with caution. If pregnant or under a doctor's care, consult physician.

Companion Oils: Basil, eucalyptus, lavender, marjoram, peppermint, and pine.

Selected Research:

Larrondo JV, et al. "Antimicrobial activity of essences from labiates." *Microbios.* 1995; 82(332):171-2.

Panizzi L, et al. "Composition and antimicrobial properties of essential oils of four Mediterranean Lamiaceae." *J Ethnopharmacol.* 1993;39(3):167-70.

Diego MA, et al. "Aromatherapy positively affects mood, EEG patterns of alertness and math computations." *Int J Neurosci.* 1998; 96(3-4):217-24.

Rosemary Verbenon *(Rosmarinus officinalis* Verbenon CT*)*

Botanical Family: Labiatae

Plant Origin: France, U.S.

Extraction Method: Steam distilled from leaves.

Chemical Constituents: Monoterpenes: α–pinene (15-34%), β–pinene, camphene, myrcene, limonene α–terpinenes, terpinolene; Sesquiterpenes: β–caryophyllene; Monoterpenols: borneol (trace to 7%); Terpene Esters: bornyl acetate; Terpene Oxides: 1,8 cineole (trace to 20%); Monoterpenones: verbenon (15-37%), camphor (1-15%).

Action: Mucolytic, expectorant, antispasmodic, antibacterial, antiseptic, and balance endocrine gland.

Found In: Clarity, En-R-Gee, JuvaFlex, Melrose, Purification, and Thieves.

Traditional Uses: The name of the oil is derived from the Latin words for dew of the sea (ros + marinus), According to folklore history, rosemary originally had white flowers; however they turned red after the Virgin Mary laid her cloak on the bush. Rosemary verbenon has been used to lower cholesterol.

Indications: Respiratory infections, bronchitis, viral hepatitis, nervous tension, cardiac arrhythmia, cystitis, arthritis, and rheumatism.

Other Uses: Because of its lower camphor and higher verbenon content, this chemotype of rosemary is milder than the cineol chemotype and so is especially well-suited for chest, lung, and sinus infections. It is ideal for skin care, and can be used to combat hair loss.

Application: Diffuse, inhale, or apply topically on location. May also be added to food or water as a dietary supplement.

Fragrant Influence: Less stimulating than rosemary cineol, rosemary verbenon can be clarifying for emotions and psychologically balancing.

Safety Data: Epileptics should use with caution. If pregnant or under a doctor's care, consult physician.

Companion Oils: Basil, eucalyptus, lavender, marjoram, peppermint, and pine.

Rosewood *(Aniba rosaeodora)*

Botanical Family: Lauraceae

Plant Origin: Brazil

Extraction Method: Steam distilled from wood.

Chemical Constituents: Monoterpenols: linalol (95%).

Action: Anti-infectious, antibacterial, antiviral, antiparasitic, antifungal, soothing to the skin. Rosewood has been researched at Weber State University for its inhibition rate against gram positive and gram negative bacterial growth.

Found In: Acceptance, Awaken, Clarity, Forgiveness, Gentle Baby, Harmony, Humility, Inspiration, Joy, Magnify Your Purpose, Sensation, Valor, and White Angelica.

Indications: Acne, candida, depression, eczema, oral infections, dry skin, and vaginitis.

Other Uses: This oil may create skin elasticity and is soothing to the skin. It is recognized for its ability to get rid of candida of the skin and slow the aging process. It may also be beneficial for cuts, nausea, tissue regeneration, and wounds. It helps to create a synergism with all other oils.

Application: Diffuse or apply topically.

Fragrant Influence: It is soothing and nourishing to the skin.

Safety Data: If pregnant or under a doctor's care, consult physician.

Sage *(Salvia officinalis)*

Botanical Family: Lamiaceae or Labiatae (mint)

Plant Origin: Spain, Croatia, France

Extraction Method: Steam distilled from leaves and flowers.

Chemical Constituents: Monoterpenes: α thujene, α pinene, β−pinene, camphene myrcene, limonene; Sesquiterpenes; Hydrocarbons; Esters; Phenols: thymol; Oxides (15%): 1,8 cineole; Monoterpenones (20-70%): α thujone (12-33%) β−-Thujone (2-14%), camphor (1-26%); Aldehydes; Coumarins.

Action: Expectorant, mucolytic, anti-infectious, fights against cholera, estrogen-like, supports menstruation, prevents and reduces scarring, regulates circulation, soothes skin conditions and is a balancer and detoxifier of the body, Sage contains camphor, which balances estrogen levels, providing support during PMS and menopause.

Found In: EndoFlex, Envision, Magnify Your Purpose, and Mister.

Traditional Uses: Known as "herba sacra" or sacred herb by the ancient Romans, sage's name, *Salvia,* is derived from the word for "salvation." Sage has been used in Europe for oral infections and skin conditions. It has been recognized for its benefits of strengthening the vital centers and supporting metabolism.

Indications: Asthma, chronic bronchitis, sluggish digestion, gingivitis, glandular disorders, menopause, and menstrual irregularity.

Other Uses: This oil may help improve estrogen, progesterone, and testosterone balance. It activates the nervous system and adrenal cortex and may help with illness that is related to digestion and liver problems. It may also be beneficial for acne, arthritis, bacterial infections, dandruff, depression, eczema, fibrosis, hair loss, low blood pressure, mental fatigue, metabolism, respiratory problems, rheumatism, skin conditions, sores, and sprains. Sage strengthens the vital centers of the body, balancing the pelvic chakra where negative emotions from denial and abuse are stored.

Application: Diffuse or apply topically mixed with massage oil. Add to food or water as a dietary supplement or flavoring.

Fragrant Influence: It is mentally stimulating and may help in coping with despair and mental fatigue.

Safety Data: If pregnant or under a doctor's care, consult your physician. Sage is an oral toxin due to thujone content. Do not use if epileptic. Use caution if suffering from high blood pressure.

Companion Oils: Bergamot, lavender, lemon, peppermint, lemongrass, pine, and rosemary.

Sandalwood *(Santalum album)*

Botanical Family: Santalaceae (sandalwood)

Plant Origin: Indonesia, India

Extraction Method: Steam distilled from wood.

Chemical Constituents: Sesquiterpenes; Sesquiterpenols: α and β−santalols (67%); Sesquiterpenals; carbonic acid.

Action: Sandalwood is high in sesquiterpenes that have been researched in Europe for their ability to stimulate the pineal gland and the limbic region of the brain, the center of emotions. The pineal gland is responsible for releasing melatonin, a powerful antioxidant that enhances deep sleep. Sandalwood is similar to frankincense oil in its support of nerves and circulation.

Found In: Acceptance, Brain Power, Dream Catcher, Forgiveness, Gathering, Harmony, Inner Child, Inspiration, Magnify Your Purpose, Passion, Release, 3 Wise Men, Trauma Life, and White Angelica.

Traditional Uses: Sandalwood has been used for centuries in Ayurvedic medicine. It was used traditionally for skin revitalization, yoga, and meditation.

Indications: Bronchitis (chronic), herpes, cystitis, skin tumors.

Other Uses: Sandalwood helps with cystitis and urinary tract infections. It may also be beneficial for acne, depression, meditation, pulmonary infections, menstrual problems, nervous tension, and skin infection. It help dry or dehydrated skin.

Application: Diffuse or apply topically. Add to food or water as a dietary supplement or flavoring.

Fragrant Influence: Enhances deep sleep, may help remove negative programming from the cells.

Safety Data: If pregnant or under a doctor's care, consult your physician.

Companion Oils: Cypress, frankincense, lemon, myrrh, patchouly, spruce, and ylang ylang.

Selected References:

Benencia F, et al. "Antiviral activity of sandalwood oil against herpes simplex viruses-1 and -2." *Phytomedicine.* 1999;6(2):119-23

Dwivedi C, et al. "Chemopreventive effects of sandalwood oil on skin papillomas in mice." *Eur J Cancer Prev.* 1997;6(4):399-401.

Spearmint *(Mentha spicata)*

Botanical Family: Lamiaceae or Labiatae (mint)

Plant Origin: Utah

Extraction Method: Steam distilled from leaves.

Chemical Constituents: Monoterpenes: α pinene, β–pinene, camphene, myrcene, limonene; Sesquiterpenes; Monoterpenols: menthol, linalol, borneol, Sesquiterpenols: farnesol: Terpene esters: Terpene oxides: 1,8 cineol: Monoterpenones: carvone (55-65%).

Action: Anti-inflammatory, calming, astringent, antiseptic, mucolytic, stimulates gallbladder, and promotes menstruation.

Found In: Citrus Fresh and EndoFlex

Traditional Uses: Spearmint oil has been used to help support the respiratory and nervous systems.

Indications: Bronchitis, candida, cystitis, and hypertension.

Other Uses: This oil may balance and increase metabolism. It may aid the glandular, nervous, and respiratory systems. It may also help with acne, stimulate poor appetite, help bad breath and balance, promote easier labor in childbirth, and help with depression, digestion, dry skin, eczema, headaches, intestines (soothes), menstruation (slow, heavy periods), nausea, sore gums, vaginitis, and excess weight.

Application: Diffuse or apply topically. Add to food or water as a dietary supplement or flavoring.

Fragrant Influence: Spearmint's hormone-like activity may help open and release emotional blocks and bring about a feeling of balance and a lasting sense of well-being.

Safety Data: If pregnant or under a doctor's care, consult your physician.

Companion Oils: Basil, lavender, peppermint, and rosemary.

Spikenard (*Nardostachys jatamansi*)

Botanical Family: Valerianaceae

Plant Origin: India

Extraction Method: Steam distilled from roots.

Chemical Constituents: Sesquiterpenes (93%): Bomyl acetate, isobornyl valerianate, borneol, terpinyl valerianate, terpineol, eugenol, pinene.

Action: Antibacterial, antifungal, anti-inflammatory, deodorant, relaxing, and skin tonic.

Found In: Exodus II and Humility

Traditional Uses: Spikenard is highly regarded in India as a perfume, medicinal herb, and skin tonic. It was the one of the most precious oils in ancient times, used only by priests, kings, or high initiates. References in the New Testament describe how Mary of Bethany used a salve of spikenard to anoint the feet of Jesus before the Last Supper.

Indications: The oil is known for helping in the treatment of allergic skin reactions.

Other Uses: Spikenard may also help with allergies, candida, flatulent indigestion, insomnia, menstrual difficulties, migraine, nausea, rashes, staph infections, stress, tachycardia, tension, and wounds that will heal. According to Dietrich Gumbel, Ph.D. it strengthens the heart and circulatory system.

Application: Apply to abdomen or on location for soothing and calming.

Fragrant Influence: Relaxing, soothing, and helps nourish and regenerate the skin.

Safety Data: If pregnant or under a doctor's care, consult physician.

Companion Oils: Cistus, lavender, patchouly, pine, and vetiver.

Bible References: (see additional Bible references in Appendix D)

Song Of Solomon 1:12—"While the king [sitteth] at his table, my spikenard sendeth forth the smell thereof."

Song Of Solomon 4:13—"Thy plants [are] an orchard of pomegranates, with pleasant fruits; camphire, with spikenard,"

Song Of Solomon 4:14—"Spikenard and saffron; calamus and cinnamon, with all trees of frankincense; myrrh and aloes, with all the chief spices:"

Spruce (*Picea mariana*)

Botanical Family: Pinaceae (pine)

Plant Origin: Canada

Extraction Method: Steam distilled from leaves, needles, and twigs.

Chemical Constituents: Monoterpenes (50-55%): camphene (10-15%), tricyclene, α pinene (13-16%); Sesquiterpenes; Monoterpenols: borneol; Terpene esters (30-37%): bornyle acetate (30-37%); Sesquiterpenols.

Action: Antispasmodic, anti-infectious, antiparasitic, antiseptic, anti-inflammatory, hormone-like, cortisone-like; general tonic, stimulates thymus, releases emotional blocks.

Found In: Abundance, Christmas Spirit, Envision, Gathering, Grounding, Harmony, Hope, Inner Child, Inspiration, Motivation, Present Time, R.C., Relieve It, Sacred Mountain, Surrender, 3 Wise Men, Trauma Life, Valor, and White Angelica

Traditional Uses: The Lakota Indians used spruce to strengthen their ability to communicate with the Great Spirit.

Indications: Arthritis, candida, hyperthyroidism, immune-depression, prostatitis and rheumatism.

Other Uses: Spruce may be beneficial for bone pain, glandular imbalances, aching joints, and sciatica pain. It may help support the nervous system and respiratory system, and can be stimulating the pineal, thymus, and adrenal glands.

Application: Diffuse or apply topically. Add to food or water as a dietary supplement or flavoring.

Fragrant Influence: Helps to open and release emotional blocks, bringing about a feeling of balance. It also helps the respiratory and nervous systems.

Safety Data: If pregnant or under a doctor's care, consult physician.

Companion Oils: Birch, eucalyptus, frankincense, helichrysum, and ravensara.

Tangerine *(Citrus nobilis)*

Botanical Family: Rutaceae (citrus)

Plant Origin: USA, South Africa

Extraction Method: Cold pressed from rind.

Chemical Constituents: Limonene, α-pinene, ß-pinene, mycene, linalol, nerol, p-cymene.

Action: Promotes happiness, helps with anxiety and nervousness.

Found In: Citrus Fresh, Dream Catcher, Inner Child, Peace & Calming.

Indications: Diffuse or apply topically. Add to food or water as a dietary supplement or flavoring.

Other Uses: Tangerine may help dissolve cellulite, improve circulation, and help digestive system disorders, dizziness, anxiety, insomnia, irritability, liver problems, parasites, stretch marks (smooths when blended with lavender), and fluid retention.

Application: Diffuse, take as dietary supplement, or apply topically.

Fragrant Influence: Calming, helps with anxiety and nervousness.

Safety Data: If pregnant or under a doctor's care, consult physician.

Companion Oils: Basil, bergamot, chamomile, clary sage, frankincense, geranium, grapefruit, lavender, lemon, orange.

Tansy (Blue) *(Tanacetum annuum)*

Botanical Family: Asteraceae or Compositae (daisy)

Plant Origin: Morocco, France

Extraction Method: Steam distilled from leaves and flowers.

Chemical Constituents: Monoterpenes: limonene; Sesquiterpenes polyinsatures: chamazulene.

Action: Anti-inflammatory, reduces pain, relieves itching, sedating to the nerves, antihistamine, hypotensive (helps with low blood pressure), hormone-like.

Found In: Acceptance, Dream Catcher, JuvaFlex, Peace & Calming, Release, SARA, and Valor.

Safety Data: If pregnant or under a doctor's care, consult physician.

Tarragon *(Artemisia dracunculus)*

Botanical Family: Asteraceae or Compositae (daisy)

Plant Origin: Slovenia, France

Extraction Method: Steam distilled from leaves.

Chemical Constituents: Methyl Chavicol (60-75%), Coumarins.

Action: Neuromuscular antispasmodic, anti-inflammatory, anti-infectious, antifermentation, and reduces allergies.

Found In: Di-Tone

Traditional Uses: Tarragon has been used in Europe for its antimicrobial and antiseptic functions.

Indications: Colitis, hiccups, intestinal spasms, parasites, rheumatic pain, sciatica.

Other Uses: Tarragon may be beneficial for abdominal discomfort and spasms, arthritis, digestive complaints, genital and urinary tract infection, nausea, premenstrual discomfort, and wounds. It may also balance the autonomic nervous system.

Application: Apply topically mixed with massage oil. Add to food or water as a dietary supplement or flavoring.

Safety Data: If pregnant or under a doctor's care, consult your physician. Do not use if epileptic.

Companion Oils: Chamomile, clary sage, fir, juniper, lavender, pine, rosewood, orange, and tangerine.

Thyme *(Thymus vulgaris)*

Botanical Family: Lamiaceae or Labiatae (mint)

Plant Origin: Utah, Idaho, France

Extraction Method: Steam distilled from leaves, stems, and flowers.

Chemical Constituents: Monoterpenols: geraniol; Terpene esters: geraniol acetate.

Action: Highly antimicrobial, antifungal, antiviral, uterine tonic, cardiotonic.

Traditional Uses: Thyme has been used for respiratory problems, digestive complaints, the prevention and treatment of infection, gastritis, bronchitis, pertussis, asthma, laryngitis, and tonsillitis. The Egyptians used thyme for embalming.

Indications: Asthma, bronchitis, colitis, cystitis, dermatitis, anthrax, fatigue (general), pleurisy, psoriasis, sciatica, tuberculosis, vaginal candida.

Other Uses: This oil is a general tonic for the nerves and stomach. It may also help with bacterial infections, respiratory infections, circulation, depression, digestion, headaches, insomnia, rheumatism, urinary infections, and viruses along the spine.

Application: Apply topically mixed with massage oil.

Fragrant Influence: It may be beneficial in helping to overcome fatigue and exhaustion after illness.

Safety Data: If pregnant or under a doctor's care, consult your physician.

Companion Oils: Bergamot, citrus oil, cedarwood, juniper, melaleuca, oregano, and rosemary.

Selected Research:

Panizzi L, et al. "Composition and antimicrobial properties of essential oils of four Mediterranean Lamiaceae." *J Ethnopharmacol.* 1993;39(3):167-70.

Youdim KA, et al. "Beneficial effects of thyme oil on age-related changes in the phospholipid C20 and C22 polyunsaturated fatty acid composition of various rat tissues." *Biochim Biophys Acta.* 1999;1438(1):140-6.

Inouye S, et al. "Antisporulating and respiration-inhibitory effects of essential oils on filamentous fungi." Mycoses. 1998;41(9-10):403-10.

Valerian *(Valeriana officinalis)*

Botanical Family: Valerianaceae

Plant Origin: Belgium, Croatia, France

Extraction Method: Steam distilled from root.

Chemical Constituents: Monoterpenes: α-pinene, camphene; Sesquiterpenes; azulene; Monoterpenols: geraniol, α-terpineol, borneol, Terpene esters: acetate formiate, butyrate and bornyle isovalerate; Sesquiterpenals L valerenal; Sesquiterpenones: valeranon; Acids: isovaleric and acetoxyvaleric acid.

Action: Sedative and tranquilizing to the central nervous system. Its warming properties can help with hypothermia.

Found In: Trauma Life

Traditional Uses: During the last three decades, valerian has been clinically investigated for its tranquilizing properties. Researchers have pinpointed the sesquiterpenes valerenic acid and valerone as the active constituents that exerts a calming effect on the central nervous system. The German Commission E have pronounced valerian to be an effective treatment for restlessness and for sleep disturbances resulting from nervous conditions.

Other Uses: Because of its effect on the nervous system, it may help with insomnia, nervous indigestion, migraine, restlessness, and tension.

Application: Diffuse or apply topically, especially in a soothing massage. May be added to food or water as a dietary supplement.

Fragrant Influence: Calming, relaxing, grounding, and emotionally balancing; sleep aid.

Safety Data: If pregnant or under a doctor's care, consult your physician. Repeated use can possibly result in contact sensitization.

Companion Oils: Cedarwood, lavender, mandarin, patchouly, petitgrain, pine, and rosemary.

Selected Research:

Wagner J, et al. "Beyond benzodiazepines: alternative pharmacologic agents for the treatment of insomnia." *Ann Pharmacother*. 1998;32(6):680-91.

Vetiver *(Vetiveria zizanioides)*

Botanical Family: Poaceae or Gramineae (grasses)

Plant Origin: Haiti, India

Extraction Method: Steam distilled from root.

Chemical Constituents: Ketones: Vitiverone; Terpenes: vitivene, cadinene; Terpene Alcohols: vetiverol.

Action: Antiseptic, antispasmodic, calming, grounding, rubefacient (locally warming), sedative (nervous system), stimulant (circulatory, production of red corpuscles).

Traditional Uses: It is well known for its anti-inflammatory properties and traditionally used for arthritic symptoms.

Other Uses: Vetiver may help acne, anxiety, arthritis, cuts, depression (including postpartum), insomnia, rheumatism, stress, skin care (oily, aging, tired, irritated).

Application: Diffuse or apply topically, especially in a soothing massage. May be added to food or water as a dietary supplement.

Fragrant Influence: Vetiver has a heavy, earthy fragrance similar to patchouly with a touch of lemon. It is psychologically grounding, calming, and stabilizing. It helps us cope with stress and recover from emotional traumas and shocks.

Safety Data: If pregnant or under a doctor's care, consult your physician.

Companion Oils: Clary sage, jasmine, lavender, patchouly, rose, sandalwood, and ylang ylang.

Vitex *(Vitex negundo)*

Botanical Family: Lamiaceae or Labiatae (mint)

Plant Origin: Turkey

Extraction Method: Steam distilled from the inner bark, small branches, and leaves of the Chaste tree.

Chemical Constituents: α-Terpinyl acetate, 1,8-Cineol, Caryophyllene Oxide, Limonene.

Traditional Uses: Vitex It has been extensively researched in Europe for its effects on Parkinson's and other neurological disorders.

Application: Diffuse or apply topically. Dilute with massage oil for massage. Put in palms and inhale. Add 2 to 4 drops to warm bath water.

Safety Data: If pregnant or under a doctor's care, consult physician.

Note: *Vitex negundo* essential oil is different from the extract of the chaste berry, which is used for PMS symptoms and hormone balance.

White Lotus *(Nymphaea lotus)*

Botanical Family: Nymphaeaceae

Plant Origin: Egypt

Extraction Method: Steam distilled from flower.

Action: Anticancerous

Traditional Uses: White lotus was traditionally used by the Egyptians for spiritual, emotional, and physical application. Research in China found that white lotus contains anticancerous and strong immune supporting properties.

Other Uses: Inflamed eyes, jaundice, kidneys, liver spots, menstruation (promotes), palpitations, rheumatism, sciatica, sprains, sunburn, toothaches, tuberculosis, and vomiting.

Fragrant Influence: Stimulates a positive attitude and a general feeling of well-being.

Safety Data: If pregnant or under a doctor's care, consult your physician.

Companion Oils: Most oils

Note: This oil is only available periodically in very small amounts.

Yarrow *(Achillea millefolium)*

Botanical Family: Asteraceae or Compositae (daisy)

Plant Origin: Utah

Extraction Method: Steam distilled from flowering top.

Chemical Constituents: Monoterpenes: α and $\beta-$ pinenes, campene, sabinene; Sesquiterpenes: chamazulene; Terpene oxides: 1,8 cineol (10%); Monoterpenones: isoartemisia ketone (9%), camphor (18%); Sesquiterpene lactones.

Action: Anti-inflammatory, reduces indigestion, reduces or prevents scarring, promotes penetration, promotes healing of wounds.

Found In: Dragon Time, Mister

Traditional Uses: The Greek Achilles, hero of the Trojan War, was said to have used yarrow herb to help cure the injury to his Achilles tendon. Yarrow was considered sacred by the Chinese, who recognized the harmony of the Yin and Yang energies within it. It has been said that the fragrance of yarrow makes possible the meeting of heaven and earth. Yarrow was used by Germanic tribes for the treatment of battle wounds.

Indications: Yarrow is a powerful decongestant of the prostate and helps to balance hormones. It may also help with acne, amenorrhea, appetite (lack of), bladder or kidney weakness, cellulite, respiratory infections, digestion (poor), menstrual problems, eczema, gallbladder inflammation, gastritis, gout, hair growth, headaches, hemorrhoids, hypertension, liver, menopause problems, neuritis, neuralgia, pelvic and urinary infections, prostitis, rheumatism, sprains, sunburn, thrombosis, ulcers, vaginitis, varicose veins, and wounds.

Application: Diffuse or apply topically.

Fragrant Influence: Balancing highs and lows, both external and internal, yarrow may allow us to have our heads in the clouds while our feet remain firm on the ground. Its balancing properties may also make it useful during meditation. It is supportive to intuitive energies and helps reduce confusion and ambivalence.

Safety Data: If pregnant or under a doctor's care, consult physician.

Ylang Ylang *(Cananga odorata)*

Botanical Family: Annonaceae (custard-apple)

Plant Origin: Commores, Indonesia, Philippines

Extraction Method: Steam distilled from flowers. Flowers are picked early in the morning to maximize oil yield. The highest quality oil is drawn from the first distillation and is known as ylang ylang. The last distillation, known as the tail, is of inferior quality and is called "cananga."

Chemical Constituents: Sesquiterpenes: α farnesene; Alcohols monoterpenes; linalol (55%); Esters; Phenols.

Action: Antispasmodic, balances blood pressure, regulates heartbeat. It is used in hair preparations to promote thick, shiny, lustrous hair (it is also reported to help control split ends).

Found In: Aroma Life, Awaken, Clarity, Dream Catcher, Forgiveness, Gathering, Gentle Baby, Grounding, Harmony, Humility, Inner Child, Into The Future, Joy, Motivation, Peace & Calming, Present Time, Release, Sacred Mountain, SARA, Sensation, White Angelica.

Traditional Use: Ylang ylang means "flower of flowers." Ylang ylang flowers have been used to cover the beds of newlywed couples on their wedding night.

Indications: Ylang ylang helps treat skin conditions, insect bites, heart arrhythmias, cardiac problems, high blood pressure, anxiety, impotence, arterial hypertension, depression, mental fatigue, hair loss, labored breathing, insomnia, palpitations, tachycardia.

Other Uses: Ylang ylang may help balance male-female energies so one can move closer towards being in spiritual attunement and allowing greater focus of thoughts, filtering out the ever-present negative frequencies. It may help lower blood pressure, rapid breathing, balance equilibrium, frustration, balance heart function, impotence, intestinal problems, shock, and skin problems.

Application: Diffuse or apply topically mixed with V-6 Mixing Oil or Massage Oil Base. Add to food or water as a dietary supplement or flavoring.

Fragrant Influence: Ylang ylang influences sexual energy and enhances relationships. It may help stimulate the adrenal glands. It is calming and relaxing and may also help with anger and possibly rage and low self-esteem. It brings back the feeling of self-love, confidence, joy and peace.

Safety Data: If pregnant or under a doctor's care, consult your physician. Repeated use can possibly result in contact sensitization.

CHAPTER 7

Floral Waters

Floral water is an exquisite by-product of the steam distillation of essential oils. It has the same properties as the essential oils, but in lower concentration. It is gentle, fragrant, and suitable for all ages. Floral water provides rehydrating, nurturing, and refreshing benefits to the skin. It is also uniquely calming, soothing, and relaxing.

Caution: DO NOT SPRAY DIRECTLY INTO EARS OR EYES!

Use

1. Spray into the air to freshen the home or office.

2. Spray in an airplane or other enclosed environment to dispel and sanitize stale air.

3. Spray on face to energize, and overcome fatigue and drowsiness.

4. Drink undiluted or diluted to taste with water or juice.

5. Spray on animals to deter pests.

6. Spray on plants to deter pests.

Basil Floral Water—stimulating, energizing, uplifting, and relaxing to the muscles.

Chamomile (German) Floral Water—soothing for sore muscles, tendons, ligaments, skin irritations, and swelling. It is also relaxing.

Clary Sage Floral Water—supports the cells and hormones. It contains natural sclareol, which stimulates the body's production of estrogen. It may also help with headaches, dry skin, or coughs.

Eucalyptus Floral Water—antiseptic and well suited for cleansing oily skin, soothing for respiratory complications, and may be used as an insect repellent.

Juniper Floral Water—stimulating to the nervous system and excellent to detoxify and cleanse the skin.

Lavender Floral Water—soothing to the skin and calming. Spray on skin or mist in air to promote sleep.

Melissa Floral Water—exquisitely relaxing and uplifting. It soothes herpe sores. In lab tests, it has been shown to be antimicrobial against *Streptococcus haemolytica*, which can colonize in the throat and esophagus.

Peppermint Floral Water—uplifting, energizing, cooling, refreshing, and soothing to digestion.

Spearmint Floral Water—cooling and refreshing. It is excellent for cleansing blemished and oily skin and soothing for digestion and headaches.

Tansy (Idaho) Floral Water—encourages an uplifting feeling, a positive attitude, and a general feeling of well-being. It is antimicrobial and supports the cleansing of the lymphatic system.

Thyme Floral Water—antiseptic, cleansing, energizing, and stimulating to the scalp.

CHAPTER 8

Oil Blends

This section describes specific blends that were formulated after years of research into both physical and emotional health. Each of these blends is formulated to maximize the synergistic effect between various oil chemistries and harmonic frequencies. When chemistry and frequency coincide harmonically, noticeable and measurable physical, spiritual, and emotional benefits can be attained.

NOTE: Please keep in mind there are many variables of frequency, based on the calibration and the type of instrument used.

Abundance

This blend was created to enhance the frequency of the energy field that surrounds us through the electrical stimulation of the somatides. Somatides transmit the frequency from the cells to the outside of the body when they are stimulated through fragrance and the thought process. This frequency, called the electrical field or the aura, creates what is called the "law of attraction," or that which we attract to ourselves. This might bring about an abundance of health, both physical and emotional. The oils in Abundance also contain tremendous antiviral and antifungal properties.

Contains:

Myrrh (*Commiphora myrrha*) is an anti-microbial oil referenced throughout the Old and New Testaments (*A bundle of myrrh is my well-beloved unto me*... Song of Solomon 1:13). It was also part of a formula the Lord gave to Moses (Exodus 30:22-27). It was used traditionally in the royal palaces by the queens as an anti-infectious agent during pregnancy and birthing. It has one of the highest levels of sesquiterpenes, a class of compounds that has direct effects on the hypothalamus, pituitary, and amygdala, the emotional center of the brain. It has been used in eastern countries to enhance the feeling of spirituality or euphoria. According to legends, myrrh, which possessed the frequency of wealth, was a trade commodity.

Cinnamon Bark (*Cinnamomum verum*) is the oil of wealth from the Orient and part of the formula the Lord gave to Moses (Exodus 30:22-27). Cinnamon oil is anti-infectious, antibacterial, anti-parasitic, antiviral, and antifungal. Researchers, including J. C. Lapraz, M.D., found that viruses could not live in the presence of cinnamon oil. Cinnamon oil was regarded by the emperors of China and India to have great value; their wealth was measured by the amount of oil they possessed. Traditionally cinnamon was thought to have a frequency that attracted wealth and abundance. Physically, it has many attributes; it is a powerful purifier and oxygenator, and it enhances the action and the activity of other oils.

Frankincense (*Boswellia carteri*) was valued more than gold during ancient times, and only those with great wealth and abundance possessed it. It is considered a holy anointing oil in the Middle East and has been used in religious ceremonies for thousands of years. High in sesquiterpenes, frankincense helps oxygenate the pineal and pituitary glands, which stimulate and elevate the mind, for overcoming stress and despair. Frankincense is presently being studied for its ability to help improve hGH (human growth hormone) receptivity. It relieves depression, builds immune function, and is antitumoral. In ancient times, it was known for its anointing and healing powers, and was reportedly used to treat every conceivable ill known to man..."

Patchouly (*Pogostemon cablin*) is used by East Indian people to fragrance their clothing and homes because of its natural insecticidal and anti-infectious properties. Legends indicate that patchouly represented money and those who possessed it were considered to be wealthy. Patchouly is very beneficial for the skin, relieving itching and preventing wrinkles or chapped skin. It is a general tonic and stimulant and helps the digestive system. It is also antimicrobial and antiseptic.

Orange (*Citrus sinensis*) was believed to bring joy, peace, and happiness to those who possessed it. It contains limonene, an antiviral compound, and citral, an antibacterial compound. It prevents the growth of bacteria and stops free radicals. Bioflavanoids enhance teh action of vitamin C. Orange is elevating to the mind and body and brings joy and peace. It has been recognized to help a dull, oily complexion.

Clove *(Syzygium aromaticum)* is another oil from the Orient associated with great abundance; those who possessed it were considered wealthy. Clove is one of the most antimicrobial and antiseptic of all essential oils. It is antifungal, antiviral, anti-infectious, and antibacterial.

Ginger *(Zingiber officinale)* fights motion sickness and has been studied for its gentle, stimulating effects. It aids digestion and has been used for rheumatism, bronchitis, dyspepsia, constipation, impotence, and lowered libido.

Spruce *(Picea mariana)* helps the respiratory and nervous systems. It is anti-infectious, antiseptic, and anti-inflammatory. Its aromatic influences help to open and release emotional blocks, bringing about a feeling of balance and grounding. Traditionally, spruce oil was believed to possess the frequency of prosperity.

Safety Data: May be irritating to those with sensitive skin. Avoid eye contact. In case of accidental contact, put a few drops of any pure vegetable oil in the eye and call your doctor if necessary. Never use water. Avoid exposure to direct sunlight for 3 to 6 hours after use.

Application: Diffuse, wear on the wrists, behind ears, or as a perfume. Individuals with sensitive skin may want to dilute with V-6 Mixing Oil, Massage Oil Base, or Satin Body Lotion. Put a drop on your checkbook, car dash, computer, phone, or wallet, or put a drop on your bills when paying invoices or when expecting payment. Many people put a drop on a piece of felt attached to the back of their watch. Add a 15 ml. bottle of Abundance to 5 gallons of any color of paint to increase the attraction of abundance and success in the work area or at home.

Companion Oils: Release may be used first to help release the emotions that stop us from receiving abundance. Then follow with Acceptance, Envision, Into the Future, Joy, Magnify Your Purpose, Motivation, and Passion.

Fragrant Influence: When focusing on issues of abundance and inhaling this oil, a memory link to the RNA template is created' where the memory is blueprinted and then passed to and stored in the DNA memory bank. Then every time you smell the oil the mental energy for abundance is created. The frequency of this blend is believed to create a harmonic magnetic energy field around oneself.

Frequency: Approximately 78 MHz—which is the same approximate frequency as the brain.

Acceptance

This blend stimulates the mind, compelling it to open and accept new things in life, allowing one to reach a higher potential. It also helps to overcome procrastination and denial.

Contains:

Neroli *(Citrus aurantium)* was highly regarded by ancient Egyptians for its ability to heal and calm the mind, body, and spirit. It is stabilizing and strengthening to the emotions, promoting peace, confidence, and awareness. It is antimicrobial and works both topically and by diffusing. It brings everything into focus at the moment.

Sandalwood *(Santalum album)* is high in sesquiterpenes, which have been researched for their ability to stimulate the pineal gland and the limbic region of the brain, the center of our emotions. The pineal gland is responsible for releasing melatonin, a hormone that enhances deep sleep. Used traditionally for skin revitalization, yoga, and meditation, sandalwood is similar to frankincense oil in its support of nerves and circulation.

Blue Tansy *(Tanacetum annuum)* may help cleanse the liver and calm the lymphatic system helping overcome anger and negative emotions which promotes a feeling of self-control. Its primary constituents are limonene and sesquiterpenes. European research shows that blue tansy works as an antihistamine, anti-inflammatory, and stimulant for the thymus gland reducing dermatitis, arthritis, sciatica, tuberculosis, and allergies.

Rosewood (*Aniba rosaeodora*) is soothing and nourishing to the skin. It has been researched at Weber State University for its inhibition rate against gram positive and gram negative bacterial growth. This oil is soothing, creates elasticity, and helps the skin rid itself of irritations and problems, such as candida. It is anti-infectious, antibacterial, antifungal, anti-viral, and antiparasitic.

Geranium (*Pelargonium graveolens*) has been used for centuries for skin care. Its strength lies in its ability to revitalize tissue. It may help with hormonal balance and the discharge of toxins from the liver, the gland where fear and anger are stored.

Frankincense (*Boswellia carteri*) is considered a holy anointing oil in the Middle East and has been used in religious ceremonies for thousands of years. High in sesquiterpenes, it helps stimulate the limbic part of the brain, which elevates the mind, helping to overcome stress and despair.

Carrier Oil: Almond oil.

Safety Data: May be irritating to those with sensitive skin. Avoid eye contact. In case of accidental contact, put a few drops of any pure vegetable oil in the eye and call your doctor if necessary. Never use water. Avoid exposure to direct sunlight for 3 to 6 hours after use.

Application: Diffuse, apply over heart and thymus, on the wrists, behind the ears, on the neck, temples, and on the face. May be worn as a perfume or cologne.

Fragrant Influence: May help calm a troubled mind and promote feelings of strength and confidence compelling one to accept new things in life striving toward a higher potential.

Frequency: Approximately 102 MHz.

Aroma Life

This blend may support cardiovascular, lymphatic, and circulatory systems helping to lower high blood pressure, reduce stress, and alleviate hemorrhoids.

Contains:

Helichrysum (*Helichrysum italicum*) has been researched in Europe for regenerating tissue and nerves and improving circulation. It is anticoagulant, prevents phlebitis, helps regulate cholesterol, stimulates liver cell function, and may help clean plaque and debris from the veins and arteries. Helichrysum is mucolytic, expectorant, antispasmodic, and reduces scarring and discoloration. It may also stimulate nerve endings and improve conditions such as hearing loss. It may help release feelings of anger promoting forgiveness.

Ylang Ylang (*Cananga odorata*) has been used traditionally to balance heart function, having been used to treat tachycardia (rapid heart beat) and high blood pressure.

Marjoram (*Origanum majorana*) is used for calming the respiratory system and soothing sore and aching muscles. Marjoram helps regenerate smooth muscle tissue, and assists in relieving spasms, sprains, bruises, migraine headaches, and calms nervous tension. It is antimicrobial, anti-infectious, antibacterial, antiseptic, and may work as a diuretic.

Cypress (*Cupressus sempervirens*) is one of the oils used most for the circulatory and lymphatic systems. It may help alleviate edema, cellulite, varicose veins, and water retention. It is anti-infectious, antibacterial, antimicrobial, mucolytic, antiseptic, refreshing, and relaxing. It may help improve the cardiovascular system and circulation as well as help relieve other lymphatic and capillary problems.

Carrier Oil: Sesame seed oil.

Safety Data: May be irritating to those with sensitive skin. Avoid eye contact. In case of accidental contact, put a few drops of any pure vegetable oil in the eye and call your doctor if necessary. Never use water. Avoid exposure to direct sunlight for 3 to 6 hours after use.

Application: Apply over the heart, on the feet, on the life line of the hand and under the ring finger, above the elbow, behind the ring toe on the left foot. Dilute with V-6 Mixing Oil or Massage Oil Base for a full body massage. It may also help to apply this blend along the spine from the first to the fourth thoracic vertebrae, which correspond to the cardiopulmonary nerves.

Companion Oils: Helichrysum, Rosemary, Joy, Valor, and Ylang Ylang.

Frequency: Approximately 84 MHz.

Aroma Siez

This special blend may help relax, calm, and relieve tight, sore, tired, and aching muscles resulting from sports injuries, fatigue, and stress. It may also help to relieve headaches.

Contains:

Basil *(Ocimum basilicum)* can be relaxing to smooth muscles (the involuntary muscles including the heart and digestive system). It may soothe insect bites such as, bees, wasps, and spiders, and may also help with snakebites. Basil has been found to alleviate mental fatigue, muscle spasms and rhinitis, and help when there is a loss of smell due to nasal congestion.

Cypress *(Cupressus sempervirens)* is one of the oils most used for the circulatory and lymphatic systems. It may help with edema, cellulite, varicose veins, and water retention. It is anti-infectious, antibacterial, antimicrobial, mucolytic, antiseptic, refreshing, and relaxing. It may help improve the cardiovascular system and circulation as well as help relieve other lymphatic and capillary problems.

Marjoram *(Origanum majorana)* is used for calming the respiratory system and soothing sore and aching muscles. Marjoram helps regenerate smooth muscle tissue, and assists in relieving spasms, sprains, bruises, migraine headaches and calming the nerves. It is antimicrobial, anti-infectious, antibacterial, antiseptic and may work as a diuretic.

Lavender *(Lavandula angustifolia)* is known as the universal oil because of its wide range of usage. It is beneficial for skin conditions such as, burns, rashes, and psoriasis. It is antispasmodic, hypotensive, anti-inflammatory, anti-infectious, and anticoagulant. It prevents scarring, stretch marks, and relieves headaches and PMS symptoms.

Peppermint *(Mentha piperita)* is one of the oldest and most highly regarded herbs for soothing digestion. Jean Valnet, M.D. studied the beneficial effects of peppermint on the liver and respiratory systems. Other scientists have researched its effect on impaired taste and smell as well as improved concentration and mental accuracy. Alan Hirsch, M.D., studied peppermint's ability to directly affect the brain's satiety center, triggering a sensation of fullness after meals, which may help in weight loss by curbing the appetite (Hirsch, 1997). Daniel Penöél, M.D., reports that it may help to reduce fevers, candida, nausea, vomiting, and strengthen the respiratory system. Adding peppermint to drinking water helps cool body temperature during hot weather.

Safety Data: May be irritating to those with sensitive skin. Avoid eye contact. In case of accidental contact, put a few drops of any pure vegetable oil in the eye and call your doctor if necessary. Never use water. Avoid exposure to direct sunlight for 3 to 6 hours after use.

Application: Apply on location for muscles, neck, feet, and to relax during stress headaches. Add to water or dilute with V-6 Mixing Oil or Massage Oil Base for a full body massage. Peppermint oil is also a great addition to foods and desserts.

Companion Oils: Basil, Elemi, Spruce, Birch, Helichrysum, Idaho Tansy, Marjoram, Ortho Ease Massage Oil and Ortho Sport Massage Oil.

Frequency: Approximately 64 MHz.

Awaken

This combination of several other blends brings one to inner knowing in order to make changes and desirable transitions helping to reach one's highest potential.

Contains:

Joy is an exotic blend that produces a magnetic energy to enhance the frequency of self-love and bring joy to the heart. It inspires romance and may help overcome grief and depression.

Forgiveness is a blend that may help release negative memories. It may help people move past emotional barriers, enabling them to achieve higher awareness and compelling them to forgive and let go.

Present Time has an empowering fragrance, which gives a feeling of being in the moment. One can only go forward and progress when in the present time.

Dream Catcher is an exotic formula that may help open the mind and enhance dreams and visualization, promoting greater potential for realizing your dreams and staying on your path. It also protects you from negative dreams that might cloud your vision.

Harmony is an exquisite blend of oils for promoting physical and emotional healing by bringing about a harmonic balance to the energy centers of the body, allowing the energy to flow more efficiently. Harmony has been found to negate allergy symptoms. It is also beneficial in reducing stress and creating a general overall feeling of well-being.

Carrier Oil: Almond oil.

Safety Data: May be irritating to those with sensitive skin. Avoid eye contact. In case of accidental contact, put a few drops of any pure vegetable oil in the eye and call your doctor if necessary. Never use water. Avoid exposure to direct sunlight for 3 to 6 hours after use.

Application: Diffuse, add to bath water, diluted with V-6 Mixing Oil or Massage Oil Base for a full-body massage. Wear over the heart, the wrists, on the neck, and use as an aftershave. For clearing allergies, rub over sternum.

Companion Oils: Live with Passion, Into The Future, Dream Catcher, Envision, Motivation, Harmony, Joy, Valor, and En-R-Gee.

Fragrant Influence: Stimulates the creativity of the right brain, enhancing the function of pineal and pituitary glands in balancing the energy centers of the body and bringing about a harmonious feeling that increases all body functions.

Frequency: Approximately 89 MHz.

Brain Power

The oils in this blend contain high sesquiterpene compounds that have been shown to increase oxygen around receptor sites around the pineal glands, pituitary, and hypothalamus. They are responsible for the secretion of human growth hormone (hGH). Research indicates that they play a major role in dissolving petrochemicals known to plug the receptor sites and prevent receptivity. Brain Power may help clear the brain fog that people experience due to exposure to synthetic petrochemicals in food, skin and hair care products, and heavy chemical-laden air. Brain Power may increase mental potential, mental clarity, and long-term use may retard the aging process. It may also support and strengthen immune function.

Contains:

Frankincense *(Boswellia carteri)* is considered a holy anointing oil in the Middle East and has been used in religious ceremonies for thousands of years. High in sesquiterpenes, it helps stimulate the limbic part of the brain, which elevates the mind, helping to overcome stress and despair.

Sandalwood *(Santalum album)* is high in sesquiterpenes, which have been researched for their ability to stimulate the pineal gland and the limbic region of the brain, the center of our emotions. The pineal gland is responsible for releasing melatonin, a hormone that enhances deep sleep. Used traditionally for skin revitalization, yoga, and meditation, sandalwood is similar to frankincense oil in its support of nerves and circulation.

Melissa *(Melissa officinalis)* is a powerful, antimicrobial oil, yet it is very gentle and delicate because of the nature of the plant, and helps to bring out those characteristics within the individual. It is calming and balancing to the emotions. Melissa is one of the oils highest in sesquiterpenes, much like cedarwood. It is very stimulating to the anterior pituitary and immune system.

Cedarwood *(Cedrus atlantica)* has calming and purifying properties. High in sesquiterpenes which can stimulate the limbic part of the brain (the center of our emotions), this conifer oil has been used by North American Indians to enhance spiritual awareness and communication. It also may help stimulate the pineal gland, which releases melatonin, a hormone that enhances deep sleep.

Blue Cypress, Australian *(Callitris intratropica)* improves circulation and increases the flow of oxygen to the brain, stimulating the amygdala, pineal gland, pituitary gland, and hypothalamus.

Lavender *(Lavandula angustifolia)* has calming and relaxing properties that can improve concentration and mental acuity. High in sedating aldehydes and esters, its ability to help overcome insomnia, headaches, stress, and nervous tension can lead to a heightened ability to reason and remember.

Helichrysum *(Helichrysum italicum)* helps improve circulation and stimulate optimum nerve function, properties which can lead to enhanced awareness and cognition. On an emotional level, its ability to help release feelings of anger, can allow the mind to gain focus and concentration.

Safety Data: May be irritating to those with sensitive skin. Avoid eye contact. In case of accidental contact, put a few drops of any pure vegetable oil in the eye and call your doctor if necessary. Never use water. Avoid exposure to direct sunlight for 3 to 6 hours after use.

Carrier Oil: Almond oil.

Application: Diffuse, wear as a perfume or cologne, apply on neck, throat, and under nose. Massage 1 or 2 drops with a finger on the insides of cheeks in the mouth. Doing this 1 or 2 times

a day will immediately improve the smell sensory cortex.

Companion Oils: Clarity, Envision, RC, and Raven.

Fragrant Influence: Perfect for promoting deep concentration and channeling physical energy into mental energy.

Frequency: Approximately 78 MHz.

Christmas Spirit

This blend contains the oils of evergreens and spices, reminiscent of Christmas, bringing joy, happiness, and security.

Contains:

Orange *(Citrus sinensis)* was believed to bring joy, peace, and happiness to those who possessed it. It contains limonene, an antiviral compound, and citral, an antibacterial compound. It prevents the growth of bacteria. It is elevating to the mind and body, bringing joy and peace. It has been recognized to help a dull, oily complexion.

Cinnamon Bark *(Cinnamomum cassia)* is the oil of wealth from the Orient and part of the formula the Lord gave Moses (Exodus 30:22-27). Emperors of China and India measured their wealth partly by the amount of cinnamon they possessed. Traditionally, it was thought to have a frequency that attracted wealth and abundance. It is highly antiviral, antifungal, and antibacterial.

Spruce *(Picea mariana)* helps the respiratory and nervous systems. It is anti-infectious, antiseptic, and anti-inflammatory. Its aromatic influences help to open and release emotional blocks, bringing about a feeling of balance and grounding. Traditionally, spruce oil was believed to possess the frequency of prosperity.

Safety Data: May be irritating to those with sensitive skin. Avoid eye contact. In case of accidental contact, put a few drops of any pure vegetable oil in the eye and call your doctor if necessary. Never use water. Avoid exposure to direct sunlight for 3 to 6 hours after use.

Application: Diffuse, sprinkle on logs in fireplace, on Christmas trees, on cedar chips for dresser drawers, or on potpourri. Use all year.

Companion Oils: Mandarin, Clove, and Nutmeg.

Fragrant Influence: This blend of oils has a delightful fragrance and is wonderful for creating the feeling of peace that usually accompanies the holiday season. It is also nice for air purification.

Frequency: Approximately 104 MHz.

Citrus Fresh

This fragrance stimulates the right brain, bringing about more creativity, a sense of well-being, and joy. It has been found to be relaxing and calming, especially for children, and works well as an air purifier.

Contains:

Orange *(Citrus sinensis)* was believed to bring joy, peace, and happiness to those who possessed it. It contains limonene, an antiviral compound, and citral, an antibacterial compound. It prevents the growth of bacteria. It is elevating to the mind and body and brings joy and peace. It has been recognized to help a dull, oily complexion.

Tangerine *(Citrus nobilis)* contains esters and aldehydes that are sedating and calming, helping with anxiety and nervousness. It is anti-inflammatory, anticoagulant, may help decongest the lymphatic system, and works as a diuretic.

Lemon *(Citrus limon)* has antiseptic-like properties and contains compounds that have been studied for their effects on immune function. It increases microcirculation, which may improve vision. It may serve as an insect repellent and may be beneficial for the skin. It has been found to promote leukocyte formation, dissolve cellulite, increase lymphatic function, and promote a sense of well-being. Its fragrance is stimulating and invigorating.

Mandarin *(Citrus reticulata)* is appealing, gentle, and promotes happiness. Apply topically or diffuse, especially at meal time and before sleep. Because of its sedative and slightly hypnotic properties, mandarin may help with insomnia and is good for stress and irritability. It is antispasmodic, antiseptic, antifungal, supports hepatic duct function, and works as a digestive tonic.

Grapefruit *(Citrus paradisi)* works as a mild disinfectant. Like many cold-pressed citrus oils, it has unique fat-dissolving characteristics. It may be beneficial for digestion, obesity, reducing water retention, and cellulite.

Spearmint *(Mentha spicata)* oil helps support the respiratory, glandular, and nervous systems. With its hormone-like activity, it may help open and release emotional blocks and bring about a feeling of balance. It is antispasmodic, anti-infectious, antiparasitic, antiseptic, and anti-inflammatory. It has also been used to increase metabolism to burn fat.

Safety Data: May be irritating to those with sensitive skin. Avoid eye contact. In case of accidental contact, put a few drops of any pure vegetable oil in the eye and call your doctor if necessary. Never use water. Avoid exposure to direct sunlight for 3 to 6 hours after use.

Application: Diffuse, put in bath water, and dilute with V-6 Mixing Oil or Massage Base Oil for full body massage. Citrus Fresh may be worn as a perfume or cologne and be applied over the heart, on the wrists, and on the ears. It is excellent for children, although dilution with V-6 Mixing Oil is recommended.

Fragrant Influence: This blend creates an enjoyable aromatic fragrance at home or at work. Simple diffusion can be achieved by putting a few drops on a cotton ball and placing it on a desk or table.

Frequency: Approximately 90 MHz.

Note: A university in Japan experimented with diffusing different oils in the office. When they diffused lemon there were 54 percent fewer errors, with jasmine there were 33 percent fewer errors, and with lavender there were 20 percent fewer errors. When oils were diffused while studying and taking a test, test scores increased by as much as 50 percent. Different oils should be used for different tests, but the same oil should be used during the test as was used while studying for that particular test. The smell of the oil may help bring back the memory of what was studied.

Clarity

This blend has been used to promote a clear mind and mental alertness. Rosemary and peppermint, found in this blend, have been used for years to improve mental activity and vitality. Dr. Dember of the University of Cincinnati discovered in his research that inhaling peppermint oil increased the mental accuracy of the students tested by 28 percent. Clarity may help keep one awake while driving and also keep one from going into shock during times of trauma.

Clarity Oil Reveals Toxic Buildup

Those who get headaches from diffusing Clarity may be suffering from significant petrochemical or heavy metal accumulation in the brain. Clarity is rich in the essential oil of cardamom, which contains high levels of transphenol—a powerful molecule which tends to generate headaches in the presence of petro-chemicals or heavy metals.

Contains:

Cardamom (*Elettaria cardamomum*) is uplifting, refreshing, and invigorating. It may be beneficial for clearing confusion.

Rosemary (*Rosmarinus officinalis*) is antiseptic and antimicrobial and may be beneficial for skin conditions and dandruff. It may help fight candida and is anti-infectious, antispasmodic, balances the endocrine system, and is an expectorant. It helps overcome mental fatigue stimulating memory and opening the conscious mind.

Peppermint (*Mentha piperita*) is one of the oldest and most highly regarded herbs for soothing digestion. Jean Valnet, M.D., studied the beneficial effects of peppermint on the liver and respiratory systems. Daniel Penöél, M.D., reports that it may help to reduce fevers, candida, nausea, vomiting, and strengthen the respiratory system. Adding peppermint to drinking water helps cool body temperature during hot weather.

Basil (*Ocimum basilicum*) can be relaxing to smooth muscles as well as those involuntary muscles of the heart and digestive system. It may soothe insect bites such as, bees, wasps, and spiders, and may also help with snake bites. It has been found to alleviate mental fatigue, spasms, rhinitis, and help when there is a loss of smell due to nasal congestion.

Bergamot (*Citrus bergamia*) is one of the most uplifting fragrances, simultaneously energizing and calming, with a unique ability to relieve anxiety, stress, and tension.

Geranium (*Pelargonium graveolens*) assists in balancing hormones. It is antispasmodic, relaxant, anti-inflammatory, anti-infectious, antibacterial, antifungal, and stimulates the liver and pancreas.

Jasmine (*Jasminum officinale*) is beneficial for dry, greasy, irritated, or sensitive skin. It is used for muscle spasms, sprains, coughs, laryngitis, frigidity, depression, and nervous exhaustion.

Lemon (*Citrus limon*) has antiseptic-like properties and contains compounds that have been studied for their effects on immune function. It increases microcirculation, which may improve vision. It may serve as an insect repellent and may be beneficial for the skin. It has been found to promote leukocyte formation, dissolve cellulite, increase lymphatic function, and promote a sense of well-being. Its fragrance is stimulating and invigorating.

Palmarosa (*Cymbopogon martinii*) is helpful for all types of skin problems, such as candida, rashes, and scaly and flaky skin. It stimulates new cell growth, moisturizes and speeds the healing process. It is antimicrobial, antibacterial, antifungal, and antiviral. It is supportive to the nervous and cardiovascular system.

Roman Chamomile (*Chamaemelum nobile*) may calm and relieve restlessness, tension, insomnia, muscle tension, cuts, scrapes, bruises and is anti-infectious. It may relieve allergies and expel toxins from the liver. It is used extensively in Europe for the skin.

Rosewood *(Aniba rosaeodora)* is soothing and nourishing to the skin. It has been researched at Weber State University for its inhibition rate against gram positive and gram negative bacterial growth. This oil is soothing, creates elasticity, and helps the skin rid itself of irritations and problems, such as candida. It is anti-infectious, antibacterial, antifungal, antiviral, and antiparasitic.

Ylang Ylang *(Cananga odorata)* helps bring about a sense of relaxation.

Safety Data: May be irritating to those with sensitive skin. Avoid eye contact. In case of accidental contact, put a few drops of any pure vegetable oil in the eye and call your doctor if necessary. Never use water. Avoid exposure to direct sunlight for 3 to 6 hours after use.

Application: Diffuse, put in bath water, put two to five drops on a cotton ball and put in home and car air vents. Apply on temples, wrists, neck, and feet.

Companion Oils: En-R-Gee (when overly tired), Brain Power, Lemon, and Peppermint.

Fragrant Influence: The oils in this blend are known for their ability to help increase mental alertness.

Frequency: Approximately 101 MHz.

Note: This blend contains cardamom and high levels of transphenol, which may cause headaches when inhaled or topically applied.

Di-Tone

These oils are blended to assist in relieving digestive problems, such as an upset stomach, belching, heartburn, and bloating. Massage a drop or two on the outer ear to help alleviate morning sickness. Di-Tone has been found to rid animals of parasites by applying it to their feet. It may also help dispel parasites by massaging and placing a compress across the stomach.

Contains:

Tarragon *(Artemisia dracunculus)* has been used in Europe for its antimicrobial and antiseptic functions. It helps to reduce dyspepsia, intestinal spasms, and urinary tract infection. It may reduce premenstrual discomfort and nerve pain.

It is antispasmodic, anti-inflammatory, anti-infectious, antiviral, antibacterial, and prevents fermentation.

Ginger *(Zingiber officinale)* is used for relief from motion sickness, arthritis, rheumatism, sprains, muscle aches and pains, congestion, coughs, sinusitis, sore throats, diarrhea, colic, indigestion, loss of appetite, fever, flu, chills, and infectious disease.

Juniper *(Juniperus osteosperma* and/or *J. scopulorum)* may work as a detoxifier and cleanser, and promotes improved nerve and kidney function. It is also beneficial for the skin reducing dermatitis, eczema, and acne.

Anise *(Pimpinella anisum)* is antispasmodic, antiseptic, stimulates the increase of bile from the liver, expels worms, increases lactation, and helps calm gall bladder contractions. It may help with painful menstruation and irregularity, problems with menopause, dyspepsia, spastic colitis, flatulence, indigestion, lung congestion, asthmatic bronchitis, and intestinal pain.

Fennel *(Foeniculum vulgare)* is antiseptic and stimulating to the circulatory and respiratory systems. It is antispasmodic, antiseptic, and stimulating to the cardiovascular and respiratory systems. With its hormone-like activity, it may help facilitate childbirth and increase lactation after birthing.

Patchouly *(Pogostemon cablin)* was used in India in ancient times as a trade commodity because of its earthy, musty fragrance and its ability to mask many different odors. East Indian people use patchouly to fragrance their clothing and their homes because of its natural insecticidal and anti-infectious properties. Legends indicate that it represented money, and those who possessed it were considered to be wealthy. Patchouly is very beneficial for the skin and may help prevent wrinkles or chapped skin. It is a general tonic and stimulant and helps the digestive system. It is also antimicrobial, antiseptic, and helps relieve itching.

Peppermint *(Mentha piperita)* is one of the oldest and most highly regarded herbs for soothing digestion. Jean Valnet, M.D., studied the beneficial effects of peppermint on the liver and respiratory systems. Daniel Penoël, M.D., reports that it may help to reduce fevers, candida, nausea, vomiting, and strengthen the respiratory system. Adding peppermint to drinking water helps cool body temperature during hot weather.

Lemongrass *(Cymbopogon flexuosus)* works well for purification. It is powerful in the regeneration of connective tissue. It is a vasodilator, anti-inflammatory, sedative, and supportive to the digestive system. A study in *Phytotherapy Research* showed that lemongrass had strong antifungal properties when applied topically. It may also help increase the flow of oxygen and uplift the spirit.

Safety Data: May be irritating to those with sensitive skin. Avoid eye contact. In case of accidental contact, put a few drops of any pure vegetable oil in the eye and call your doctor if necessary. Never use water. Avoid exposure to direct sunlight for 3 to 6 hours after use.

Application: May be applied to the Vita Flex points on the feet and ankles. Massage a drop or two on outer ear to help alleviate morning sickness. Massage 2 or 3 drops on the paws of your animals to expel parasites. Parasites may also be dispelled by massaging or placing a compress across the stomach. Add 1 or 2 drops to 8 ounces of water and sip slowly as a dietary supplement.

Companion Oils: Peppermint and Spearmint.

Companion Products: ComforTone, Megazyme, and JuvaTone.

Frequency: Approximately 102 MHz.

Dragon Time

This blend helps relieve PMS symptoms and menstrual discomforts including cramping and irregular periods.

Contains:

Clary Sage *(Salvia sclarea)* balances the hormones. It contains natural sclareol, a phytoestrogen that mimics estrogen function. It may help with menstrual cramps, PMS, and pre-menopause symptoms and may help with circulatory problems.

Yarrow *(Achillea millefolium)* is a decongestant of the prostate and balances hormones. It is anti-inflammatory and reduces scarring. It also helps with nerve inflammation.

Lavender *(Lavandula angustifolia)* is known as the universal oil because of its wide range of usage. It helps relieve headaches and PMS symptoms.

Jasmine *(Jasminum officinale)* is beneficial for dry, greasy, irritated, or sensitive skin. It is used for muscle spasms, sprains, coughs, laryngitis, frigidity, depression, and nervous exhaustion.

Fennel *(Foeniculum vulgare)* is antiseptic and stimulating to the circulatory and respiratory systems. It is antispasmodic, and stimulating to the cardiovascular system. With its hormone-like activity, fennel may help facilitate childbirth and increase lactation after birthing.

Marjoram *(Origanum majorana)* is used for calming the respiratory system and soothing sore and aching muscles. Marjoram helps regenerate smooth muscle tissue, and also assists in relieving spasms and migraine headaches and calming the nerves. It is antimicrobial, anti-infectious, antibacterial, antiseptic and may work as a diuretic.

Safety Data: May be irritating to those with sensitive skin. Avoid eye contact. In case of accidental contact, put a few drops of any pure vegetable oil in the eye and call your doctor if necessary. Never use water. Avoid exposure to direct sunlight for 3 to 6 hours after use.

Application: Apply to the Vita Flex points on the feet and around the ankles, both inside and out. It may be diluted with V-6 Mixing Oil or Massage Oil Base for application on the other Vita Flex points on the body. It may be applied as a hot compress over the lower abdomen, across the lower back, or anywhere it hurts.

Companion Oil: EndoFlex may help alleviate hot flashes in women.

Fragrant Influence: This blend of oils may be beneficial in times of hormonal stress. It may be diffused in the home, the office, or put a few drops on a cotton ball and place in the car vent.

Frequency: Approximately 72 MHz.

Dream Catcher

This exotic formula may help open the mind and enhance dreams and visualization, promoting greater potential for realizing your dreams and staying on your path. It also protects you from negative dreams that might cloud your vision.

Contains:

Sandalwood *(Santalum album)* is high in sesquiterpenes, which have been researched for their ability to stimulate the pineal gland and the limbic region of the brain, the center of our emotions. The pineal gland is responsible for releasing melatonin, a hormone that enhances deep sleep. Used traditionally for skin revitalization, yoga, and meditation, sandalwood is similar to frankincense oil in its support of nerves and circulation.

Blue Tansy *(Tanacetum annuum)* may help cleanse the liver and calm the lymphatic system helping one to overcome anger and negative emotions promoting a feeling of self-control. Its primary constituents are limonene and sesquiterpenes. European research shows that it works as an antihistamine, anti-inflammatory, and stimulant for the thymus gland reducing dermatitis, arthritis, sciatica, tuberculosis, and allergies.

Juniper *(Juniperus osteosperma* and/or *J. scopulorum)* may work as a detoxifier and cleanser, and promotes improved nerve and kidney function. It is also beneficial for the skin reducing dermatitis, eczema, and acne.

Bergamot *(Citrus bergamia)* is one of the most uplifting fragrances, simultaneously energizing and calming, with a unique ability to relieve anxiety, stress, and tension.

Anise *(Pimpinella anisum)* is antispasmodic, antiseptic, stimulates the increase of bile from the liver, expels worms, increases lactation, and helps calm gall bladder contractions. It may help with painful menstruation and irregularity, problems with menopause, dyspepsia, spastic colitis, flatulence, indigestion, lung congestion, asthmatic bronchitis, and intestinal pain.

Tangerine *(Citrus nobilis)* contains esters and aldehydes that are sedating and calming, helping with anxiety and nervousness. It is anti-inflammatory, anticoagulant, may help decongest the lymphatic system, and works as a diuretic.

Ylang Ylang *(Cananga odorata)* helps bring about a sense of relaxation and may help balance male and female energies. It balances equilibrium and restores confidence and self-love.

Pepper, Black *(Piper nigrum)* stimulates the endocrine system and increases energy while increasing cellular oxygenation. It is anti-inflammatory and may soothe deep tissue muscle aches. Black pepper is expectorant, supportive to the digestive glands, and has been traditionally used for rheumatoid arthritis.

Safety Data: May be irritating to those with sensitive skin. Avoid eye contact. In case of accidental contact, put a few drops of any pure vegetable oil in the eye and call your doctor if necessary. Never use water. Avoid exposure to direct sunlight for 3 to 6 hours after use.

Application: Diffuse, apply on forehead, ears, throat, under nose, eyebrow, and base of neck. Place a couple of drops on the pillow. This blend may be useful during meditation in sweat lodges, and in bath water.

Companion Oils: Envision, Passion, Motivation, Awaken, Gathering, and Into the Future.

Fragrant Influence: This blend may be diffused during the day, but seems to be most effective during sleep.

Frequency: Approximately 98 MHz.

Note: If unpleasant dreams occur, continue to use this oil, as something in the subconscious may need to be processed. Hold onto your dreams and visualize them into reality.

EndoFlex

This blend may help overall vitality. It contains oils associated with hormonal balance, improving and balancing metabolism and weight control.

Contains:

Spearmint *(Mentha spicata)* helps support the respiratory and nervous systems. With its hormone-like activity, it may help open and release emotional blocks and bring about a feeling of balance. This oil may aid the respiratory, nervous, and glandular systems. Spearmint is antispasmodic, anti-infectious, antiparasitic, antiseptic, and anti-inflammatory. It has also been used to increase metabolism to burn fat.

Myrtle *(Myrtus communis)* may help normalize hormonal imbalances of the thyroid and ovaries. It may help the respiratory system with chronic coughs and tuberculosis. Myrtle is suitable to use for coughs and chest complaints with children, and may support immune function infighting cold, flu, and infectious disease.

Nutmeg *(Myristica fragrans)* helps support the adrenal glands for increased energy. It may help with difficulties related to circulation, and aches and pains in muscles and joints related to stress, arthritis, and gout. Nutmeg may also help with digestive problems such as flatulence, indigestion, and nausea. It is antiseptic, antiparasitic, and a neurotonic.

German Chamomile *(Matricaria recutita)* has been a highly respected oil for over 3,000 years and has been used to help skin conditions, such as dermatitis, boils, acne, rashes, and eczema. It is also used for hair care, burns, cuts, toothaches, teething pains, inflamed joints, menopausal problems, insomnia, migraine headaches, and stress-related complaints. It has an electrical frequency that promotes peace and harmony, bringing about a feeling of security.

Geranium *(Pelargonium graveolens)* assists in balancing hormones. It is antispasmodic, relaxant, anti-inflammatory, anti-infectious, antibacterial, antifungal, and stimulates the liver and pancreas.

Sage *(Salvia officinalis)* has been used in Europe for skin conditions such as eczema, acne, dandruff, and hair loss. It has been recognized for its ability to strengthen the vital centers. It may help in relieving depression and mental fatigue. Sage contains sclareol, which stimulates the body to produce its own estrogen. It contains natural estrogenic compounds that help relieve PMS symptoms. The Lakota Indians used it for purification and healing and to dispel negative emotions from denial and sexual abuse, as well as a complete body tonic for healing and strength.

Carrier Oil: Sesame seed oil.

Safety Data: May be irritating to those with sensitive skin. Avoid eye contact. In case of accidental contact, put a few drops of any pure vegetable oil in the eye and call your doctor if necessary. Never use water. Avoid exposure to direct sunlight for 3 to 6 hours after use.

Application: Apply over lower back, thyroid, kidneys, liver, feet, and glandular areas. It may also be applied to the Vita Flex points on the feet for these same areas of the body.

Frequency: Approximately 138 MHz.

En-R-Gee

Traditionally, the oils in this blend were used for increasing vitality, circulation, and alertness in the body.

Contains:

Clove *(Syzygium aromaticum)* was another oil from the Orient hailed as an oil of great abundance; those who possessed it were considered wealthy. This oil is one of the most antimicrobial and antiseptic of all essential oils. It is antifungal, antiviral, anti-infectious, and antibacterial. It works as a general stimulant and is used to treat sinusitis, bronchitis, cystitis, and cholera.

Juniper *(Juniperus osteosperma* and/or *J. scopulorum)* may work as a detoxifier and cleanser, and promotes improved nerve and kidney function. It is also beneficial for the skin reducing dermatitis, eczema, and acne. It elevates spiritual awareness creating feelings of love and peace.

Fir *(Abies alba)* is antimicrobial. It has been researched for its ability to kill airborne germs and bacteria. It is antiseptic, antiarthritic, and stimulating. It supports the body and reduces the symptoms of arthritis, rheumatism, bronchitis, coughs, sinusitis, cold, flu, and fevers. As a conifer oil, it creates a feeling of grounding, anchoring and empowerment.

Pepper, Black *(Piper nigrum)* stimulates the endocrine system and increases energy while increasing cellular oxygenation. It is anti-inflammatory which may soothe deep tissue muscle aches. It is expectorant, supportive to the digestive glands, and has been traditionally used for rheumatoid arthritis.

Nutmeg *(Myristica fragrans)* has adrenal cortex-like activity, which helps support the adrenal glands for increased energy. It may help with difficulties related to circulation, aches, and pains in muscles and joints related to stress, arthritis, and gout. Nutmeg may also help with digestive problems. It is antiseptic, antiparasitic, analgesic, and a neurotonic.

Rosemary *(Rosmarinus officinalis* - Camphor, 1,8 Cineol) is antiseptic and antimicrobial and may be beneficial for skin conditions and dandruff. It may help fight candida and is anti-infectious, antispasmodic, balances the endocrine system, and is an expectorant. It helps overcome mental fatigue stimulating memory and opening the conscious mind.

Lemongrass *(Cymbopogon flexuosus)* works well for purification. It is powerful in the regeneration of connective tissue. It is a vasodilator, anti-inflammatory, sedative, and supportive to the digestive system. A study in *Phytotherapy Research* showed that lemongrass essential oil had strong antifungal properties when applied topically. It may also help increase the flow of oxygen and uplift the spirit.

Safety Data: May be irritating to those with sensitive skin. Avoid eye contact. In case of accidental contact, put a few drops of any pure vegetable oil in the eye and call your doctor if necessary. Never use water. Avoid exposure to direct sunlight for 3 to 6 hours after use.

Application: Diffuse, apply 2 drops on the wrists or temples, back of neck, behind ears, or add to warm bath water with Bath Gel Base. Dilute with V-6 Mixing Oil or Massage Oil Base for an uplifting body massage. Massage on Vita Flex points of the feet. It may be worn as a perfume or cologne.

Companion Oils: One may feel like they have had eight hours of sleep by rubbing this blend on the feet and Awaken on the temples. This blend and Clarity together may help one stay awake while driving late at night.

Fragrant Influence: This blend of oils may help boost one's energy when diffused. It is also purifying when diffused. Simple diffusion can be achieved by applying a few drops on a cotton ball and placing in the air vent of a car or on the heat registers of the home or hotel room.

Frequency: Approximately 106 MHz.

Envision

This blend helps bring renewed faith in the future and maintain the emotional fortitude to achieve your goals and dreams. Many people suppress their own internal drive and creativity and can become a doormat or they may shut down out of fear of the unknown and fear of the responsibility that comes with getting out of the rut. Some people are in relationships where the spouse is very dominating. Envision helps in awakening and renewing your drive and independence, and overcoming the fear of experiencing new dimensions and letting the creativity flow, which will help you become a self-made person.

Contains:

Sage *(Salvia officinalis)* has been used in Europe for skin conditions such as eczema, acne, dandruff, and hair loss. It has been recognized for its benefits of strengthening the vital centers. It may help in relieving depression and mental fatigue. Sage contains sclareol, which stimulates the body to produce its own estrogen. It may nutritionally support the body during PMS and menopause. The Lakota Indians used it for purification and healing and to dispel negative emotions from denial and sexual abuse, as well as a complete body tonic for healing and strength.

Geranium *(Pelargonium graveolens)* helps release negative memories, thereby opening and elevating the mind.

Orange *(Citrus sinensis)* was believed to bring joy, peace, and happiness to those who possessed it. It contains limonene, an antiviral compound, and citral, an antibacterial compound. It prevents the growth of bacteria. It is elevating to the mind and body and brings joy and peace. Orange has been recognized to help a dull, oily complexion.

Rose *(Rosa damascena)* possesses the highest frequency of the oils. It brings balance and harmony, and elevates the mind, creating a sense of well-being. It is antihemorrhaging, anti-infectious, and prevents scarring. Rose may help with chronic bronchitis, asthma, tuberculosis, sexual disabilities, frigidity, impotency, skin disease, ulcers, sprains, wrinkles, thrush, and gingivitis. It also promotes healthy skin.

Lavender *(Lavandula angustifolia)* has sedative and calming properties that help overcome insomnia, headaches, stress, and nervous tension.

Spruce *(Picea mariana)* helps to open and release emotional blocks, bringing about a feeling of balance and grounding. Traditionally, spruce oil was believed to possess the frequency of prosperity.

Safety Data: May be irritating to those with sensitive skin. Avoid eye contact. In case of accidental contact, put a few drops of any pure vegetable oil in the eye and call your doctor if necessary. Never use water. Avoid exposure to direct sunlight for 3 to 6 hours after use.

Application: Diffuse, apply 2 drops on wrists or temples, or add to warm bath water with bath Gel Base. Dilute with V-6 Mixing Oil or Massage Oil Base for an uplifting massage.

Companion Oils: Motivation, Acceptance, Valor, Magnify Your Purpose, Into the Future, and Clarity.

Fragrant Influence: This blend stimulates one's creative and intuitive abilities in a positive and progressive way moving one to take action.

Frequency: Approximately 90 MHz.

Exodus II

Some researchers believe that these aromatics were used by Moses to protect the Israelites from a plague. Modern science shows that these oils contain either immune-stimulating or antiviral compounds or both, which may explain why these oils were used in ancient times. Today viruses and bacteria are beginning to mutate and become resistant to conventional drugs. Because of the complex chemistry of essential oils, viruses and bacteria have a more difficult time acquiring resistance. This blend was designed to work with the Exodus food supplement to help build the body's natural defenses.

Contains:

Cassia *(Cinnamomum cassia)* is anti-infectious, antibacterial, and anticoagulant. It was part of the formula the Lord gave Moses (Exodus 30:22-27) for protecting the Israelites.

Hyssop *(Hyssopus officinalis)* is anti-inflammatory and antiviral, supporting the respiratory system. It is antiparasitic, mucolytic, decongestant, antiasthmatic, anti-infectious, regulates lipid metabolism, and prevents scarring.

Frankincense *(Boswellia carteri)* is considered a holy anointing oil in the Middle East and has been used in religious ceremonies for thousands of years. High in sesquiterpenes, it helps stimulate the hypothalamus which can lead to heightened immune function. Frankincense is being researched and used therapeutically in European hospitals to build immunity and treat cancer. In ancient times, it was well-known for its healing powers, and was reportedly used to treat every conceivable ill known to man.

Spikenard *(Nardostachys jatamansi)* was highly prized at the time of Christ and was used by Mary of Bethany to anoint the feet of Jesus. High in sesquiterpenes, spikenard is very supporting to the immune system. It strengthens and calms the cardiovascular system, stimulates under-active ovaries, and helps with tachycardia, anemia, psoriasis, and hemorrhoids.

Galbanum *(Ferula gummosa)* was used for both medicinal and spiritual purposes. It is antimicrobial. When combined with frankincense and sandalwood, its frequency increases dramatically. *(And the Lord said unto Moses, Take unto thee sweet spices, stacte, and onycha, and galbanum; sweet spices with pure with frankincense*: Exodus 30:34).

Myrrh *(Myrtus communis)* is an antimicrobial oil referenced throughout the Old and New Testaments *(A bundle of myrrh is my well-beloved unto me... Song of Solomon 1:13)*. It was used traditionally in the royal palaces by the queens as an anti-infectious agent during pregnancy and birthing. It has one of the highest levels of sesquiterpenes, which is a class of compounds having direct effects on the hypothalamus and the pituitary, glands responsible for activating hormone and immune response. Today, myrrh is widely used in oral hygiene products.

Cinnamon Bark *(Cinnamomum verum)* is the oil of wealth from the Orient and part of the formula the Lord gave Moses (Exodus 30:22-27). Cinnamon oil is anti-infectious, antibacterial, antiparasitic, antiviral, and antifungal. Cinnamon oil was regarded by the emperors of China and India to have great value; their wealth was measured by the amount of oil they possessed. Traditionally, it was thought to have a frequency that attracted wealth and abundance. Physically, it has many attributes; it is a powerful purifier, it is a powerful oxygenator, and it enhances the action and the activity of other oils. Researchers, including J. C. Lapraz, M.D., found that viruses could not live in the presence of cinnamon oil.

Calamus *(Acorus calamus)* is part of the formula the Lord gave Moses (Exodus 30:22-27). It is antispasmodic, anti-inflammatory (gastrointestinal), and supportive for stomach disorders. Calamus also helps inflammation of the small intestine and colon, gastritis and spasms, asthmatic bronchitis, kidney congestion after intoxication, cystitis, gout, and arterial hypotension (low blood pressure). It is highly regarded as an aromatic stimulant and a tonic for the digestive system.

Carrier Oil: Olive oil.

Safety Data: May be irritating to those with sensitive skin. Avoid eye contact. In case of accidental contact, put a few drops of any pure vegetable oil in the eye and call your doctor if necessary. Never use water. Avoid exposure to direct sunlight for 3 to 6 hours after use.

Application: Apply to Vita Flex points on feet and/or directly on area of concern. Put 2 drops on wrists, feet, or other non-sensitive areas of the body. Diffuse, apply to palms of hands, cup hands over nose and mouth, and inhale. It may also be applied along the spine raindrop-style. However, dilution may be necessary because of the high levels of sesquiterpenes and phenols.

Companion Supplements: Exodus and Immune Tune.

Frequency: Approximately 180 MHz.

Forgiveness

The electrical frequencies of the oils in this blend may help release negative memories. This may have powerful effects in helping people move past emotional barriers, enabling them to achieve higher awareness, and compelling them to forgive and let go.

Contains:

Rose *(Rosa damascena)* possesses the highest frequency of the oils. It creates a sense of balance, harmony, and well-being and elevates the mind. Rose oil promotes healthy skin, reduces scarring, and may help with chronic bronchitis, asthma, tuberculosis, sexual disabilities, frigidity, impotency, skin disease, ulcers, sprains, wrinkles, thrush, and gingivitis.

Melissa *(Melissa officinalis)* is a powerful, antimicrobial oil, yet it is very gentle and delicate because of the nature of the plant, and helps to bring out those characteristics within the individual. It is calming and balancing to the emotions. Melissa is one of the highest in sesquiterpenes, much like cedarwood. It is very stimulating to the anterior pituitary and immune system.

Helichrysum *(Helichrysum italicum)* may help release feelings of anger promoting forgiveness.

Angelica *(Angelica archangelica)* helps to calm emotions and to bring memories back to the point of origin before trauma or anger was experienced, helping us to let go of negative feelings.

Frankincense *(Boswellia carteri)* is considered a holy anointing oil in the Middle East and has been used in religious ceremonies for thousands of years. High in sesquiterpenes, it helps oxygenate the pineal and pituitary glands, which stimulate and elevate the mind, helping to overcome stress and despair.

Sandalwood *(Santalum album)* is high in sesquiterpenes, which have been researched for their ability to stimulate the pineal gland and the limbic region of the brain, the center of our emotions. The pineal gland is responsible for releasing melatonin, a hormone that enhances deep sleep. Used traditionally for skin revitalization, yoga, and meditation, sandalwood is similar to frankincense oil in its support of nerves and circulation.

Lavender (*Lavandula angustifolia*) has sedative and calming properties that help overcome insomnia, headaches, stress, and nervous tension.

Bergamot (*Citrus bergamia*) is one of the most uplifting fragrances, simultaneously energizing and calming, with a unique ability to relieve anxiety, stress, and tension.

Geranium (*Pelargonium graveolens*) assists in balancing hormones. It is antispasmodic, relaxant, anti-inflammatory, anti-infectious, antibacterial, antifungal, and stimulates the liver and pancreas.

Jasmine (*Jasminum officinale*) is beneficial for dry, greasy, irritated, or sensitive skin. It is used for muscle spasms, sprains, coughs, laryngitis, frigidity, depression, and nervous exhaustion.

Lemon (*Citrus limon*) has antiseptic-like properties and contains compounds that have been studied for their effects on immune function. It increases microcirculation, which may improve vision. It may serve as an insect repellent and may be beneficial for the skin. It has been found to promote leukocyte formation, dissolve cellulite, increase lymphatic function, and promote a sense of well-being. Its fragrance is stimulating and invigorating.

Palmarosa (*Cymbopogon martinii*) is helpful for all types of skin problems, such as candida, rashes, and scaly and flaky skin. It stimulates new cell growth, moisturizes and speeds the healing process. It is antimicrobial, antibacterial, antifungal, and antiviral. It is supportive to the nervous and cardiovascular system.

Roman Chamomile (*Chamaemelum nobile*) may calm and relieve restlessness, tension, insomnia, muscle tension, cuts, scrapes, bruises and is anti-infectious. It may relieve allergies and expel toxins from the liver. It is used extensively in Europe for the skin.

Rosewood (*Aniba rosaeodora*) is soothing and nourishing to the skin. It has been researched at Weber State University for its inhibition rate against gram positive and gram negative bacterial growth. This oil is soothing, creates elasticity, and helps the skin rid itself of irritations and problems, such as candida. It is anti-infectious, antibacterial, antifungal, antiviral, and antiparasitic.

Ylang Ylang (*Cananga odorata*) helps bring about a sense of relaxation.

Safety Data: May be irritating to those with sensitive skin. Avoid eye contact. In case of accidental contact, put a few drops of any pure vegetable oil in the eye and call your doctor if necessary. Never use water. Avoid exposure to direct sunlight for 3 to 6 hours after use.

Carrier Oil: Sesame seed oil

Application: Massage over the navel and the heart. It may be worn as a perfume or cologne or added to Pharaoh or Rawhide Aftershave.

Companion Oils: Valor on feet, Joy, and Gathering.

Fragrant Influence: Diffused or worn, this blend may stimulate the desire to forgive and let go of hurt feelings, insults, and negative emotions.

Frequency: Approximately 192 MHz.

Gathering

This blend was created to help us overcome the bombardment of chaotic energy that alters our focus and takes us off our path toward higher achievements. Galbanum, a favorite oil of Moses, has a strong effect when blended with frankincense and sandalwood in gathering our emotional and spiritual thoughts, helping us to achieve our potential. These oils may help increase the oxygen around the pineal and pituitary gland, bringing greater harmonic frequency to receive the communication we desire. This blend may help bring people together on a physical, emotional, and spiritual level for greater focus and clarity. It may help one stay focused, grounded, and clear in gathering ones potential for self-improvement.

Contains:

Galbanum *(Ferula gummosa)* was used for both medicinal and spiritual purposes. It is antimicrobial and supporting to the body. When combined with frankincense and sandalwood, its frequency increases dramatically. *(And the Lord said unto Moses, Take unto thee sweet spices, stacte, and onycha, and galbanum; sweet spices with pure with frankincense*: Exodus 30:34).

Frankincense *(Boswellia carteri)* is considered a holy anointing oil in the Middle East and has been used in religious ceremonies for thousands of years. It elevates the mind and helps overcome stress and despair. It is high in sesquiterpenes, which stimulate the limbic region of the brain, the center of emotions. In ancient times, it was known for its anointing and healing powers, and was reportedly used to treat every conceivable ill known to man.

Sandalwood *(Santalum album)* is high in sesquiterpenes, which have been researched for their ability to stimulate the pineal gland and the limbic region of the brain, the center of our emotions. The pineal gland is responsible for releasing melatonin, a hormone that enhances deep sleep. Used traditionally for skin revitalization, yoga, and meditation, sandalwood is similar to frankincense oil in its support of nerves and circulation.

Rose *(Rosa damascena)* possesses the highest frequency of the oils. It creates a sense of balance, harmony, and well-being and elevates the mind. Rose promotes healthy skin, reduces scarring, and may help with chronic bronchitis, asthma, tuberculosis, sexual disabilities, frigidity, impotency, skin disease, ulcers, sprains, wrinkles, thrush, and gingivitis. It also promotes healthy skin.

Lavender *(Lavandula angustifolia)* has sedative and calming properties that help overcome insomnia, headaches, stress, and nervous tension.

Cinnamon Bark *(Cinnamomum verum)* is the oil of wealth from the Orient and part of the formula the Lord gave Moses (Exodus 30:22-27). Cinnamon oil is anti-infectious, antibacterial, antiparasitic, antiviral, and antifungal.

Cinnamon oil was regarded by the emperors of China and India to have great value; their wealth was measured by the amount of oil they possessed. Traditionally, it was thought to have a frequency that attracted wealth and abundance. Physically, it has many attributes; it is a powerful purifier and oxygenator, and it enhances the action and the activity of other oils. Researchers, including J. C. Lapraz, M.D., found that viruses could not live in the presence of cinnamon oil.

Spruce *(Picea mariana)* helps to open and release emotional blocks, bringing about a feeling of balance and grounding. Traditionally, spruce oil was believed to possess the frequency of prosperity.

Ylang Ylang *(Cananga odorata)* helps bring about a sense of relaxation and may help balance male and female energies. It balances equilibrium and restores confidence and self-love.

Geranium *(Pelargonium graveolens)* stimulates nerves and assists in balancing hormones. Its aromatic influence helps release negative memories, thereby opening and elevating the mind.

Safety Data: May be irritating to those with sensitive skin. Avoid eye contact. In case of accidental contact, put a few drops of any pure vegetable oil in the eye and call your doctor if necessary. Never use water. Avoid exposure to direct sunlight for 3 to 6 hours after use.

Application: Diffuse, wear on temples, neck, wrists, or where needed. It may be worn as a perfume or cologne.

Companion Oils: Forgiveness on navel, Sacred Mountain on crown (to clear negative attitudes), Valor on crown or feet, Three Wise Men on the crown, Clarity on the temples, and Dream Catcher.

Fragrant Influence: A feeling of coming together for a higher purpose.

Frequency: Approximately 99 MHz.

Gentle Baby

This is a beautiful combination of therapeutic-grade essential oils for mothers and babies. It is comforting, soothing, relaxing, and may be beneficial during the birthing process and for reducing stress during pregnancy. It helps reduce stretch marks and scar tissue. Gentle Baby enhances a youthful appearance of the skin, improving skin elasticity and smoothing wrinkles. It is particularly soothing to dry, chapped skin, and even diaper rash (dilute 1-3 drops in 1/2 tsp. carrier oil).

Contains:

Palmarosa (*Cymbopogon martinii*) is helpful for all types of skin problems, such as candida, rashes, and scaly and flaky skin. It stimulates new cell growth, moisturizes and speeds the healing process. It is antimicrobial, antibacterial, antifungal, and antiviral. It is supportive to the nervous and cardiovascular system.

Geranium (*Pelargonium graveolens*) has been used for centuries for skin care, especially the skin of pregnant mothers. It revitalizes tissue and nerves and assists in balancing hormones. It is antispasmodic, relaxant, anti-inflammatory, anti-infectious, antibacterial, antifungal and supports the liver, pancreas, and kidneys. Its aromatic influence helps release negative memories, thus opening and elevating the mind.

Roman Chamomile (*Chamaemelum nobile*) may calm and relieve restlessness, tension, insomnia, muscle tension, cuts, scrapes, bruises and is anti-infectious. It may relieve allergies and expel toxins from the liver. It is used extensively in Europe for the skin.

Rose (*Rosa damascena*) possesses the highest frequency of the oils. It creates a sense of balance, harmony, and well-being and elevates the mind. Rose promotes healthy skin, reduces scarring, and may help with chronic bronchitis, asthma, tuberculosis, sexual disabilities, frigidity, impotency, skin disease, ulcers, sprains, wrinkles, thrush, and gingivitis. It also promotes healthy skin.

Lavender (*Lavandula angustifolia*) is known as the universal oil because of its wide range of usage. It is beneficial for skin conditions, such as burns, rashes, and psoriasis. Lavender's sedative and calming properties help overcome insomnia, headaches, stress, and nervous tension. It is antispasmodic, hypotensive, anti-inflammatory, anti-infectious, and anticoagulant. It prevents scarring and stretch marks and relieves headaches and PMS symptoms.

Rosewood (*Aniba rosaeodora*) is soothing and nourishing to the skin. It has been researched at Weber State University for its inhibition rate against gram positive and gram negative bacterial growth. This oil is soothing, creates elasticity, and helps the skin rid itself of irritations and problems, such as candida. It is anti-infectious, antibacterial, antifungal, antiviral, and antiparasitic.

Ylang Ylang (*Cananga odorata*) helps bring about a sense of relaxation.

Bergamot (*Citrus bergamia*) is one of the most uplifting fragrances, simultaneously energizing and calming, with a unique ability to relieve anxiety, stress, and tension.

Jasmine (*Jasminum officinale*) is beneficial for dry, greasy, irritated, or sensitive skin. It is used for muscle spasms, sprains, coughs, laryngitis, frigidity, depression, and nervous exhaustion.

Lemon (*Citrus limon*) has antiseptic-like properties and contains compounds that have been studied for their effects on immune function. It increases microcirculation, which may improve vision. It may serve as an insect repellent and may be beneficial for the skin. It has been found to promote leukocyte formation, dissolve cellulite, increase lymphatic function, and promote a sense of well-being. Its fragrance is stimulating and invigorating.

Safety Data: May be irritating to those with sensitive skin. Avoid eye contact. In case of accidental contact, put a few drops of any pure vegetable oil in the eye and call your doctor if necessary. Never use water. Avoid exposure to direct sunlight for 3 to 6 hours after use.

Application: Diffuse, apply over mother's abdomen, on feet, lower back, face and neck areas. Dilute with V-6 Mixing Oil or Massage Oil Base for full-body massage and for applying on baby's skin.

Fragrant Influence: Relaxing, calming, creating memories of childhood.

Frequency: Approximately 152 MHz.

Note: For Baby: Dilute by 1/2 with V-6 Mixing Oil. Apply to the feet, abdomen, back, face and neck.

For Pregnancy and Delivery: Use for massage throughout entire pregnancy for relieving stress and anxiety, and to prevent scarring and create a calm and peaceful feeling. Massage on the perineum to help it stretch for easier birthing.

Grounding

This blend helps stabilize and ground us in order to deal logically with reality in a peaceful manner. When we're hurting emotionally we sometimes wish to leave this physical existence. When this happens, it is easy to make choices that lead to unfortunate circumstances, such as bad relationships and bad business decisions. We escape because we do not have anchoring or awareness to know how to deal with the emotions.

Contains:

Spruce *(Picea mariana)* helps to open and release emotional blocks, bringing about a feeling of balance and grounding. Traditionally, spruce oil was believed to possess the frequency of prosperity.

Fir *(Abies alba)* creates a feeling of grounding, anchoring, and empowerment.

Ylang Ylang *(Cananga odorata)* helps bring about a sense of relaxation and it may help balance male and female energies. It balances equilibrium, restores confidence, and self-love.

Pine *(Pinus sylvestris)* may help reduce stress, relieve anxiety, and energize the entire body.

Cedarwood *(Cedrus atlantica)* is high in sesquiterpenes which can stimulate the limbic part of the brain (the center of our emotions). This conifer oil has been used by North American Indians to enhance spiritual awareness and communication. It also may help stimulate the pineal gland, which releases melatonin, a hormone that enhances deep sleep.

Angelica *(Angelica archangelica)* helps to bring memories back to the point of origin before trauma or anger was experienced, helping us to release negative feelings.

Juniper *(Juniperus osteosperma* and/or *J. scopulorum)* may work as a detoxifier and cleanser, and promotes improved nerve and kidney function. It is also beneficial for the skin reducing dermatitis, eczema, and acne. It elevates spiritual awareness creating feelings of love and peace.

Safety Data: May be irritating to those with sensitive skin. Avoid eye contact. In case of accidental contact, put a few drops of any pure vegetable oil in the eye and call your doctor if necessary. Never use water. Avoid exposure to direct sunlight for 3 to 6 hours after use.

Application: Diffuse, wear on back of neck and on temples.

Fragrant Influence: Creates a feeling of solidity and balance.

Frequency: Approximately 140 MHz.

Harmony

This is an exquisite blend of oils promoting physical and emotional healing by bringing about a harmonic balance to the energy centers of the body, allowing the energy to flow more efficiently through the body. It is also beneficial in reducing stress and creating a general overall feeling of well-being. Harmony has also been found to stop allergy attacks and symptoms.

Contains:

Hyssop *(Hyssopus officinalis)* is very balancing for emotions.

Spruce *(Picea mariana)* helps to open and release emotional blocks, bringing about a feeling of balance and grounding. Traditionally, spruce oil was believed to possess the frequency of prosperity.

Lavender *(Lavandula angustifolia)* has sedative and calming properties that help overcome insomnia, headaches, stress, and nervous tension.

Geranium *(Pelargonium graveolens)* stimulates nerves and assists in balancing hormones. Its aromatic influence helps release negative memories, thereby opening and elevating the mind.

Frankincense (*Boswellia carteri*) is considered a holy anointing oil in the Middle East and has been used in religious ceremonies for thousands of years. High in sesquiterpenes, frankincense helps stimulate the limbic part of the brain, which elevates the mind, helping to overcome stress and despair. It is used in European medicine to combat depression.

Ylang Ylang (*Cananga odorata*) helps bring about a sense of relaxation and may help balance male and female energies. It balances equilibrium and restores confidence and self-love.

Sandalwood (*Santalum album*) is high in sesquiterpenes, which have been researched for their ability to stimulate the pineal gland and the limbic region of the brain, the center of our emotions. The pineal gland is responsible for releasing melatonin, a hormone that enhances deep sleep. Used traditionally for skin revitalization, yoga, and meditation, sandalwood is similar to frankincense oil in its support of nerves and circulation.

Angelica (*Angelica archangelica*) helps to bring memories back to the point of origin before trauma or anger was experienced, helping us to release negative feelings.

Rose (*Rosa damascena*) possesses the highest frequency of the oils. It creates a sense of balance, harmony, and well-being and elevates the mind. It promotes healthy skin, reduces scarring, and may help with chronic bronchitis, asthma, tuberculosis, sexual problems or disabilities, impotency, skin disease, ulcers, sprains, wrinkles, thrush, and gingivitis. It also promotes healthy skin.

Orange (*Citrus sinensis*) was believed to bring joy, peace, and happiness to those who possessed it. It contains limonene, an antiviral compound, and citral, an antibacterial compound. Orange is elevating to the mind and body and brings joy and peace. It has been recognized to help a dull, oily complexion.

Bergamot (*Citrus bergamia*) is one of the most uplifting fragrances, simultaneously energizing and calming, with a unique ability to relieve anxiety, stress, and tension.

Jasmine (*Jasminum officinale*) is beneficial for dry, greasy, irritated, or sensitive skin. It is used for muscle spasms, sprains, coughs, laryngitis, frigidity, depression, and nervous exhaustion.

Lemon (*Citrus limon*) has antiseptic-like properties and contains compounds that have been studied for their effects on immune function. It increases microcirculation, which may improve vision. It may serve as an insect repellent and may be beneficial for the skin. It has been found to promote leukocyte formation, dissolve cellulite, increase lymphatic function, and promote a sense of well-being. Its fragrance is stimulating and invigorating.

Palmarosa (*Cymbopogon martinii*) is helpful for all types of skin problems, such as candida, rashes, and scaly and flaky skin. It stimulates new cell growth, moisturizes and speeds the healing process. It is antimicrobial, antibacterial, antifungal, and antiviral. It is supportive to the nervous and cardiovascular system.

Roman Chamomile (*Chamaemelum nobile*) may calm and relieve restlessness, tension, insomnia, muscle tension, cuts, scrapes, bruises and is anti-infectious. It may relieve allergies and expel toxins from the liver. It is used extensively in Europe for the skin.

Rosewood (*Aniba rosaeodora*) is soothing and nourishing to the skin. It has been researched at Weber State University for its inhibition rate against gram positive and gram negative bacterial growth. This oil is soothing, creates elasticity, and helps the skin rid itself of irritations and problems, such as candida. It is anti-infectious, antibacterial, antifungal, antiviral, and antiparasitic.

Safety Data: May be irritating to those with sensitive skin. Avoid eye contact. In case of accidental contact, put a few drops of any pure vegetable oil in the eye and call your doctor if necessary. Never use water. Avoid exposure to direct sunlight for 3 to 6 hours after use.

Application: Diffuse, wear on ears, feet, over the heart, on areas of poor circulation, and over or around the energy centers of the body. Wear it as a perfume or cologne or aftershave. If there is an irritation or allergic reaction to any oil or blend, the following may help: Rub a few drops of Harmony over the thymus gland (at the base of the neck) with one hand and hold the other hand over the navel for about one minute. For allergies, rub three drops on sternum, breathing deeply.

Fragrant Influence: Uplifting and elevating to the mind creating a happy, positive attitude.

Frequency: Approximately 101 MHz.

Hope

Everyone needs hope in order to go forward in life. Hopelessness can cause a loss of vision of goals and dreams. This blend helps to reconnect with a feeling of strength and grounding, restoring hope for tomorrow and helping us to go forward. It may help overcome suicidal depression.

Contains:

Melissa *(Melissa officinalis)* is a powerful, antimicrobial oil, yet it is very gentle and delicate because of the nature of the plant, and helps to bring out those characteristics within the individual. It is calming and balancing to the emotions. Melissa is one of the highest in sesquiterpenes, much like cedarwood. It is very stimulating to the anterior pituitary and immune system.

Spruce *(Picea mariana)* helps to open and release emotional blocks, bringing about a feeling of balance and grounding. Traditionally, spruce oil was believed to possess the frequency of prosperity. Spruce is anti-infectious, antiseptic, and anti-inflammatory.

Juniper *(Juniperus osteosperma* and/or *J. scopulorum)* may work as a detoxifier and cleanser, and promotes improved nerve and kidney function. It is also beneficial for the skin reducing dermatitis, eczema, and acne. It elevates spiritual awareness creating feelings of love and peace.

Myrrh *(Commiphora myrrha)* is referenced throughout the Old and New Testaments constituting a part of a holy anointing formula given Moses (Exodus 30:22-27). It has one of the highest levels of sesquiterpenes, a class of compounds that can stimulate the hypothalamus, pituitary, and amygdala, the control center for emotions and hormones in the brain. It has been used in eastern countries to enhance the feeling of spirituality or euphoria.

Carrier Oil: Almond oil.

Safety Data: May be irritating to those with sensitive skin. Avoid eye contact. In case of accidental contact, put a few drops of any pure vegetable oil in the eye and call your doctor if necessary. Never use water. Avoid exposure to direct sunlight for 3 to 6 hours after use.

Application: Diffuse, massage 1 or 2 drops on outer edge of ears. Apply to wrists, neck, or wear as a perfume or cologne.

Fragrant Influence: A feeling of peace and security and the ability to live life.

Frequency: Approximately 98 MHz.

Humility

Having humility and forgiveness helps us to heal ourselves and our earth (Chronicles 7:14). Humility is an integral ingredient in obtaining forgiveness and a closer relationship with God. Through the frequency and fragrance of this blend, you may find that special place where your own healing may begin.

Contains:

Frankincense *(Boswellia carteri)* is considered a holy anointing oil in the Middle East and has been used in religious ceremonies for thousands of years. High in sesquiterpenes, frankincense helps stimulate the pineal gland, which secretes melatonin, a hormone that enhances deep sleep. It also helps to overcome stress and despair, and is used in European medicine to combat depression.

Rose *(Rosa damascena)* possesses the highest frequency of the oils. It creates a sense of balance, harmony, and well-being and elevates the mind. Rose promotes healthy skin, reduces scarring, and may help with chronic bronchitis, asthma, tuberculosis, sexual disabilities, frigidity, impotency, skin disease, ulcers, sprains, wrinkles, thrush, and gingivitis. It also promotes healthy skin.

Rosewood *(Aniba rosaeodora)* is soothing and nourishing to the skin. It has been researched at Weber State University for its inhibition rate against gram positive and gram negative bacterial growth. This oil is soothing, creates elasticity, and helps the skin rid itself of irritations and problems, such as candida. It is anti-infectious, antibacterial, antifungal, antiviral, and antiparasitic.

Ylang Ylang *(Cananga odorata)* helps bring about a sense of relaxation and may help balance male and female energies. It balances equilibrium and restores confidence and self-love.

Geranium *(Pelargonium graveolens)* stimulates nerves and assists in balancing hormones. Its aromatic influence helps release negative memories, thereby opening and elevating the mind.

Melissa *(Melissa officinalis)* is a powerful, antimicrobial oil, yet it is very gentle and delicate because of the nature of the plant, and helps to bring out those characteristics within the individual. It is calming and balancing to the emotions. Melissa is one of the highest in sesquiterpenes, much like cedarwood. It is very stimulating to the anterior pituitary and immune system.

Spikenard *(Nardostachys jatamansi)* was highly prized at the time of Christ and was used by Mary of Bethany to anoint the feet of Jesus. High in sesquiterpenes, it is very supporting to the immune system. It strengthens and calms the cardiovascular system, stimulates under active ovaries, and helps with tachycardia, anemia, psoriasis, and hemorrhoids.

Myrrh *(Commiphora myrrha)* is referenced throughout the Bible and was part of a holy anointing formula given Moses (Exodus 30:22-27). It has one of the highest levels of sesquiterpenes, a class of compounds that can stimulate the hypothalamus, pituitary, and amygdala, the control center for emotions and hormone release in the brain. Myrrh has been used in eastern countries to enhance the feeling of spirituality or euphoria.

Neroli *(Citrus aurantium)* was highly regarded by the Egyptian people for its great attributes of healing and calming the mind, body, and spirit. It is stabilizing and strengthening to the emotions, promoting peace, confidence and awareness, thereby bringing everything into focus at the moment.

Carrier Oil: Sesame seed oil.

Application: Diffuse, rub over the heart, on neck, temples, or as needed.

Companion Oils: Inspiration, Inner Child, Peace & Calming, Envision, Acceptance, and Forgiveness.

Safety Data: May be irritating to those with sensitive skin. Avoid eye contact. In case of accidental contact, put a few drops of any pure vegetable oil in the eye and call your doctor if necessary. Never use water. Avoid exposure to direct sunlight for 3 to 6 hours after use.

Fragrant Influence: Peaceful healing.

Frequency: Approximately 88 MHz.

ImmuPower

This is a powerful blend for building, strengthening, and protecting the body and supporting its defense mechanism. Diffusing ImmuPower protects the home environment especially during the seasons of cold and flu. ImmuPower has been found to reverse symptoms of lupus and inner ear infections.

Contains:

Cistus *(Cistus ladaniferus),* also known as rock rose, has been studied for its effects on cell regeneration. It is anti-infectious, antiviral, antibacterial, and prevents hemorrhaging and scarring. It is a tonic to the parasympathetic nervous system and may help with viral problems and auto-immune disorders, such as rheumatoid arthritis.

Frankincense *(Boswellia carteri)* is considered a holy anointing oil in the Middle East and has been used in religious ceremonies for thousands of years. High in sesquiterpenes, frankincense helps stimulate the hypothalamus which can lead to heightened immune function. Frankincense is being researched and used therapeutically in European hospitals to build immunity and treat cancer. In ancient times, it was well-known for its healing powers, and was reportedly used to treat every conceivable ill known to man.

Oregano *(Origanum compactum)* is one of the most powerful antimicrobial essential oils. Laboratory research as Weber State University showed it to have a 99 percent kill rate against *in vitro* colonies of *Streptococcus pneumoniae*, a microorganism responsible for many kinds of lung and throat infections. This oil is antiviral, antibacterial, antifungal, and antiparasitic.

Idaho Tansy *(Tanacetum vulgare)* is antiviral, anti-infectious, antibacterial, and fights cold and flu and infections. According to E. Joseph Montagna's *Herbal Desk Reference*, tansy may improve weakness of the kidneys, heart, joints, digestive system, and may help tone the entire system.

Cumin *(Cuminum cyminum)*, commonly found in Egypt, helps with digestion and supports the immune system. It is antiseptic, antispasmodic, and carminative.

Clove *(Syzygium aromaticum)* was another oil from the Orient hailed as an oil of great abundance; those who possessed it were considered wealthy. This oil is one of the most antimicrobial and antiseptic of all essential oils. It is antifungal, antiviral, anti-infectious, and antibacterial. It works as a general stimulant and is used to treat sinusitis, bronchitis, cystitis, and cholera.

Hyssop *(Hyssopus officinalis)* has anti-inflammatory and antiviral properties and is antiparasitic, mucolytic, decongestant, antiasthmatic, and anti-infectious.

Ravensara *(Ravensara aromatica)* is referred to by the people of Madagascar as the oil that heals. It is antiseptic, anti-infectious, antiviral, antibacterial, antifungal, expectorant and supporting to the nerves. Similar to clove and nutmeg, ravensara may aid the respiratory system and support the adrenal glands. It has been shown to help with flu, sinusitis, bronchitis, viral hepatitis, cholera, herpes, infectious mononucleosis, insomnia, muscle fatigue and rhinopharyngitis.

Mountain Savory *(Satureja montana)* is antimicrobial and immune stimulating. It is antiviral, antibacterial, antifungal, antiparasitic, and a general tonic for the body.

Safety Data: May be irritating to those with sensitive skin. Avoid eye contact. In case of accidental contact, put a few drops of any pure vegetable oil in the eye and call your doctor if necessary. Never use water. Avoid exposure to direct sunlight for 3 to 6 hours after use.

Application: Diffuse daily for 15 to 30 minutes every 3 or 4 hours or as needed. Massage on bottom of feet and use in Raindrop application along the spine as needed. It may be necessary to dilute with V-6 Mixing Oil or Massage Oil Base as this blend may be too warming to the skin. May also be rubbed on throat and chest. Apply 2 to 3 drops on thymus. Put 1 to 2 drops on a piece of cotton and place in the ear for earaches.

Companion Oils: Alternate with Thieves and Exodus II. Other single oils may be added for extra strength: Rosewood, Melissa, Oregano, Clove, Cistus, Frankincense, and Mountain Savory.

Companion Supplements: ImmuneTune, Exodus, Radex, Super C, ImmuGel, Megazyme, and ComforTone.

Frequency: Approximately 89 MHz.

Inner Child

This blend was created for those suffering from abuse. When children are abused, they become disconnected from their inner child, or identity, which causes confusion. This can contribute to multiple personality disorder. Sometimes these problems do not manifest themselves until early- to mid-adult years, often labeled as a mid-life crisis. This fragrance may stimulate memory response and help one reconnect with the inner-self or identity. This is one of the first steps to finding emotional balance.

Contains:

Orange *(Citrus sinensis)* was believed to bring joy, peace, and happiness to those who possessed it. It contains limonene, an antiviral compound, and citral, an antibacterial compound. It prevents the growth of bacteria. It is elevating to the mind and body and brings joy and peace. It has been recognized to help a dull, oily complexion.

Tangerine *(Citrus nobilis)* contains esters and aldehydes that are sedating and calming, helping with anxiety and nervousness. It is anti-inflammatory, anticoagulant, may help decongest the lymphatic system and works as a diuretic.

Jasmine *(Jasminum officinale)* is beneficial for dry, greasy, irritated, or sensitive skin. It is used for muscle spasms, sprains, coughs, laryngitis, frigidity, depression, and nervous exhaustion.

Ylang Ylang *(Cananga odorata)* helps bring about a sense of relaxation and may help balance male and female energies. It balances equilibrium and restores confidence and self-love.

Sandalwood *(Santalum album)* is high in sesquiterpenes, which have been researched for their ability to stimulate the pineal gland and the limbic region of the brain, the center of our emotions. The pineal gland is responsible for releasing melatonin, a hormone that enhances deep sleep. Used traditionally for skin revitalization, yoga, and meditation, sandalwood is similar to frankincense oil in its support of nerves and circulation.

Spruce *(Picea mariana)* helps to open and release emotional blocks, bringing about a feeling of balance and grounding. Traditionally, spruce oil was believed to possess the frequency of prosperity. Spruce is anti-infectious, antiseptic, and anti-inflammatory.

Lemongrass *(Cymbopogon flexuosus)* works well for purification. It is powerful in the regeneration of connective tissue. It is a vasodilator, anti-inflammatory, sedative, and supportive to the digestive system. Research published in *Phytotherapy Research* showed that lemongrass oil had strong antifungal properties when applied topically. It may also help increase the flow of oxygen and uplift the spirit.

Neroli *(Citrus aurantium)* has been highly regarded by the Egyptian people for its great attributes of healing and calming the mind, body and spirit. It is stabilizing and strengthening to the emotions, promoting peace, confidence, and awareness. Neroli brings everything into focus at the moment.

Safety Data: May be irritating to those with sensitive skin. Avoid eye contact. In case of accidental contact, put a few drops of any pure vegetable oil in the eye and call your doctor if necessary. Never use water. Avoid exposure to direct sunlight for 3 to 6 hours after use.

Application: Apply around navel, chest, temples, and nose.

Companion Oils: Citrus Fresh, Gentle Baby, Acceptance, Envision, Awaken, Surrender, and Forgiveness.

Fragrant Influence: Calming to the nerves with a feeling of inner peace.

Frequency: Approximately 98 MHz.

Inspiration

This blend combines oils traditionally used by the Native Americans to increase spirituality, enhancing prayer and inner awareness. Inspiration brings us closer to our spiritual connection. It can also reverse bladder and kidney infections.

Contains:

Frankincense *(Boswellia carteri)* is considered a holy anointing oil in the Middle East and has been used in religious ceremonies for thousands of years. High in sesquiterpenes, frankincense helps stimulate the limbic part of the brain, which elevates the mind, helping to overcome stress and despair. It is used in European medicine to combat depression.

Cedarwood *(Cedrus atlantica)* has calming and purifying properties. High in sesquiterpenes which can stimulate the limbic part of the brain (the center of our emotions), this conifer oil has been used by North American Indians to enhance spiritual awareness and communication. Cedarwood may also help stimulate the pineal gland, which releases melatonin, a hormone that enhances deep sleep.

Spruce *(Picea mariana)* helps to open and release emotional blocks, bringing about a feeling of balance and grounding. Traditionally, spruce oil was believed to possess the frequency of prosperity. Spruce is anti-infectious, antiseptic, and anti-inflammatory.

Rosewood (*Aniba rosaeodora*) is soothing and nourishing to the skin. It has been researched at Weber State University for its inhibition rate against gram positive and gram negative bacterial growth. This oil is soothing, creates elasticity, and helps the skin rid itself of irritations and problems, such as candida. Rosewood is anti-infectious, antibacterial, antifungal, antiviral, and antiparasitic.

Sandalwood (*Santalum album*) is high in sesquiterpenes, which have been researched for their ability to stimulate the pineal gland and the limbic region of the brain, the center of our emotions. The pineal gland is responsible for releasing melatonin, a hormone that enhances deep sleep. Used traditionally for skin revitalization, yoga, and meditation, sandalwood is similar to frankincense oil in its support of nerves and circulation.

Myrtle (*Myrtus communis*) may help normalize hormonal imbalances of the thyroid and ovaries as well as balance an under-active thyroid. It may help the respiratory system with chronic coughs and tuberculosis. It is suitable to use for coughs and chest complaints with children, and may support immune function in fighting colds, flu and infectious disease.

Mugwort (*Artemisia vulgaris*)

Safety Data: May be irritating to those with sensitive skin. Avoid eye contact. In case of accidental contact, put a few drops of any pure vegetable oil in the eye and call your doctor if necessary. Never use water. Avoid exposure to direct sunlight for 3 to 6 hours after use.

Application: Diffuse during times of meditation and prayer, put 2 or 3 drops on a cotton ball and put in car vent, wear on back of neck, sides of forehead, crown of head, bottom of feet, or along spine.

Companion Oils: Humility, Surrender, Acceptance, Forgiveness, and 3 Wise Men.

Fragrant Influence: A feeling of being wrapped in a cocoon of spiritual quietness.

Frequency: Approximately 141 MHz.

Into the Future

This helps one leave the past behind in order to go forward with vision and excitement. So many times we find ourselves settling for mediocrity and sacrificing our own potential and success because of fear of the unknown and the future. This blend was formulated to inspire determination and a pioneering spirit and support the emotions in helping us create the feeling of moving forward. Living on the edge with tenacity and integrity brings the excitement of the challenge and the joy of success.

Contains:

Frankincense (*Boswellia carteri*) is considered a holy anointing oil in the Middle East and has been used in religious ceremonies for thousands of years. High in sesquiterpenes, frankincense helps stimulate the limbic part of the brain, which elevates the mind, helping to overcome stress and despair. It is used in European medicine to combat depression.

Clary Sage (*Salvia sclarea*) regulates the cells and balances the hormones. It contains natural sclareol, a phytoestrogen that mimics estrogen function. Clary sage may help with menstrual cramps, PMS, and pre-menopause symptoms and may help with circulatory problems.

Jasmine (*Jasminum officinale*) is beneficial for dry, greasy, irritated, or sensitive skin. It is used for muscle spasms, sprains, coughs, laryngitis, frigidity, depression, and nervous exhaustion.

Juniper (*Juniperus osteosperma* and/or *J. scopulorum*) may work as a detoxifier and cleanser, and promotes improved nerve and kidney function. It is also beneficial for the skin reducing dermatitis, eczema, and acne. Juniper elevates spiritual awareness creating feelings of love and peace.

Fir (*Abies alba*) is antimicrobial. It has been researched for its ability to kill airborne germs and bacteria. Fir is antiseptic, antiarthritic, and stimulating. It supports the body and reduces the symptoms of arthritis, rheumatism bronchitis, coughs, sinusitis, cold, flu, and fevers. As a conifer oil, fir creates a feeling of grounding, anchoring, and empowerment.

Orange *(Citrus sinensis)* was believed to bring joy, peace, and happiness to those who possessed it. It contains limonene, an antiviral compound, and citral, an antibacterial compound. Orange is elevating to the mind and body and brings joy and peace. It has been recognized to help a dull, oily complexion.

Cedarwood *(Cedrus atlantica)* has calming and purifying properties. High in sesquiterpenes which can stimulate the limbic part of the brain (the center of our emotions), this conifer oil has been used by North American Indians to enhance spiritual awareness and communication. Cedarwood may also help stimulate the pineal gland, which releases melatonin, a hormone that enhances deep sleep.

Ylang Ylang *(Cananga odorata)* helps bring about a sense of relaxation and may help balance male and female energies. It balances equilibrium and restores confidence and self-love.

Idaho Tansy *(Tanacetum vulgare)* is antiviral, anti-infectious, antibacterial, and fights colds, flu, and infections. According to E. Joseph Montagna's PDR on herbal formulas, tansy may help skin problems, strengthen the kidneys, heart, joints, digestive system.

Carrier Oil: Almond oil.

Safety Data: May be irritating to those with sensitive skin. Avoid eye contact. In case of accidental contact, put a few drops of any pure vegetable oil in the eye and call your doctor if necessary. Never use water. Avoid exposure to direct sunlight for 3 to 6 hours after use.

Application: Diffuse, put in bath water, over the heart, on wrists, neck, as a compress, and dilute with V-6 Mixing Oil or Massage Oil Base for full body massage.

Companion Oils: Envision, Awaken, Passion, Magnify Your Purpose, Clarity, Dream Catcher, and Inspiration.

Fragrant Influence: A strong emotional feeling of being able to reach one's potential.

Frequency: Approximately 88 MHz.

Joy

Joy is an exotic blend that produces a magnetic energy to enhance the frequency of self-love and bring joy to the heart. It inspires romance and may help overcome grief and depression.

Contains:

Rose *(Rosa damascena)* possesses the highest frequency of the oils. It creates a sense of balance, harmony, and well-being and elevates the mind. Rose promotes healthy skin, reduces scarring, and may help with chronic bronchitis, asthma, tuberculosis, sexual disabilities, frigidity, impotency, skin disease, ulcers, sprains, wrinkles, thrush, and gingivitis. It also promotes healthy skin.

Bergamot *(Citrus bergamia)* has been used in the Middle East for hundreds of years for acne, boils, cold sores, eczema, insect bites, psoriasis, scabies, spot varicose veins, ulcers, sore throat, thrush, oily complexion, infectious disease, and depression. It balances hormones, calms emotions, and relieves anxiety, stress, and tension.

Mandarin *(Citrus reticulata)* is appealing, gentle, and promotes happiness. Diffuse or apply topically, especially around meals and before sleep. Because of its sedative and slightly hypnotic properties, it may help with insomnia and is good for stress and irritability. It is antispasmodic, antiseptic, antifungal, supports hepatic-duct function, and works as a digestive tonic.

Ylang Ylang *(Cananga odorata)* helps bring about a sense of relaxation and may help balance male and female energies. It balances equilibrium and restores confidence and self-love.

Lemon *(Citrus limon)* has antiseptic-like properties and contains compounds that have been studied for their effects on immune function. It increases microcirculation, which may improve vision. It may serve as an insect repellent and may be beneficial for the skin. It has been found to promote leukocyte formation, dissolve cellulite, increase lymphatic function, and promote a sense of well-being. Its fragrance is stimulating and invigorating.

Geranium *(Pelargonium graveolens)* assists in balancing hormones. It is antispasmodic, relaxant, anti-inflammatory, anti-infectious, antibacterial, antifungal, and stimulates the liver and pancreas.

Jasmine *(Jasminum officinale)* is beneficial for dry, greasy, irritated, or sensitive skin. It is used for muscle spasms, sprains, coughs, laryngitis, frigidity, depression, and nervous exhaustion.

Palmarosa *(Cymbopogon martinii)* is helpful for all types of skin problems, such as candida, rashes, and scaly and flaky skin. It stimulates new cell growth, moisturizes and speeds the healing process. It is antimicrobial, antibacterial, antifungal, and antiviral. It is supportive to the nervous and cardiovascular system.

Roman Chamomile *(Chamaemelum nobile)* may calm and relieve restlessness, tension, insomnia, muscle tension, cuts, scrapes, bruises and is anti-infectious. It may relieve allergies and expel toxins from the liver. It is used extensively in Europe for the skin.

Rosewood *(Aniba rosaeodora)* is soothing and nourishing to the skin. It has been researched at Weber State University for its inhibition rate against gram positive and gram negative bacterial growth. This oil is soothing, creates elasticity, and helps the skin rid itself of irritations and problems, such as candida. It is anti-infectious, antibacterial, antifungal, antiviral, and antiparasitic.

Safety Data: May be irritating to those with sensitive skin. Avoid eye contact. In case of accidental contact, put a few drops of any pure vegetable oil in the eye and call your doctor if necessary. Never use water. Avoid exposure to direct sunlight for 3 to 6 hours after use.

Application: Diffuse, use as a perfume or cologne, apply over heart, thymus, temples, and wrists. Add to bath water or put a few drops in Pharaoh or Rawhide Aftershave. Dilute with V-6 Mixing Oil or Massage Oil Base for a full-body massage. Put two drops on a wet cloth and put in the dryer for fragrancing.

Companion Oils: Hope, Valor, Motivation, Passion, Clarity, and Magnify Your Purpose.

Fragrant Influence: Feelings of self-love and confidence.

Frequency: Approximately 188 MHz.

JuvaFlex

These oils have been known to support liver and lymphatic system detoxification as well. Anger and hate are stored in the liver, creating toxicity and leading to sickness and disease. JuvaFlex helps break addictions to substances such as coffee, alcohol, drugs, and tobacco.

Contains:

Geranium *(Pelargonium graveolens)* helps improve the flow of bile to and from the liver. It is antispasmodic, antibacterial, antifungal, and supports the liver, pancreas, and kidneys.

Rosemary *(Rosmarinus officinalis)* is antiseptic and antimicrobial and may be beneficial for skin conditions and dandruff. It may help fight candida and is anti-infectious, antispasmodic, balances the endocrine system, and is an expectorant. It helps overcome mental fatigue stimulating memory and opening the conscious mind.

Roman Chamomile *(Chamaemelum nobile)* may calm and relieve restlessness, tension, insomnia, muscle tension, cuts, scrapes, bruises, and is anti-infectious. It may relieve allergies and expel toxins from the liver. It is used extensively in Europe for the skin.

Fennel *(Foeniculum vulgare)* is antiseptic and stimulating to the circulatory and respiratory systems. It is antispasmodic, antiseptic, and stimulating to the cardiovascular and respiratory systems. With its hormone-like activity, it may help facilitate childbirth and increase lactation after birthing.

Helichrysum *(Helichrysum italicum)* has been researched in Europe for regenerating tissue and nerves and improving circulation. It is anticoagulant, prevents phlebitis, helps regulate cholesterol, stimulates liver cell function, and may help to clean plaque and debris from the veins and arteries. It is mucolytic, expectorant, antispasmodic, and reduces scarring and discoloration. It may also stimulate nerve endings and improve conditions such as hearing loss. It may help release feelings of anger and promote forgiveness.

Blue Tansy (*Tanacetum annuum*) may help cleanse the liver and calm the lymphatic system, helping one to overcome anger and negative emotions and promote a feeling of self-control. Its primary constituents are limonene and sesquiterpenes. European research shows that it works as an antihistamine, anti-inflammatory, and stimulant for the thymus gland reducing dermatitis, arthritis, sciatica, tuberculosis, and allergies.

Carrier Oil: Sesame seed oil.

Safety Data: May be irritating to those with sensitive skin. Avoid eye contact. In case of accidental contact, put a few drops of any pure vegetable oil in the eye and call your doctor if necessary. Never use water. Avoid exposure to direct sunlight for 3 to 6 hours after use.

Application: Apply over liver neat or use a hot compress. Massage the Vita Flex points on the feet or use Raindrop Technique on the spine and dilute with V-6 Mixing Oil or Massage Oil Base.

Companion Oils: Di-Tone.

Companion Supplements: Combine JuvaTone and ComforTone for maximum results. Best taken an hour apart. Add Megazyme to digest toxic waste.

Frequency: Approximately 82 MHz.

Magnify Your Purpose

The oils in this blend were specifically chosen to stimulate the endocrine system, creating energy flow to the brain that activates the right hemisphere of creativity, desire, motivation, and focus. These characteristics are required to bring about commitment to purpose, and magnify your desire and pure intentions until they become reality.

Contains:

Sandalwood (*Santalum album*) is high in sesquiterpenes, which have been researched for their ability to stimulate the pineal gland and the limbic region of the brain, the center of our emotions. The pineal gland is responsible for releasing melatonin, a hormone that enhances deep sleep. Used traditionally for skin revitalization, yoga, and meditation, sandalwood is similar to frankincense oil in its support of nerves and circulation.

Nutmeg (*Myristica fragrans*) has adrenal cortex-like activity, which helps support the adrenal glands for increased energy. It may help with difficulties related to circulation, aches, and pains in muscles and joints related to stress, arthritis and gout. It may also help with digestive problems such as flatulence, indigestion, sluggish digestion, and nausea. It is antiseptic, antiparasitic, analgesic, and a neurotonic.

Patchouly (*Pogostemon cablin*) was used in India in ancient times as a trade commodity because of its earthy, musty fragrance and its ability to mask many different odors. East Indian people use it to fragrance their clothing and their homes because of its natural insecticidal and anti-infectious properties. Legends indicate that patchouly represented money and those who possessed it were considered to be wealthy. Patchouly is very beneficial for the skin and may help prevent wrinkles or chapped skin. It is a general tonic and stimulant and helps the digestive system. It is also antimicrobial, antiseptic, and helps relieve itching.

Rosewood (*Aniba rosaeodora*) is soothing and nourishing to the skin. It has been researched at Weber State University for its inhibition rate against gram positive and gram negative bacterial growth. This oil is soothing, creates elasticity, and helps the skin rid itself of irritations and problems, such as candida. It is anti-infectious, antibacterial, antifungal, antiviral, and antiparasitic.

Cinnamon Bark (*Cinnamomum verum*) is the oil of wealth from the Orient and part of the formula the Lord gave Moses (Exodus 30:22-27). Cinnamon oil is anti-infectious, antibacterial, antiparasitic, antiviral, and antifungal. Cinnamon oil was regarded by the emperors of China and India to have great value; their wealth was measured by the amount of oil they possessed. Traditionally, cinnamon bark oil was thought to have a frequency that attracted wealth and abundance. Physically, it has many attributes; it is a powerful purifier, it is a powerful oxygenator, and it enhances the action and the activity of other oils. Researchers, including J. C. Lapraz, M.D., found that viruses could not live in the presence of cinnamon oil.

Ginger *(Zingiber officinale)* is used for relief from motion sickness, arthritis, rheumatism, sprains, muscular aches and pains, congestion, coughs, sinusitis, sore throats, diarrhea, colic, indigestion, loss of appetite, fever, flu, chills, and infectious disease.

Sage *(Salvia officinalis)* has been used in Europe for skin conditions such as eczema, acne, dandruff, and hair loss. It has been recognized for its benefits of strengthening the vital centers. It may help in relieving depression and mental fatigue. Sage contains sclareol, which stimulates the body to produce its own estrogen. It may nutritionally support the body during PMS and menopause. The Lakota Indians used sage for purification and healing and to dispel negative emotions from denial and sexual abuse, as well as a complete body tonic for healing and strength.

Safety Data: May be irritating to those with sensitive skin. Avoid eye contact. In case of accidental contact, put a few drops of any pure vegetable oil in the eye and call your doctor if necessary. Never use water. Avoid exposure to direct sunlight for 3 to 6 hours after use.

Application: Diffuse, use as a perfume or cologne, apply over heart, thymus, temples, and wrists. Add to bath water or put a few drops in Pharaoh or Rawhide Aftershave. Dilute with V-6 Mixing Oil or Massage Oil Base for a full body massage. Put two drops on a wet cloth and put in the dryer for fragrancing.

Companion Oils: Into the Future, Gathering, Clarity, Passion, Sensation, and Harmony.

Frequency: Approximately 99 MHz.

Melrose

This blend has antiseptic-like properties when used topically for cleansing cuts, scrapes, burns, rashes, and bruised tissue. It may also help prevent growth of bacteria, fungus, or infection. Melrose is very strong in the regeneration of damaged tissue and helps fight infection and fungus. It is very beneficial for animals such as horses, dogs and cats in the same way it benefits humans.

Contains:

Melaleuca *(Melaleuca alternifolia)* is antiseptic, anti-infectious, antibacterial, antifungal, antiviral, antiparasitic, antiseptic, anti-inflammatory, immune-stimulating, decongestant, neurotonic, and protects against radiation.

Melaleuca *(Melaleuca quinquenervia)* is anti-inflammatory to the respiratory system and urinary tract, tonic to digestive system, antihypertensive, anti-infectious, antiviral, antiparasitic, and antibacterial. It has been used by European doctors for liver and pancreas deficiencies in children, viral hepatitis, colitis, ulcers, rheumatoid arthritis, hypertension of the arteries, and eczema.

Rosemary *(Rosmarinus officinalis)* has been researched for its antiseptic and antimicrobial properties. It may be beneficial for skin conditions and dandruff. It may help fight candida and is anti-infectious, antispasmodic, balances the endocrine system, and is an expectorant. Rosemary helps overcome mental fatigue stimulating memory and opening the conscious mind.

Clove *(Syzygium aromaticum)* was another oil from the Orient hailed as an oil of great abundance; those who possessed it were considered wealthy. This oil is one of the most antimicrobial and antiseptic of all essential oils. It is antifungal, antiviral, anti-infectious, and antibacterial. Clove works as a general stimulant and is used to treat sinusitis, bronchitis, cystitis, and cholera.

Safety Data: May be irritating to those with sensitive skin. Avoid eye contact. In case of accidental contact, put a few drops of any pure vegetable oil in the eye and call your doctor if necessary. Never use water. Avoid exposure to direct sunlight for 3 to 6 hours after use.

Application: Diffuse to dispel odors, apply topically on areas where the skin is broken, including cuts, scrapes, burns, rashes, and infection. Put 1 to 2 drops on a piece of cotton and place in the ear for earaches.

Companion Products: Rose Ointment (to keep wounds soft and promote healing).

Fragrant Influence: Dispels odors.

Frequency: Approximately 48 MHz.

Mister

This blend is beneficial for both men and women. It may help to decongest the prostate and promote greater hormonal balance. Some women have found it reduces hot flashes. Generally, Mister helps women age 30 and older, and Dragon Time is for teenagers and young women.

Contains:

Yarrow *(Achillea millefolium)* is a decongestant of the prostate and balances hormones. It is anti-inflammatory, and reduces scarring. It also helps with nerve inflammation.

Sage *(Salvia officinalis)* has been used in Europe for skin conditions such as eczema, acne, dandruff, and hair loss. It has been recognized for its benefits of strengthening the vital centers. It may help in relieving depression and mental fatigue. Sage contains sclareol, which stimulates the body to produce its own estrogen. It may nutritionally support the body during PMS and menopause. The Lakota Indians used sage for purification and healing and to dispel negative emotions from denial and sexual abuse, as well as a complete body tonic for healing and strength.

Myrtle *(Myrtus communis)* may help normalize hormonal imbalances of the thyroid and ovaries. It may help the respiratory system with chronic coughs and tuberculosis. It is suitable to use for coughs and chest complaints with children, and may support immune function in fighting cold, flu, and infectious disease.

Fennel *(Foeniculum vulgare)* is antiseptic and stimulating to the circulatory and respiratory systems. It is antispasmodic, antiseptic, and stimulating to the cardiovascular and respiratory systems. With its hormone-like activity, it may help facilitate childbirth and increase lactation after birthing.

Lavender *(Lavandula angustifolia)* is known as the universal oil because of its wide range of usage. It is antispasmodic, hypotensive, anti-inflammatory, anti-infectious, and anticoagulant. It relieves headaches and PMS symptoms.

Peppermint *(Mentha piperita)* is one of the oldest and most highly regarded herbs for soothing digestion. Jean Valnet, M.D., studied the beneficial effects of peppermint on the liver and respiratory systems. Daniel Penöél, M.D., reports that it may help to reduce fevers, candida, nausea, vomiting, and strengthen the respiratory system. Adding peppermint oil to drinking water helps cool body temperature during hot weather.

Carrier Oil: Sesame seed oil.

Safety Data: May be irritating to those with sensitive skin. Avoid eye contact. In case of accidental contact, put a few drops of any pure vegetable oil in the eye and call your doctor if necessary. Never use water. Avoid exposure to direct sunlight for 3 to 6 hours after use.

Application: This blend is effective for both men and women. Apply to Vita Flex points on ankles. Massage over lower pelvis, apply as a hot compress. Use directly on areas of concern. May be used diluted on prostate.

Companion Oils: Dragon Time, Clary Sage, and Sage.

Companion Supplements: FemiGen (capsule), Femalin (tincture), and Estro (tincture).

Frequency: Approximately 147 MHz.

Motivation

This blend has an electrical frequency which may enable one to overcome feelings of fear and procrastination and help stimulate feelings of moving forward and accomplishing new things.

Contains:

Roman Chamomile *(Chamaemelum nobile)* may calm and relieve restlessness, tension, insomnia, muscle tension, cuts, scrapes, bruises and is anti-infectious. It may relieve allergies and expel toxins from the liver. It is used extensively in Europe for the skin.

Spruce *(Picea mariana)* helps to open and release emotional blocks, bringing about a feeling of balance and grounding. Traditionally, spruce oil was believed to possess the frequency of prosperity. Spruce is anti-infectious, antiseptic, and anti-inflammatory.

Ylang Ylang *(Cananga odorata)* helps bring about a sense of relaxation and may help balance male and female energies. It balances equilibrium and restores confidence and self-love.

Lavender *(Lavandula angustifolia)* is known as the universal oil because of its wide range of usage. It has sedative and calming properties that help overcome insomnia, tension, and stress.

Safety Data: May be irritating to those with sensitive skin. Avoid eye contact. In case of accidental contact, put a few drops of any pure vegetable oil in the eye and call your doctor if necessary. Never use water. Avoid exposure to direct sunlight for 3 to 6 hours after use.

Application: Diffuse, apply on ears, feet (big toe), on chest or the nape of the neck, behind ears, wrists, around navel, or as needed. May be worn as a perfume or cologne.

Fragrant Influence: Creates a feeling of action and accomplishment.

Frequency: Approximately 103 MHz.

M-Grain

This blend contains oils that were traditionally used to relieve headaches, nausea, depression, and problems related to severe migraine headaches.

Contains:

Marjoram *(Origanum majorana)* is used for calming the respiratory system and soothing sore and aching muscles. Marjoram helps regenerate smooth muscle tissue, and also assists in relieving spasms and migraine headaches and calming the nerves. It is antimicrobial, anti-infectious, antibacterial, antiseptic, and may work as a diuretic.

Lavender *(Lavandula angustifolia)* is relaxing and calming, helping to overcome insomnia, nervous tension, headaches, and stress. It is antispasmodic, hypotensive, anti-inflammatory, anti-infectious, and anticoagulant. It relieves headaches and PMS symptoms.

Peppermint *(Mentha piperita)* is one of the oldest and most highly regarded herbs for soothing digestion. Jean Valnet, M.D., studied the beneficial effects of peppermint on the liver and respiratory systems. Other scientists have researched its effect on impaired taste and smell as well as improved concentration and mental accuracy. Alan Hirsch, M.D., studied its ability to directly affect the brain's satiety center, triggering a sensation of fullness after meals, which may help in weight loss by curbing the appetite. Daniel Penöél, M.D., reports that it may help to reduce fevers, candida, nausea, vomiting, and strengthen the respiratory system. Adding peppermint oil to drinking water helps cool body temperature during hot weather.

Basil *(Ocimum basilicum)* can be relaxing to smooth muscles as well as those involuntary muscles of the heart and digestive system. It may soothe insect bites such as, bees, wasps, and spiders, and may also help with snakebites. Basil has been found to alleviate mental fatigue, spasms, rhinitis, and help when there is a loss of smell due to nasal congestion.

Roman Chamomile *(Chamaemelum nobile)* may calm and relieve restlessness, tension, insomnia, muscle tension, cuts, scrapes, bruises, and is anti-infectious. It may relieve allergies and expel toxins from the liver. It is used extensively in Europe for the skin.

Helichrysum *(Helichrysum italicum)* has been researched in Europe for regenerating tissue and nerves and improving circulation. It is anticoagulant, prevents phlebitis, helps regulate cholesterol, stimulates liver cell function, and may help clean plaque and debris from the veins and arteries. It is mucolytic, expectorant, antispasmodic, and reduces scarring and discoloration. It may also stimulate nerve endings and improve conditions such as hearing loss. It may help release feelings of anger promoting forgiveness.

Safety Data: May be irritating to those with sensitive skin. Avoid eye contact. In case of accidental contact, put a few drops of any pure vegetable oil in the eye and call your doctor if necessary. Never use water. Avoid exposure to direct sunlight for 3 to 6 hours after use.

Application: It is most effective when inhaled. Place 2 drops in palm of hand and cup over nose and inhale. Massage along the brain stem. Apply on forehead, crown, shoulders, back of neck, temples, and Vita Flex points on the feet.

Companion Oils: Aroma Siez, Clarity, and PanAway.

Frequency: Approximately 72 MHz.

PanAway

This blend was created to help heal an injury where the ligaments in a leg were severely torn. It helps reduce inflammation, increasing circulation and healing thus reducing pain. Many people have had relief from arthritis symptoms, sports injuries, sprains, muscle spasms, bumps, and bruises.

Contains:

Helichrysum *(Helichrysum italicum)* has been researched in Europe for regenerating tissue and nerves and improving circulation. It is anticoagulant, prevents phlebitis, helps regulate cholesterol, stimulates liver cell function, and may help clean plaque and debris from the veins and arteries. Helichrysum is mucolytic, expectorant, antispasmodic, and reduces scarring and discoloration. It may also stimulate nerve endings and improve conditions such as hearing loss. It may help release feelings of anger promoting forgiveness.

Birch *(Betula alleghaniensis)* contains 99 percent methyl salicylate that has a cortisone-like activity. It is beneficial for bone, muscle, and joint discomfort. It has been helpful in decreasing pain from arthritis, tendonitis and rheumatism.

Clove *(Syzygium aromaticum)* was another oil from the Orient hailed as an oil of great abundance; those who possessed it were considered wealthy. This oil is one of the most antimicrobial and antiseptic of all essential oils. It is antifungal, antiviral, anti-infectious, and antibacterial. It works as a general stimulant and is used to treat sinusitis, bronchitis, cystitis, and cholera.

Peppermint *(Mentha piperita)* is one of the oldest and most highly regarded herbs for soothing digestion. Jean Valnet, M.D., studied the beneficial effects of peppermint on the liver and respiratory systems. Daniel Penoël, M.D., reports that it may help to reduce fevers, candida, nausea, vomiting, and strengthen the respiratory system. Adding peppermint oil to drinking water helps cool body temperature during hot weather.

Safety Data: May be irritating to those with sensitive skin. Avoid eye contact. In case of accidental contact, put a few drops of any pure vegetable oil in the eye and call your doctor if necessary. Never use water. Avoid exposure to direct sunlight for 3 to 6 hours after use.

Application: Apply to bottom of the feet first, working the Vita Flex points, and then topically on location. Rub on temples, back of neck, forehead or use as a compress on back. Apply on location for sore muscles, cramps, bruises, or wherever it may hurt.

Companion Oils: Relieve It (deep tissue pain), Melrose, add Helichrysum (to enhance), Birch (bone pain), or use with Ortho Ease or Ortho Sport Massage Oil.

Frequency: Approximately 112 MHz.

Live with Passion

One of the reasons people fail to be successful in business, work, or personal accomplishment, is due to a lack of passion. The oils in this blend stimulate a feeling of passion. It has often been said that the lack of passion is the creation of disease in the body. The feeling of passion overcomes depression, mood swings, and loss of drive. Live life with passion and make a difference in the world.

Contains:

Melissa *(Melissa officinalis)* is a powerful, antimicrobial oil, yet it is very gentle and delicate because of the nature of the plant, and helps to bring out those characteristics within the individual. It is calming and balancing to the emotions. Melissa is one of the oils highest in sesquiterpenes, much like cedarwood. It is very stimulating to the anterior pituitary and immune system.

Helichrysum (*Helichrysum italicum*) has been researched in Europe for regenerating tissue and nerves and improving circulation. It is anticoagulant, prevents phlebitis, helps regulate cholesterol, stimulates liver cell function, and may help to clean plaque and debris from the veins and arteries. Helichrysum is mucolytic, expectorant, antispasmodic, and reduces scarring and discoloration. It may also stimulate nerve endings and improve conditions such as hearing loss. It may help release feelings of anger, promoting forgiveness.

Clary Sage (*Salvia sclarea*) regulates the cells and balances the hormones. It contains natural sclareol, a phytoestrogen that mimics estrogen function. It may help with menstrual cramps, PMS, and pre-menopause symptoms and may help with circulatory problems.

Cedarwood (*Cedrus atlantica*) has calming and purifying properties. High in sesquiterpenes, which can stimulate the limbic part of the brain (the center of our emotions), this conifer oil has been used by North American Indians to enhance spiritual awareness and communication.

Angelica (*Angelica archangelica*) helps to bring memories back to the point of origin before trauma or anger was experienced, helping us to release negative feelings.

Ginger (*Zingiber officinale*) is used for relief from motion sickness, arthritis, rheumatism, sprains, muscular aches and pains, congestion, coughs, sinusitis, sore throats, diarrhea, colic, indigestion, loss of appetite, fever, flu, chills, and infectious disease.

Neroli (*Citrus aurantium*) was highly regarded by the Egyptian people for its great attributes of healing and calming the mind, body, and spirit. It is stabilizing and strengthening to the emotions, promoting peace, confidence, and awareness. It brings everything into focus at the moment.

Sandalwood (*Santalum album*) is high in sesquiterpenes, which have been researched for their ability to stimulate the pineal gland and the limbic region of the brain, the center of our emotions. Used traditionally for skin revitalization, yoga, and meditation, sandalwood is similar to frankincense oil in its support of nerves and circulation.

Patchouly (*Pogostemon cablin*) was used in India in ancient times as a trade commodity because of its earthy, musty fragrance and its ability to mask many different odors. Its fragrance reestablishes equilibrium while simultaneously quieting emotion and energizing the mind.

Jasmine (*Jasminum officinale*) exudes an exquisite fragrance that revitalizes spirits.

Safety Data: May be irritating to those with sensitive skin. Avoid eye contact. In case of accidental contact, put a few drops of any pure vegetable oil in the eye and call your doctor if necessary. Never use water. Avoid exposure to direct sunlight for 3 to 6 hours after use.

Application: Diffuse, use as a perfume or cologne, apply over heart, thymus, temples, and wrists. Add to bath water or put a few drops in Pharaoh or Rawhide Aftershave. Dilute with V-6 Mixing Oil or Massage Oil Base for a full-body massage. Put two drops on a wet cloth and put in the dryer for fragrancing.

Companion Oils: Acceptance, Motivation, Clarity, Gathering, Harmony, Inspiration, 3 Wise Men, Magnify Your Purpose.

Frequency: Approximately 89 MHz.

Peace & Calming

This gentle fragrance is specifically designed for diffusing. It promotes relaxation and a deep sense of peace, helping to dampen tensions and uplift spirits. When massaged on the bottom of the feet, it can be a wonderful prelude to a peaceful night's rest. It may calm overactive and hard-to-manage children. The oils in this blend have historically been used to help reduce depression, anxiety, stress, and insomnia. This blend along with Mineral Essence may be a healthy alternative to Ritalin.

Contains:

Blue Tansy (*Tanacetum annuum*) may help cleanse the liver and calm the lymphatic system, helping one to overcome anger and negative emotions promoting a feeling of self-control. It contains sesquiterpenes that can stimulate the pineal gland, which secretes the hormone melatonin, a hormone that enhances deep sleep.

Patchouly *(Pogostemon cablin)* was used in India in ancient times as a trade commodity because of its earthy, musty fragrance and its ability to mask many different odors. Its fragrance reestablishes equilibrium while simultaneously quieting emotion and energizing the mind.

Tangerine *(Citrus nobilis)* contains esters and aldehydes that are sedating and calming, helping with anxiety and nervousness.

Orange *(Citrus sinensis)* was believed to bring joy, peace, and happiness to those who possessed it. It is elevating to the mind and body.

Ylang Ylang *(Cananga odorata)* helps bring about a sense of relaxation and may help balance male and female energies. It balances equilibrium and inspires confidence and self-love.

Safety Data: May be irritating to those with sensitive skin. Avoid eye contact. In case of accidental contact, put a few drops of any pure vegetable oil in the eye and call your doctor if necessary. Never use water. Avoid exposure to direct sunlight for 3 to 6 hours after use.

Application: Diffuse, wear as a perfume, apply on bottom of the feet, on wrists, and outside of ears. Put in bath water. Dilute with V-6 Mixing Oil or Massage Oil Base for a full-body massage.

Companion Oils: Lavender (for insomnia) and chamomile (for calming).

Fragrant Influence: A feeling of calming and emotional well-being.

Frequency: Approximately 105 MHz.

Present Time

This blend has an empowering fragrance, which gives a feeling of being in the moment. Disease develops when we live in the past and with regret. One can only go forward and progress when in the present time.

Contains:

Neroli *(Citrus aurantium)* has been highly regarded for its ability to heal the mind, body,

and spirit. It is stabilizing and strengthening to the emotions, promoting peace, confidence, and awareness. It brings everything into focus at the moment.

Ylang Ylang *(Cananga odorata)* helps bring about a sense of relaxation and may help balance male and female energies. It balances equilibrium and restores confidence and self-love.

Spruce *(Picea mariana)* helps to open and release emotional blocks, bringing about a feeling of balance and grounding. Traditionally, spruce oil was believed to possess the frequency of prosperity.

Carrier Oil: Almond oil.

Safety Data: May be irritating to those with sensitive skin. Avoid eye contact. In case of accidental contact, put a few drops of any pure vegetable oil in the eye and call your doctor if necessary. Never use water. Avoid exposure to direct sunlight for 3 to 6 hours after use.

Application: Rub over the sternum and thymus area, neck and forehead. Add a few drops to Pharaoh and Rawhide as an aftershave.

Companion Oils: Harmony and Hope.

Frequency: Approximately 98 MHz.

Purification

This is an antiseptic blend formulated for diffusing to help purify the home and work environment. It cleanses the air and neutralizes mildew, cigarette smoke, and disagreeable odors. When applied directly to the skin, Purification may be used to cleanse cuts and scrapes and may help neutralize the poison of bites from spiders, bees, hornets, wasps, scorpions, and rattlesnakes.

Contains:

Citronella *(Cymbopogon nardus)* is antiseptic, antibacterial, antispasmodic, anti-inflammatory, insecticidal, antispasmodic, and soothing to the tissues.

Lemongrass *(Cymbopogon flexuosus)* has strong antifungal properties when applied topically.

Lavandin (*Lavandula* x *hybrida*) is antifungal, antibacterial, a strong antiseptic, and a tissue regenerator.

Rosemary (*Rosmarinus officinalis*) is antiseptic and antimicrobial and may be beneficial for skin conditions and dandruff. It may help fight candida and is anti-infectious and antispasmodic.

Melaleuca (*Melaleuca alternifolia*) is antiseptic, anti-infectious, antibacterial, antifungal, antiviral, antiparasitic, antiseptic, anti-inflammatory, immune-stimulating, decongestant, neurotonic, and protects against radiation.

Myrtle (*Myrtus communis*) is antibacterial and may support immune function in fighting cold, flu, and infectious disease.

Safety Data: May be irritating to those with sensitive skin. Avoid eye contact. In case of accidental contact, put a few drops of any pure vegetable oil in the eye and call your doctor if necessary. Never use water. Avoid exposure to direct sunlight for 3 to 6 hours after use.

Application: Diffuse 15 to 30 minutes every 3 to 4 hours. Apply topically to disinfect and cleanse. Put on cotton balls to place in air vents in the home, car, hotel room, office, enclosed areas, etc. Put on cotton balls in air vents for purifying and repelling insects at home or at work.

Companion Products: Melrose, Citrus Fresh, and Thieves.

Frequency: Approximately 46 MHz.

Raven

This combination gives strength in fighting respiratory disease and infections; and may help alleviate symptoms of tuberculosis, asthma, and pneumonia.

Contains:

Ravensara (*Ravensara aromatica*) is referred to by the people of Madagascar as the oil that heals. It is antiseptic, anti-infectious, antiviral, antibacterial, antifungal, expectorant, and supporting to the nerves. Similar to clove and nutmeg, ravensara may aid the respiratory system. It has been shown to help with flu, sinusitis, bronchitis, herpes, infectious mononucleosis, and rhinopharyngitis.

Eucalyptus (*Eucalyptus radiata*) may have a profound antiviral effect upon the respiratory system. It may also help reduce inflammation of the nasal mucous membrane.

Peppermint (*Mentha piperita*) is useful for many kinds of respiratory conditions, including bronchitis and pneumonia. High in menthol and menthone, it helps suppress coughs and clears lung and nasal congestion.

Birch (*Betula alleghaniensis*) contains 99 percent methyl salicylate that has a cortisone-like activity.

Lemon (*Citrus limon*) has antiseptic-like properties and contains compounds that have been studied for their effects on immune function. It increases microcirculation.

Safety Data: May be irritating to those with sensitive skin. Avoid eye contact. In case of accidental contact, put a few drops of any pure vegetable oil in the eye and call your doctor if necessary. Never use water. Avoid exposure to direct sunlight for 3 to 6 hours after use.

Application: Diffuse, massage on Vita Flex points on the feet. Apply topically over throat and lung area. Put on pillow at night. Use in a suppository with V-6 Mixing Oil and retain during the night. With this method, the benefits go directly to the lungs in seconds.

Companion Oils: R.C., Thieves, and Melrose.

Frequency: Approximately 70 MHz.

R.C.

This blend was formulated to help give relief from colds, bronchitis, sore throats, sinusitis, and respiratory congestion. Diffusing may help decongest and relieve allergy symptoms, such as coughs and sore throats. R.C. has also been reported to help dissolve bone spurs when applied topically.

Contains:

Eucalyptus (*Eucalyptus globulus*) has shown to be a powerful antimicrobial agent containing a high percentage of eucalyptol (a key ingredient in many antiseptic mouth rinses.) It is expectorant, mucolytic, antimicrobial, antibacterial, antifungal, antiviral, and antiseptic. It helps reduce infections in the throat and lungs, such as rhinopharyngitis, laryngitis, flu, sinusitis, bronchitis, bronchial asthma, and bronchial pneumonia.

Eucalyptus *(Eucalyptus radiata)* is anti-infectious, antibacterial, antiviral, expectorant, and anti-inflammatory. It has strong action against bronchitis and sinusitis.

Eucalyptus *(Eucalyptus australiana)* is antiviral, antibacterial, and antifungal.

Eucalyptus *(Eucalyptus citriodora)* helps decongest and disinfect the sinuses and lungs. It is anti-inflammatory, anti-infectious, and mildly antispasmodic.

Myrtle *(Myrtus communis)* supports the respiratory system and help treat chronic coughs and tuberculosis. It is suitable to use for coughs and chest complaints with children.

Pine *(Pinus sylvestris)* opens and disinfects the respiratory system, particularly the bronchial tract. It has been used since the time of Hippocrates to support respiratory function and fight infection. According to Daniel Penöel, M.D., pine is one of the best oils for bronchitis and pneumonia.

Spruce *(Picea mariana)* helps the respiratory and nervous systems. It is anti-infectious, antiseptic, and anti-inflammatory.

Marjoram *(Origanum majorana)* supports the respiratory system and reduces spasms. It is antimicrobial, anti-infectious, antibacterial, antiseptic, and may work as a diuretic.

Lavender *(Lavandula angustifolia)* is antispasmodic, hypotensive, anti-inflammatory, and anti-infectious. It prevents scarring, stretch marks, and relieves headaches and PMS symptoms.

Cypress *(Cupressus sempervirens)* promotes blood circulation and lymph flow. It is anti-infectious, antibacterial, antimicrobial, mucolytic, antiseptic, refreshing, and relaxing.

Peppermint *(Mentha piperita)* is one of the oldest and most highly regarded herbs for soothing digestion. Jean Valnet, M.D., studied the beneficial effects of peppermint on the liver and respiratory systems. Other scientists have researched its effect on impaired taste and smell as well as improved concentration and mental

accuracy. Daniel Penöel, M.D., reports that it may help to reduce fevers, candida, nausea, vomiting, and strengthen the respiratory system. Adding peppermint oil to drinking water helps cool body temperature during hot weather.

Safety Data: May be irritating to those with sensitive skin. Avoid eye contact. In case of accidental contact, put a few drops of any pure vegetable oil in the eye and call your doctor if necessary. Never use water. Avoid exposure to direct sunlight for 3 to 6 hours after use.

Application: Diffuse, apply on chest, neck, ears, bottom of feet, or use in a humidifier. Dilute with V-6 Mixing Oil or Massage Oil Base and massage on chest and back and Vita Flex points on the body. Use as a hot compress. Put on sinuses or up nasal passages with a cotton swab. Rub around ears and on feet, neck, and throat. May help with headache if deeply inhaled. Run hot, steaming water in sink, put Raven, R.C., or birch in water, put towel over head, and inhale to open sinuses. May help relieve difficulties breathing related to flu, colds, and pneumonia.

Companion Oils: Raven (alternating morning and night) and Thieves.

Fragrant Influence: Diffusing R.C. helps to decongest and relieve allergy symptoms such as coughs, sore throat, and lung congestion.

Frequency: Approximately 75 MHz

Release

This oil blend may stimulate a sense of harmony and balance within the mind and body, and help release anger and memory trauma from the cells of the liver bringing about a sense of peace and emotional well-being. Letting go of negative emotions and releasing frustration enables one to progress in a positive way.

Contains:

Ylang Ylang *(Cananga odorata)* helps bring about a sense of relaxation and may help balance male and female energies. It balances equilibrium and restores confidence and self-love.

Lavandin (*Lavandula* x *hybrida*) is antifungal, antibacterial, a strong antiseptic, and a tissue regenerator.

Geranium *(Pelargonium graveolens)* stimulates nerves and assists in balancing hormones. Its aromatic influence helps release negative memories, thereby opening and elevating the mind.

Sandalwood *(Santalum album)* is high in sesquiterpenes, which have been researched for their ability to stimulate the pineal gland and the limbic region of the brain, the center of our emotions. The pineal gland is responsible for releasing melatonin, a hormone that enhances deep sleep. Used traditionally for skin revitalization, yoga, and meditation, sandalwood is similar to frankincense oil in its support of nerves and circulation.

Blue Tansy *(Tanacetum annuum)* may help cleanse the liver and calm the lymphatic system helping one to overcome anger and negative emotions promoting a feeling of self-control. Its primary constituents are limonene and sesquiterpenes. European research shows that it works as an antihistamine, anti-inflammatory, and stimulant for the thymus gland reducing dermatitis, arthritis, sciatica, tuberculosis, and allergies.

Carrier Oil: Olive oil.

Safety Data: May be irritating to those with sensitive skin. Avoid eye contact. In case of accidental contact, put any vegetable oil or cream in the eye and call your doctor if necessary. Never use water. Avoid exposure to direct sunlight for 3 to 6 hours after use.

Application: Apply over liver or as a compress. Massage on bottom of feet and put behind ears. May be worn as a perfume or cologne.

Companion Oils: Valor, Harmony, and JuvaFlex on the feet.

Fragrant Influence: A feeling of being free and unburdened.

Frequency: Approximately 102 MHz.

Relieve It

This blend contains high anti-inflammatory compounds to relieve deep tissue pain. It is calming to the nerves and alleviates skin and muscle soreness.

Contains:

Spruce *(Picea mariana)* helps the respiratory and nervous systems. High in terpenes, it is anti-infectious, antiseptic, and anti-inflammatory.

Pepper, Black *(Piper nigrum)* stimulates the endocrine system and increases energy while increasing cellular oxygenation. It is anti-inflammatory which may soothe deep tissue muscle aches. It has been traditionally used to treat rheumatoid arthritis.

Peppermint *(Mentha piperita)* is one of the oldest and most highly regarded herbs for soothing digestion. Jean Valnet, M.D., studied the beneficial effects of peppermint on the liver and respiratory systems. Daniel Penöel, M.D., reports that it may help to reduce fevers, candida, nausea, vomiting, and strengthen the respiratory system. Adding peppermint to drinking water helps cool body temperature during hot weather.

Hyssop *(Hyssopus officinalis)* is anti-inflammatory and anti-infectious.

Safety Data: May be irritating to those with sensitive skin. Avoid eye contact. In case of accidental contact, put a few drops of any pure vegetable oil in the eye and call your doctor if necessary. Never use water. Avoid exposure to direct sunlight for 3 to 6 hours after use.

Application: Apply on location, wherever there is pain.

Companion Oils: PanAway, Melrose, Aroma Siez, Cypress, and Helichrysum.

Frequency: Approximately 56 MHz.

Sacred Mountain

This is a blend of oils extracted from the conifer trees representing the sacred feeling of the mountains. They bring about a feeling of protection, strength, grounding, empowerment, and security. Sacred Mountain is antibacterial and soothing to the respiratory system.

Contains:

Spruce (*Picea mariana*) helps to open and release emotional blocks, bringing about a feeling of balance and grounding. Traditionally, spruce oil was believed to possess the frequency of prosperity. Spruce is anti-infectious, antiseptic, and anti-inflammatory.

Fir (*Abies alba*) has been researched for its ability to kill airborne germs and bacteria. As a conifer oil, it creates a feeling of grounding, anchoring, and empowerment.

Cedarwood (*Cedrus atlantica*) has calming and purifying properties. High in sesquiterpenes which can stimulate the limbic part of the brain (the center of our emotions), this conifer oil has been used by North American Indians to enhance spiritual awareness and communication. It also may help stimulate the pineal gland, which releases melatonin, a hormone that enhances deep sleep.

Ylang Ylang (*Cananga odorata*) helps bring about a sense of relaxation and may help balance male and female energies. It balances equilibrium and restores confidence and self-love.

Safety Data: May be irritating to those with sensitive skin. Avoid eye contact. In case of accidental contact, put a few drops of any pure vegetable oil in the eye and call your doctor if necessary. Never use water. Avoid exposure to direct sunlight for 3 to 6 hours after use.

Application: Diffuse, put on crown of head, back of neck, behind ears, on thymus and wrists. Wear as a perfume or cologne.

Fragrant Influence: A feeling of strength, empowerment, grounding, and protection.

Frequency: Approximately 176 MHz.

SARA

The blend produces a beautiful fragrance that may enable one to relax into a mental state whereby one may be able to release the trauma of Sexual And/or Ritual Abuse. SARA also helps unlock other traumatic experiences such as physical and emotional abuse.

Contains:

Geranium (*Pelargonium graveolens*) helps release negative memories, thereby opening and elevating the mind.

Lavender (*Lavandula angustifolia*) has sedative and calming properties that help overcome headaches, stress, and nervous tension.

Rose (*Rosa damascena*) possesses the highest frequency of the oils. It creates a sense of balance, harmony, and well-being and elevates the mind.

Blue Tansy (*Tanacetum annuum*) may help cleanse the liver and calm the lymphatic system helping one to overcome anger and negative emotions promoting a feeling of self-control. Its primary constituents are limonene and sesquiterpenes.

Orange (*Citrus sinensis*) was believed to bring joy, peace, and happiness to those who possessed it. It is elevating to the mind and body and brings joy and peace.

Cedarwood (*Cedrus atlantica*) has calming and purifying properties. This conifer oil was used by North American Indians to enhance their spiritual awareness and communication. It may help stimulate the pineal gland which is responsible for releasing melatonin, a hormone associated with deep sleep.

Ylang Ylang (*Cananga odorata*) helps bring about a sense of relaxation and may help balance male and female energies. It balances equilibrium and restores confidence and self-love.

Carrier Oil: Almond oil.

Safety Data: May be irritating to those with sensitive skin. Avoid eye contact. In case of accidental contact, put a few drops of any pure vegetable oil in the eye and call your doctor if necessary. Never use water. Avoid exposure to direct sunlight for 3 to 6 hours after use.

Application: Apply over energy centers and areas of abuse, on Vita Flex points, navel, lower abdomen, temples, and nose.

Companion Oils: Hope, Forgiveness, Valor, Inner Child, Trauma Life, White Angelica, Joy, Inspiration, Magnify Your Purpose, and 3 Wise Men.

Fragrant Influence: Peace to the soul and freedom to go forward in life with joy.

Frequency: Approximately 102 MHz.

Sensation

This blend has a beautiful and romantic fragrance that is extremely uplifting, refreshing, and arousing. Sensation is also very nourishing and hydrating for the skin and is beneficial for various skin problems.

Contains:

Ylang Ylang *(Cananga odorata)* helps bring about a sense of relaxation and may help balance male and female energies. It balances equilibrium and restores confidence and self-love.

Rosewood *(Aniba rosaeodora)* is soothing and nourishing to the skin. It has been researched at Weber State University for its inhibition rate against gram positive and gram negative bacterial growth. This oil is soothing, creates elasticity, and helps the skin rid itself of irritations and problems, such as candida. Rosewood is anti-infectious, antibacterial, antifungal, antiviral, and antiparasitic.

Jasmine *(Jasminum officinale)* is beneficial for dry, oily, irritated, or sensitive skin. It is used for muscle spasms, sprains, coughs, laryngitis, frigidity, depression, and nervous exhaustion.

Safety Data: May be irritating to those with sensitive skin. Avoid eye contact. In case of accidental contact, put a few drops of any pure vegetable oil in the eye and call your doctor if necessary. Never use water. Avoid exposure to direct sunlight for 3 to 6 hours after use.

Application: Apply on location, use for massage, and add to Sensation Bath and Shower Gel. May also be used with a compress over the abdomen, or worn as a perfume or cologne.

Companion Oils: Passion, Into the Future, Joy, Dream Catcher, and Awaken.

Fragrant Influence: Excitement of experiencing new heights of self-expression and awareness.

Frequency: Approximately 88 MHz.

Surrender

This blend is a combination of oils that may help one surrender aggression and a controlling attitude. Stress and tension are released very quickly when we surrender our own will.

Contains:

Lavender *(Lavandula angustifolia)* has sedative and calming properties to help overcome insomnia, headaches, stress, and nervous tension.

Roman Chamomile *(Chamaemelum nobile)* may calm and relieve restlessness, tension, insomnia, muscle tension, cuts, scrapes, bruises and is anti-infectious. It may relieve allergies and expel toxins from the liver. It is used extensively in Europe for the skin.

German Chamomile *(Matricaria recutita)* has been a highly respected oil for over 3,000 years and has been used for helping skin conditions, such as dermatitis, boils, acne, rashes, and eczema. It is also used for hair care, burns, cuts, toothaches, teething pains, inflamed joints, menopausal problems, insomnia, migraine headaches, and stress-related complaints. German chamomile has an electrical frequency that promotes peace and harmony bringing about a feeling of security.

Angelica *(Angelica archangelica)* helps to calm emotions and brings memories back to the point of origin before trauma or anger was experienced, helping us to let go of negative feelings.

Mountain Savory *(Satureja montana)* is antimicrobial and immune stimulating. It is antiviral, antibacterial, antifungal, antiparasitic, and a general tonic for the body.

Lemon (*Citrus limon*) has antiseptic-like properties and contains compounds that have been studied for their effects on immune function. It increases microcirculation, which may improve vision. Lemon may serve as an insect repellent and may be beneficial for the skin. It has been found to promote leukocyte formation, dissolve cellulite, increase lymphatic function, and promote a sense of well-being. Its fragrance is stimulating and invigorating.

Spruce (*Picea mariana*) helps to open and release emotional blocks, bringing about a feeling of balance and grounding. Traditionally, spruce oil was believed to possess the frequency of prosperity. Spruce is anti-infectious, antiseptic, and anti-inflammatory.

Safety Data: May be irritating to those with sensitive skin. Avoid eye contact. In case of accidental contact, put a few drops of any pure vegetable oil in the eye and call your doctor if necessary. Never use water. Avoid exposure to direct sunlight for 3 to 6 hours after use.

Application: Diffuse. Apply on forehead, solar plexus, along the ear rim, on the chest and nape of the neck. Add 2 to 4 drops to warm bath water with or without Bath Gel Base.

Companion Oils: Peace & Calming, Forgiveness, Grounding, Sacred Mountain, and Clarity.

Fragrant Influence: Let go of the need to control. Allow the need to be alone.

Frequency: Approximately 98 MHz.

Thieves

This blend was created from research about a group of 15th-century thieves who rubbed oils on themselves to avoid contracting the plague while they robbed the bodies of the dead and dying. When apprehended, these thieves disclosed the formula of herbs, spices, and oils they used to protect themselves in exchange for more lenient punishment.

This blend of therapeutic-grade essential oils was tested at Weber State University for its potent antimicrobial properties. Thieves was found to have a 99.96 percent kill rate against airborne bacteria. The oils are highly antiviral, antiseptic, antibacterial, anti-infectious and help to protect the body against such illnesses as flu, colds, sinusitis, bronchitis, pneumonia, sore throats, cuts, etc.

Contains:

Clove (*Syzygium aromaticum*) was another oil from the Orient hailed as an oil of great abundance; those who possessed it were considered wealthy. This oil is one of the most antimicrobial and antiseptic of all essential oils. Clove is antifungal, antiviral, anti-infectious, and antibacterial. It works as a general stimulant and is used to treat sinusitis, bronchitis, cystitis, and cholera.

Lemon (*Citrus limon*) has antiseptic-like properties and contains compounds that have been studied for their effects on immune function. It increases microcirculation, which may improve vision. It may serve as an insect repellent and may be beneficial for the skin. Lemon has been found to promote leukocyte formation, dissolve cellulite, increase lymphatic function, and promote a sense of well-being. Its fragrance is stimulating and invigorating.

Cinnamon Bark (*Cinnamomum verum*) is the oil of wealth from the Orient and part of the formula the Lord gave Moses (Exodus 30:22-27). Cinnamon oil is anti-infectious, antibacterial, antiparasitic, antiviral, and antifungal. Cinnamon oil was regarded by the emperors of China and India to have great value; their wealth was measured by the amount of oil they possessed. Traditionally, it was thought to have a frequency that attracted wealth and abundance. Physically, cinnamon bark oil has many attributes; it is a powerful purifier,' it is a powerful oxygenator, and it enhances the action and the activity of other oils. Researchers, including J. C. Lapraz, M.D., found that viruses could not live in the presence of cinnamon oil.

Eucalyptus (*Eucalyptus radiata*) is anti-infectious, antibacterial, antiviral, expectorant, and anti-inflammatory. It has strong action against conjunctivitis, vaginitis, endometriosis, acne, bronchitis, and sinusitis.

Rosemary (*Rosmarinus officinalis*) is antiseptic and antimicrobial and may be beneficial for skin conditions and dandruff. It may help fight candida and is anti-infectious, antispasmodic, balances the endocrine system, and is an expectorant. It helps overcome mental fatigue, stimulating memory and opening the conscious mind.

Safety Data: May be irritating to those with sensitive skin. Avoid eye contact. In case of accidental contact, put a few drops of any pure vegetable oil in the eye and call your doctor if necessary. Never use water. Avoid exposure to direct sunlight for 3 to 6 hours after use.

Application: Diffuse for 15 to 30 minutes every 3 to 4 hours in work or home environment. Apply to bottom of feet, or rub over feet, throat, stomach, and abdomen. Dilute one drop of Thieves in 15 drops of V-6 Mixing Oil or Massage Oil Base and massage over thymus. It is best applied to the bottom of the feet as it may be caustic to the skin. It is best to dilute with V-6 Mixing Oil. For headaches put one drop on tongue and push tongue against the roof of the mouth.

Companion Oils: Immupower and Exodus II (to be alternated).

Frequency: Approximately 150 MHz.

Note: Studies conducted at Weber State University (Ogden, UT) during 1997 showed the antibacterial effectiveness of the Thieves blend against airborne microorganisms. One analysis showed a 90 percent reduction in the number of gram positive *Micrococcus luteus* organisms after diffusing Thieves for 12 minutes. After diffusing Thieves for a total of 20 minutes, there was a 99.3 percent reduction. Another study against the gram negative *Pseudomonas aeruginosa* showed a kill rate of 99.96 percent after just 12 minutes of diffusion.

3 Wise Men

This blend was formulated to open the subconscious mind through pineal stimulation to help release deep-seated trauma. The oils bring a sense of grounding and uplifting through emotional releasing and elevated spiritual consciousness.

Contains:

Sandalwood (*Santalum album*) is high in sesquiterpenes, which have been researched for their ability to stimulate the pineal gland and the limbic region of the brain, the center of our emotions. The pineal gland is responsible for releasing melatonin, a hormone that enhances deep sleep. Used traditionally for skin revitalization, yoga, and meditation, sandalwood is similar to frankincense oil in its support of nerves and circulation.

Juniper (*Juniperus osteosperma* and/or *J. scopulorum*) may work as a detoxifier and cleanser, and promotes improved nerve and kidney function. It is also beneficial for the skin reducing dermatitis, eczema, and acne. It elevates spiritual awareness creating feelings of love and peace.

Frankincense (*Boswellia carteri*) is considered a holy anointing oil in the Middle East and has been used in religious ceremonies for thousands of years. High in sesquiterpenes, it helps stimulate the limbic part of the brain, which elevates the mind, helping to overcome stress and despair. It is used in European medicine to combat depression.

Myrrh (*Commiphora myrrha*) is referenced throughout the Bible, constituting a part of a holy anointing formula given to Moses (Exodus 30:22-27). It has one of the highest levels of sesquiterpenes, a class of compounds that can stimulate the hypothalamus, pituitary, and amygdala, the control center for emotions and hormone release in the brain. Myrrh has been used in eastern countries to enhance the feeling of spirituality or euphoria.

Spruce (*Picea mariana*) helps to open and release emotional blocks, bringing about a feeling of balance and grounding. Traditionally, this conifer oil was believed to possess the frequency of prosperity. Spruce is anti-infectious, antiseptic, and anti-inflammatory.

Carrier Oil: Almond oil.

Safety Data: May be irritating to those with sensitive skin. Avoid eye contact. In case of accidental contact, put a few drops of any pure vegetable oil in the eye and call your doctor if necessary. Never use water. Avoid exposure to direct sunlight for 3 to 6 hours after use.

Application: Apply 2 drops on the crown of the head, behind the ears, over the eyebrows, on the chest, over the thymus, and at the back of the neck. It may also be diffused.

Companion Oils: Frankincense, Myrrh, Sandalwood, Juniper, and Spruce.

Fragrant Influence: A feeling of reverence and spiritual awareness.

Frequency: Approximately 72 MHz.

Trauma Life

This blend was created at the request of Steven Seagal, renowned actor, director, and producer, for his volunteer work in hospital trauma centers. Trauma Life may help release buried emotional trauma as well as upsets, such as accidents, the death of a loved one, assault, abuse, etc. This blend of calming, grounding essential oils can help purge stress and uproot traumas that cause fatigue, anger, restlessness, and a weakened immune response. Seven Seagal is extremely pleased with the results that he has seen with this blend, using it even to help bring victims out of a coma.

Contains:

Valerian *(Valeriana officinalis)* has been used for calming, relaxing, grounding, and emotionally balancing influences. It has been clinically researched for its tranquilizing properties. German health authorities have pronounced valerian to be an effective treatment for restlessness and for sleep disturbances resulting from nervous conditions. It may help minimize shock, anxiety, and stress that accompanies traumatic situations.

Lavender *(Lavandula angustifolia)* has sedative and calming properties that can help overcome insomnia, headaches, stress, and nervous tension.

Frankincense *(Boswellia carteri)* elevates the mind and helps overcome stress and despair. It is high in sesquiterpenes, which stimulate the limbic region of the brain, the center of emotions. In ancient times, frankincense was known for its anointing and healing powers, and was used to treat every conceivable ill known to man.

Sandalwood *(Santalum album)* is high in sesquiterpenes, which have been researched for their ability to stimulate the pineal gland and the limbic region of the brain, the center of our emotions. The pineal gland is responsible for releasing melatonin, a hormone that enhances deep sleep. Used traditionally for skin revitaliza-tion, yoga, and meditation, sandalwood is similar to frankincense oil in its support of nerves and circulation.

Rose *(Rosa damascena)* possesses the highest frequency of the oils. It creates a sense of balance, harmony, and well-being and elevates the mind. Rose creates a magnetic energy that attracts love and brings joy to the heart.

Helichrysum *(Helichrysum italicum)* has been researched in Europe for regenerating tissue and nerves and improving circulation. It is anti-coagulant, prevents phlebitis, helps regulate cholesterol, stimulates liver cell function, and may help to clean plaque and debris from the veins and arteries. Helichrysum is mucolytic, expectorant, antispasmodic, and reduces scarring and discoloration. It may also stimulate nerve endings and improve conditions such as hearing loss. It may help release feelings of anger promoting forgiveness.

Spruce *(Picea mariana)* helps to open and release emotional blocks, bringing about a feeling of balance and grounding. Traditionally, spruce oil was believed to possess the frequency of prosperity. Spruce is anti-infectious, antiseptic, and anti-inflammatory.

Geranium *(Pelargonium graveolens)* stimulates nerves and assists in balancing hormones. Its aromatic influence helps release negative memories, thereby opening and elevating the mind.

Davana *(Artemisia pallens)* is high in sesquiterpenes which are supporting to the immune system. It is mucolytic, antispasmodic, works to reduce painful scarring, and helps overcome anxiety.

Citrus hystrix is anti-infectious, antiseptic, neurotonic, and a liver decongestant. With its hormone-like properties, it helps underactive sexual glands. The constituents of aldehydes, esters, and coumarins make it calming and sedating.

Safety Data: May be irritating to those with sensitive skin. Avoid eye contact. In case of accidental contact, put a few drops of any pure vegetable oil in the eye and call your doctor if necessary. Never use water. Avoid exposure to direct sunlight for 3 to 6 hours after use.

Application: Diffuse, apply a few drops to the bottom of the feet, on the chest, behind the ears, on the forehead, and at the back of the neck. May also be applied along the spine using Raindrop Technique.

Companion Oils: Peace and Calming, Joy, Hope, and Into the Future.

Fragrant Influence: Promotes a feeling of calmness and a sense of awareness.

Frequency: Approximately 92 MHz.

Valor

Valor helps balance electrical energies within the body, giving courage, confidence, and self-esteem. It has been found to help the body self-correct its balance and alignment giving relief of pain. The oils in this blend empower the physical and spiritual bodies to overcome fear and opposition when facing adversity. It helps build courage, confidence, and self-esteem. Valor has been touted as a chiropractor in a bottle. It has improved scoliosis for some in as little as 30 minutes, while other individuals require several applications. Valor has also been shown to change anaerobic-mutated cells back to their aerobic natural state.

Contains:

Rosewood *(Aniba rosaeodora)* is soothing and nourishing to the skin. It has been researched at Weber State University for its inhibition rate against gram positive and gram negative bacterial growth. This oil is soothing, creates elasticity, and helps the skin rid itself of irritations and problems, such as candida. It is anti-infectious, antibacterial, antifungal, antiviral, and antiparasitic.

Blue Tansy *(Tanacetum annuum)* may help cleanse the liver and calm the lymphatic system helping one to overcome anger and negative emotions promoting a feeling of self-control. Its primary constituents are limonene and sesquiterpenes. European research shows that it works as an antihistamine, anti-inflammatory, and stimulant for the thymus gland reducing dermatitis, arthritis, sciatica, tuberculosis, and allergies.

Frankincense *(Boswellia carteri)* is considered a holy anointing oil in the Middle East and has been used in religious ceremonies for thousands of years. High in sesquiterpenes, it helps stimulate the limbic part of the brain, which elevates the mind, helping to overcome stress and despair. It is used in European medicine to combat depression.

Spruce *(Picea mariana)* helps to open and release emotional blocks, bringing about a feeling of balance and grounding. Traditionally, spruce oil was believed to possess the frequency of prosperity. Spruce is anti-infectious, antiseptic, and anti-inflammatory.

Carrier Oil: Almond oil.

Safety Data: May be irritating to those with sensitive skin. Avoid eye contact. In case of accidental contact, put a few drops of any pure vegetable oil in the eye and call your doctor if necessary. Never use water. Avoid exposure to direct sunlight for 3 to 6 hours after use.

Application: Apply 4 to 6 drops on bottom of feet. Put on wrists, chest, and at the back of the neck, or along the spine in a Raindrop application. When using a series of oils, as in the Raindrop application, apply Valor first and let it work for 5 to 10 minutes before applying other oils. This blend may be worn as a perfume or cologne. (For more detailed instruction, see Raindrop Technique.)

Fragrant Influence: Gives a feeling of strength, courage, and protection.

Frequency: Approximately 47 MHz. (Low to work with the physical body.)

White Angelica

This blend is a combination of 10 essential oils, some of which were used during ancient times to increase the aura around the body. It brings a delicate sense of strength and protection, creating a feeling of wholeness in the realm of one's own spirituality. Its frequency neutralizes negative energy. It is calming and soothing and brings a feeling of protection and security.

Contains:

Ylang Ylang (*Cananga odorata*) helps bring about a sense of relaxation and may help balance male and female energies. It balances equilibrium and restores confidence and self-love.

Rose (*Rosa damascena*) possesses the highest frequency of the oils. It creates a sense of balance, harmony, and well-being and elevates the mind. Rose promotes healthy skin, reduces scarring, and may help with sexual disabilities, frigidity, impotency, skin diseases, and wrinkles. It creates a magnetic energy that attracts love and brings joy to the heart.

Melissa (*Melissa officinalis*) is a powerful, antimicrobial oil, yet it is very gentle and delicate because of the nature of the plant, and helps to bring out those characteristics within the individual. It is calming and balancing to the emotions. Melissa is one of the highest in sesquiterpenes, much like cedarwood. It is very stimulating to the anterior pituitary and immune system.

Sandalwood (*Santalum album*) is high in sesquiterpenes, which have been researched for their ability to stimulate the pineal gland and the limbic region of the brain, the center of our emotions. The pineal gland is responsible for releasing melatonin, a hormone that enhances deep sleep. Used traditionally for skin revitalization, yoga, and meditation, sandalwood is similar to frankincense oil in its support of nerves and circulation.

Geranium (*Pelargonium graveolens*) stimulates nerves and assists in balancing hormones. Its aromatic influence helps release negative memories, thereby opening and elevating the mind.

Spruce (*Picea mariana*) helps to open and release emotional blocks, bringing about a feeling of balance and grounding. Traditionally, spruce oil was believed to possess the frequency of prosperity. Spruce is anti-infectious, antiseptic, and anti-inflammatory.

Myrrh (*Commiphora myrrha*) is referenced throughout the Old and New Testaments, constituting a part of a holy anointing formula given to Moses (Exodus 30:22-27). It has one of the highest levels of sesquiterpenes, a class of compounds that can stimulate the hypothalamus, pituitary, and amygdala, the control center for emotions and hormone in the brain. Myrrh has been used in eastern countries to enhance the feeling of spirituality or euphoria.

Hyssop (*Hyssopus officinalis*) is strongly balancing for emotions.

Bergamot (*Citrus bergamia*) is one of the most uplifting fragrances, simultaneously energizing and calming, with a unique ability to relieve anxiety, stress, and tension.

Rosewood (*Aniba rosaeodora*) is soothing and nourishing to the skin. It has been researched at Weber State University for its inhibition rate against gram positive and gram negative bacterial growth. This oil is soothing, creates elasticity, and helps the skin rid itself of irritations and problems, such as candida. It is anti-infectious, antibacterial, antifungal, antiviral, and antiparasitic.

Carrier Oil: Almond oil.

Safety Data: May be irritating to those with sensitive skin. Avoid eye contact. In case of accidental contact, put a few drops of any pure vegetable oil in the eye and call your doctor if necessary. Never use water. Avoid exposure to direct sunlight for 3 to 6 hours after use.

Application: Diffuse, apply on shoulders, along spine, on crown of head, on wrists, behind ears, back of neck, and may be added to bath water. Wear as perfume or cologne.

Companion Oils: Valor, Inspiration, Awaken, Sacred Mountain, Joy, and Aroma Life.

Fragrant Influence: A feeling of protection and security.

Frequency: Approximately 89 MHz.

CHAPTER 9

Dietary Supplements with Essential Oils

These supplements contain both herbs and therapeutic-grade essential oils. The essential oils act as catalysts to help deliver nutrients through the cell membranes while assisting in the removal of cellular wastes.

It is important to remember that these supplements are usually dissolved and assimilated by the body within a couple of hours. Therefore, spacing them throughout the day will provide better assimilation and nutrient value than consuming a handful all at once.

When using supplements, a general guideline is to discontinue use for at least one or two days a week to allow the body to regain homeostasis and permit its natural recuperative powers to engage.

An approximate frequency is indicated for some of the supplements. Please keep in mind that these are only estimates; and that due to the many variables involved in determining frequency, the results may be difficult to duplicate.

A.D.&E.

Contents:

Beta Carotene (Vitamin A) is converted by the body to Vitamin A.

Vitamin A (Palmitate) is a fat-soluble vitamin that helps support the function of the eyes, liver, immune system, and acts as a superb antioxidant and needed for proper growth and development.

Vitamin D3 (Cholecalciferol) stimulates the absorption of calcium, thereby helping to prevent osteoporosis, estrogen and magnesium deficiency, and cancer.

Vitamin E (d-Alpha Tocopheryl Acetate) provides many health benefits including helping to prevent acne, AIDS, cancer, diabetes, cataracts, Lupus, macular degeneration, myopathy, and works as a wonderful antioxidant.

In a base of grapeseed oil, and several tocopherols.

AlkaLime

This specially-designed alkaline mineral powder contains an array of high-alkaline salts and other yeast/fungus-fighting elements, such as citric acid and essential oils. Its precisely-balanced, acid-neutralizing mineral formulation helps preserve the body's proper pH balance—the cornerstone of health. By boosting blood alkalinity, yeast and fungus are deprived of the acidic terrain they require to flourish. The effectiveness of other essential oils is enhanced when the body's blood and tissues are alkaline.

AlkaLime may help reduce the following signs of acid-based yeast and fungus dominance: fatigue/low energy, unexplained aches and pains, overweight conditions, low resistance to illness, allergies, headaches, irritability/mood swings, indigestion, colitis/ulcers, diarrhea/constipation, urinary tract infections, and rectal/ vaginal itch.

Contents:

Calcium carbonate provides calcium, which is needed for healthy bones.

Citric acid is added to help cleanse the digestive system.

Magnesium supports healthy intestinal flora, the first-line defense against fungus overgrowth.

Potassium bicarbonate added for electrolyte balance.

Sea salts added to provide trace minerals and regulate pH balance.

Sodium bicarbonate used for electrolyte and pH balance.

Essential Oils:

Lemon (*Citrus limon*) promotes leukocyte formation and increases lymphatic function.

Lime (*Citrus aurantiifolia*) decongests the lymphatic system.

Companion Products: Megazyme, Mineral Essence, Mint Condition, Royaldophilus, and VitaGreen.

Companion Oils: Di-Tone, peppermint, Purification, spearmint, and Thieves.

Suggested Use: Stir one rounded teaspoon into six to eight oz. of distilled or purified water and drink immediately. To aid in alkalizing connective tissue, AlkaLime may be taken one to three times per day before meals or before eating. As an antacid, AlkaLime may be taken as needed. Otherwise, an ideal time to take AlkaLime would be prior to bedtime.

Arthro Plus

Arthro Plus is an herbal tincture that may be taken orally or applied topically. It works well with ArthroTune. Take one to three droppers (25-75 drops) three to six times daily in distilled or purified water with meals as a dietary supplement.

Contents:

Extracts of:

Yucca is popular in the southwest U.S. as a folklore medicine.

Alfalfa high in chlorophyll, beta carotene, calcium, and the vitamins D, E and K.

Chaparral used by Native American healers as a tonic for cancer, snake bite, infection, arthritis, and tuberculosis treatments.

Cayenne (red pepper) has been traditionally used as an aid to digestion. It also possesses the ability to break down blood clots.

Dandelion root traditionally used for arthritis and rheumatism.

Barberry (also known as Oregon grape root) is commonly recommended as a treatment for liver problems such as hepatitis and jaundice. It is also considered effective in lowering blood pressure, reducing heart rate and respiration, reducing bronchial constriction, and as a palliative for menstrual irregularities. It is also used as a topical antiseptic.

Burdock root a diuretic and believed to be useful in treating impotence and sterility.

Cascara sagrada a safe and natural laxative, it is often prescribed by herbalists to stimulate the liver, pancreas, gallbladder, and stomach and to support the digestive system.

Licorice root traditionally used for rheumatism and arthritis.

Juniper berry (*Juniperus communis*) **extract** acts as a detoxifier and is used to stimulate nerve function.

Essential Oils of:

Birch (*Betula alleghaniensis*) contains an active principle similar to cortisone and is beneficial for massage associated with bone, muscle, and joint discomfort.

Marjoram (*Origanum majorana*) used for soothing the muscles and the respiratory system. It also assists in calming the nerves. It is antimicrobial and antiseptic.

Cypress (*Cupressus sempervirens*) used to improve the circulatory system. It is antimicrobial.

Suggested Use: Take one to two droppers in 1/2 cup of distilled water, three times daily or as desired.

ArthroTune

An herbal complex that may help arthritis and rheumatoid conditions.

Contents:

Alfalfa leaf supports muscles and joints.

Butcher's broom has anti-inflammatory action.

Yucca improves blood circulation.

Cayenne has been used for pain relief and to help stimulate circulation.

Uncaria tomentosa, known as Cat's Claw, is used as an immune system stimulant and possesses anti-inflammatory properties.

Grapeseed proanthocyanidins inhibits swelling and is used as an antioxidant.

Magnesium relaxes muscles.

Alpha keto glutaric acid

Essential Oils:

Basil (*Ocimum basilicum*) relaxes both striated and smooth muscles.

Birch (*Betula alleghaniensis*) helps reduce bone, joint, and muscle pain.

Cypress (*Cupressus sempervirens*) can improve circulation.

Fir (*Abies alba*) is high in terpenes to soothe and tone the muscles.

Helichrysum (*Helichrysum italicum*) has been studied by European researchers for regenerating tissue and improving circulation.

Juniper (*Juniperus osteosperma* and/or *J. scopulorum*) has been used to stimulate nerve function.

Marjoram (*Origanum majorana*) is used extensively for soothing the muscles.

Pepper (*Piper nigrum*) has been used for soothing deep tissue muscle pain.

Spruce (*Picea mariana*) helps the respiratory and nervous systems.

Companion Products: Arthro Plus, Megazyme, Ortho Ease or Ortho Sport massage oils, Royaldophilus, Sulfurzyme (capsules or powder), and VitaGreen.

Companion Oil Blends: PanAway and Relieve It.

Suggested Use: Take one capsule, twice daily. Best taken before meals. If you have sensitive digestion, take with meals.

AuraLight

This spray nutriceutical utilizes a unique, nutrient delivery system through oral mucosa absorption (directly into the bloodstream through the dense network of blood vessels lining the mucus membrane inside the mouth). This type of delivery system is 90 percent efficient, with five times the efficiency of assimilating the nutrients in tablets or supplements. This unique product combines several natural mood-elevating compounds with the essential oils that are effective for reducing stress.

Contents:

Vitamin B6 promotes the production of mood-balancing neurotransmitters in the brain, including serotonin. It requires the presence the magnesium.

Vitamin B12 helps protect against deterioration of mental functioning, neurological damage, and other psychological disturbances.

Magnesium and **Vitamin B6** work synergistically with the neurotransmitters in the brain, which regulate mood, attitude, and emotion.

St. John's wort (*Hypericum perforatum*, standardized to 0.3 percent hypericin) has been extensively researched for its ability to promote relaxation and uplifted attitude.

Humulus lupulus (Hops extract) contains a natural sedative-like compound, which is highly effective in combating stress.

Passiflora incarnata (Passion flower extract) helps ease nervous tension and enhances feelings of relaxation.

Para aminobenzoic acid (PABA) helps the bones form red blood cells.

L-tyrosine supports the formation of neurotransmitters, such as dopamine and serotonin.

Ginkgo biloba (standardized for flavone glycosides and terpene lactones) helps improve energy levels, improve memory, helps with oxygenation and blood flow, and increases hormonal balance. It also helps to improve mood and reduce depression by increasing circulation in the brain.

Kava (*Piper methysticum*—30 percent kavalactones*) contains natural compounds that exhibit sedative, analgesic, and muscle-relaxant effects.

Essential Oils:

Lavender (*Lavandula angustifolia*) is calming and relaxing.

Orange (*Citrus sinensis*) is rich in compounds noted for their stress-reducing effects.

Roman chamomile (*Chamaemelum nobile*) is relaxing and sedating.

Sandalwood (*Santalum album*) stimulates the pineal gland, which produces melatonin, a hormone associated with deep sleep.

Companion Supplements: Mineral Essence, Power Meal, Super B, and VitaGreen.

Companion Oils: Forgiveness, Hope, Joy, Passion, Peace & Calming, and Surrender.

Suggested Use: Three sprays, three times a day, or as needed. (Vial contains approximately 30 servings). Shake gently before using. For additional benefit, take a deep diaphragmatic breath after each spray.

Be-Fit

A high-powered formula for enhancing strength and endurance and promoting muscle formation. Several ingredients are utilized in this product to help build muscle tissue.

Contents:

Wolfberry powder contains over 15 percent protein by weight. It is rich in amino acids for supporting muscle integrity.

HMB (Betahydroxy beta-methylbutyrate) well-researched nutrients for increasing muscle mass.

Siberian ginseng extract helps provide energy and reduce stress. It also has the unique ability to stimulate lymphocyte formation (an essential part of the immune system).

Ginkgo biloba extract improves energy, memory, and mood, due to its ability to enhance cerebral and peripheral circulation.

L-arginine is an amino acid that promotes circulation in the small capillaries of our tissues, allowing greater nutrient absorption and cellular metabolism.

L-lysine (HCl) works to enhance the benefits of the amino acid L-leucine found in wolfberry powder.

Creatine monohydrate is a naturally occurring compound of three amino acids, providing high-energy fuel for muscles. It helps increase muscle mass as well as muscle contraction for improved intensity and endurance.

Cayenne is excellent as a general stimulant and stamina booster.

Essential Oils:

Birch (*Betula alleghaniensis*) has a cortisone-like action for pain relief due to its high concentration of methyl salicylate.

Lemongrass (*Cymbopogon flexuosus*) is used for ligament support.

Nutmeg (*Myristica fragrans*) is used for its adrenal cortex-like activity, which helps support the adrenal glands for increased energy.

Rosemary (*Rosmarinus officinalis*) helps overcome mental fatigue.

Companion Supplements: Master HIS/HERS, Royal Essence, Power Meal, Ultra Young, and Wolfberry Power Bars.

Companion Oils: Brain Power, En-R-Gee, Endo-Flex, Envision, Live With Passion, and Valor.

Suggested Use: Two capsules in the morning and two capsules at night.

Body Balance

Body Balance is a milk and soy protein supplement fortified with vitamins, minerals, and essential oils. It helps balance the body at its ideal weight and promotes muscle formation. It contains soy solids that have been studied for their effects against breast and ovarian cancer.

Contents:

Non-fat dry milk supplies calcium and protein.

Fructose is a low-glycemic sweetener having minimal impact on blood sugar levels.

Calcium caseinate is one of the most complete sources of protein. The enzymes in these proteins are left intact, thanks to an advanced low-heat, glass-pack pasteurization technology.

Soy protein isolate is used extensively for protein without harmful side effects of the hormonal system.

Potassium citrate is needed to help prevent cancer, heart disease, strokes, and high blood pressure.

Lecithin is a part of the phospholipid membranes of almost every cell in the body.

Xanthan/Guar gum is a natural stabilizer.

Sodium chloride is needed for proper electrolyte balance.

Magnesium is needed for normal muscle contractions and heart rhythm. High intake can reduce high blood pressure, fight arteriosclerosis, and improve insulin action.

Vitamin C (ascorbic acid) helps the body manufacture collagen for connective tissue, cartilage, tendons, etc., and is used for proper immune function. It is also an antioxidant.

Vitamin E protects against cardiovascular disease and is beneficial for acne, allergies, and wound healing.

Vitamin A is an important antioxidant.

Calcium pantothenate is needed for the prevention of depression and tinnitus.

Niacinamide (vitamin B3) is essential for the production of energy, is involved in the regulation of blood sugar, and helps regulate cholesterol.

Zinc is crucial for proper immune function and is needed for proper action of many hormones, including insulin and growth hormone. It helps improve wound healing.

Iron chelation plays a central role in transporting oxygen from the lungs to the body's tissues and carbon dioxide from tissues to lungs.

Copper is necessary for proper red blood cell formation and immune function.

Vitamin D helps with the absorption of calcium and has many anticancer properties.

Vitamin B6 supports immune function and protects the heart and blood vessels. It inhibits skin cancer growth and helps prevent kidney stones and PMS symptoms. Vitamin B6 requires folic acid and magnesium to maximize its effects.

Riboflavin (vitamin B2) has shown to be crucial in the production of energy, is involved in regenerating glutathione, and may help prevent certain esophageal cancers.

Thiamin (vitamin B1) functions as part of an enzyme essential for energy production, carbohydrate metabolism, and nerve cell function.

Vitamin B12 is critical for red blood cell formation and proper immune and nerve function.

Folic acid plays an important role in cardiovascular health.

Biotin helps convert fats and amino acids into energy. It promotes healthy nails and hair and combats yeast and fungus overgrowth.

Essential Oils:

Lime (*Citrus aurantiifolia*) decongests the lymphatic system.

Tangerine (*Citrus nobilis*) is an anticoagulant and helps decongest the lymphatic system.

Orange (*Citrus sinensis*) helps reduce fluid retention and is beneficial to the skin.

Lemon (*Citrus limon*) promotes leukocyte formation and increases lymphatic function.

Cypress (*Cupressus sempervirens*) helps circulation and decongests the lymphatic system.

Grapefruit (*Citrus paradisi*) has been used for disinfection.

Mandarin (*Citrus reticulata*) is antifungal, antispasmotic, and promotes digestion.

Companion Products: Be-Fit, Cel-Lite Magic Massage Oil, Mineral Essence, Royal Essence (tincture), Super B, Super Cal, and Thyromin.

Companion Oil Blends: Citrus Fresh, EndoFlex, Envision, Live with Passion, and Magnify Your Purpose.

Suggested Use: Add one measuring scoop to eight to ten oz. purified water, juice, or low-fat milk. Blend in blender for 30 seconds. Ice cubes may be added to thicken like a shake. Body Balance works with all juices. It is a predigested protein and may be taken anytime.

For optimum results, take with Master Formula HIS or HERS and Thyromin food supplements.

Tips for Getting the Most from Body Balance

1. **For fast weight reduction:** Enjoy Body Balance as a alternative for breakfast and dinner. Eat a sensible, low-fat, well-balanced lunch, which should include vegetables, fruits, and whole grains. As with any weight balancing program, fats, sugars, and high-caloric foods should be

omitted from your diet. Raw organic vegetables and fruits are excellent snacks.

2. **For weight gain:** Enjoy Body Balance mixed with whole milk or apple juice. Add a banana or a pear and drink after each meal.

3. **For good health and weight maintenance:** After you have achieved your ideal weight, enjoy a Body Balance shake as a meal alternative daily, possibly for breakfast. Body Balance may also be used as a filling and nutritious snack for the entire family. Drink plenty of distilled or purified water.

Note: Anyone who is pregnant or nursing, has health problems, or wants to lose more than 50 pounds or more than 20 percent of his/her body weight, should consult a physician before starting this or any other weight management program.

Frequency: Approximately 87 MHz.

For optimum benefits, Body Balance may be mixed with soy or rice milk.

CardiaCare

Strengthens and supports the heart and cardiovascular system.

Contents:

Rhododendron caucasicum contains phenylpropanoids that have been shown in clinical studies to increase the efficiency of the cardiovascular system.

Wolfberry powder contains the amino acids that are vital to supporting cardiovascular function.

Magnesium is needed for normal muscle contractions and heart rhythm. High intake can reduce high blood pressure, fight arteriosclerosis, and improve insulin action.

Hawthorn berry has been used for decades in European cardiac medicine. Active constituents in the berries dilate coronary blood vessels, thereby increasing blood circulation in the heart.

Coenzyme Q10 (CoQ10) is used by every cell in the body to convert food to energy. Heart cells require more CoQ10 to maintain muscle strength because of their higher demand for energy.

Vitamin E prevents oxidative damage to low-density lipoproteins (LDLs), a primary cause of clogged coronary arteries and heart disease.

Essential Oils:

Helichrysum (*Helichrysum italicum*) helps regulate cholesterol, stimulates liver function, helps regulate blood thickness, allowing for better blood flow between vessels and tissues.

Lemon (*Citrus limon*) helps dissolve cholesterol and cellulite, increases lymphatic function.

Marjoram (*Origanum majorana*) provides support for smooth muscles of the heart, relieves spasms, and may work as a diuretic.

Ylang Ylang (*Cananga odorata*) has been used traditionally to support heart functions.

Companion Products: A.D.&E., HRT, and Mineral Essence.

Companion Oil Blends: Aroma Life, Forgiveness, Harmony, Joy, and Live with Passion.

Chelex

Chelex contains herbs that have been traditionally used to chelate and neutralize heavy metals and and disarm free radicals. Take one to three droppers three times a day.

Contents:

Extracts of:

Astragalus—used as a diuretic, a vasodilator, and respiratory infection treatment, this herb reputedly has immune-stimulating effects and increases energy.

Garlic—demonstrated by Louis Pasteur to have antibacterial properties in 1858. Albert Schweitzer used garlic to treat amoebic dysentery. Later, researchers found that garlic can protect against heart disease and cancer. Garlic juice halts the growth of more than 60 types of fungi and 20 types of bacteria.

Sarsaparilla—contains saponins, steroid-like molecules that neutralize endotoxins, poisons secreted by fungi and bacteria in the human body that contribute to many kinds of disease.

Siberian ginseng—energizes the body and boosts the immune system.

Red Clover—used to treat asthma, bronchitis, skin ailments, ulcers, and arthritis. Used in some cultures to prevent recurrence of cancer.

Royal jelly—a viscous, milky white secretion produced by the worker bee upon which future queens are continually nourished. Royal jelly's chemistry has been extensively studied and contains all the essential amino acids, unsaturated fats, natural sugars, minerals, and vitamins B5 and B6. Tests have shown that royal jelly can have an effect on the adrenal cortex, stimulating the adrenal glands to produce increased metabolism and enhanced energy.

Essential Oils of:

Roman chamomile (*Chamaemelum nobile*)—promotes bile flow and liver function.

Eucalyptus (*Eucalyptus globulus*)—is a powerful antimicrobial agent, rich in eucalyptol (a key ingredient in many antiseptic mouth rinses).

Helichrysum (*Helichrysum italicum*)—has been studied by European researchers for regenerating tissue and improving circulation. This oil has also been studied for its natural chelating action.

ComforTone

An herbal complex of bentonite, apple pectin, and herbal extracts that may relieve constipation, enhance colon function, and dispel parasites and toxins.

ComforTone can help eliminate parasites from the body, break up the encrustation along the colon wall, and relax spasms that may occur. If you experience nausea when using ComforTone, use Di-Tone or peppermint (diluted if necessary); if you experience constipation, increase your water intake and avoid using I.C.P. If you have a history of chronic constipation, do not start I.C.P. and ComforTone at the same time. First use Comfor-Tone until the system is open, and then follow with I.C.P. Drink ten glasses of water per day.

Contents:

Licorice root cleanses the blood and supports the liver, the most important organ for cleansing.

Psyllium seed helps relieve abdominal pain, constipation, diarrhea, and protects against flatulence and nausea.

Apple pectin helps with enzyme production and supports proper digestive function.

Bentonite is an intestinal cleansing agent.

Fennel is antiparasitic, antimicrobial, antispasmotic, is a digestive aid, helps regulate intestinal flora, and increases gastric secretions.

Garlic is antifungal, antiparasitic, antiviral, an immune stimulant, works as a digestive aid, and is a catalyst for the oils.

German chamomile is antimicrobial, anti-inflammatory, suppresses the parasympathetic nervous system that produces excess mucus, and relaxes spasms in the colon wall.

Echinacea is antimicrobial, antiparasitic, lowers bowel transit time, absorbs toxins in the colon, and stimulates the immune system.

Ginger root is anti-inflammatory, antispasmodic, helps lower cholesterol, and cleanses the colon.

Cascara sagrada works as an herbal laxative and as a liver cleanser.

Burdock root lowers bowel transit time, balances intestinal flora, and absorbs toxins from the bowels.

Contains therapeutic-grade essential oils of:

Rosemary (*Rosmarinus officinalis*) is antiparasitic and balances the endocrine system.

German chamomile (*Matricaria recutita*) helps prevent acne, rashes, and eczema.

Tarragon (*Artemisia dracunculus*) has been used to reduce flatulence, intestinal spasms, sluggish digestion, and to prevent fermentation.

Peppermint (*Mentha piperita*) reduces candida, nausea, and vomiting.

Ginger (*Zingiber officinale*) combats indigestion, diarrhea, loss of appetite, and congestion.

Anise (*Pimpinella anisum*) helps prevent flatulence, colon spasms, and indigestion.

Mugwort (*Artemisia vulgaris*) has been used traditionally to calm nerves.

Tangerine (*Citrus reticulata*) helps decongest the lymphatic system and is anti-inflammatory.

Companion Products: Chelex, I.C.P., JuvaTone, Megazyme, and ParaFree.

Companion Oil Blends: Di-Tone, JuvaFlex, Purification, Release, and Thieves.

Suggested Use: Start with two to five capsules first thing in the morning, and two to five capsules just before going to bed. Drink eight to ten eight-ounce glasses of purified or distilled water per day for best results. If you get cramps, skip the next morning or day and start up again with two capsules in the morning and two in the evening. After starting ComforTone, you may cut back; but do not stop completely because all the toxins that have been pulled out of the system will go back into the system. Take at least one in the morning and one in the evening, but do not stop once you start. For maximum results, use with JuvaTone and Megazyme. ComforTone may be taken every day without becoming addictive.

Safety Data: ComforTone may be taken during pregnancy, as long as you do not get diarrhea. Diarrhea might cause cramping, which could bring on labor.

Frequency: Approximately 43 MHz.

Essential Manna

This is a nutritionally dense, fiber-rich super-food that has been based on the diet of the Hunza people. The Hunza's longevity has been attributed to their consumption of a high potassium, high magnesium diet of dried fruits (especially apricots), nuts, and a variety of whole grains.

Contents:

Apricots contain high concentrations of carotinoids, a class of high-powered antioxidants that includes beta carotene (provitamin A). Apricots are also rich in rutin, which strengthens blood vessels.

Chinese wolfberry (*Lycium barbarum*) has been studied for its ability to combat cancer and improve the immunity.

Barley is exceptionally rich in soluble fiber and is an ideal food for type II diabetics.

Buckwheat is high in potassium, magnesium, and other essential minerals. It helps improves cholesterol levels and glucose tolerance.

Amaranth is rich in lysine, an amino acid lacking in many traditional grains, such as wheat and corn.

Almonds contain high amounts of magnesium and vitamin E, which enhance immune support.

Millet contains over 12 percent protein and is a source of 12 essential minerals, including magnesium, potassium, zinc, and iodine.

Brown rice is rich in protein with high concentrations of the muscle-building amino acids, L-leucine, L-isoleucine, and L-valine. Brown rice is packed with a fiber content necessary for proper digestion.

Coconut is rich in potassium and low in sodium.

Rolled oats contain high amounts of manganese, selenium, and magnesium.

Pineapples are rich in potassium and contain bromelain, a protein-digesting enzyme.

Sesame seeds are rich in linoleic and oleic acid and contain unusual antioxidant compounds, used to prevent free radical damage.

Stevia is an all-natural supplement. (*See Stevia*).

Also contains pumpkin seeds, filberts, pecans, cashews, and papaya.

Essential Manna comes in carob and spice flavors.

Use: Eat throughout the day when desired.

Companion Products: JuvaTone, Megazyme, Mineral Essence, Power Meal, and Sulfurzyme (capsules or powder).

Companion Oils: En-R-Gee, EndoFlex, Envision, JuvaFlex, Magnify Your Purpose, and Valor.

Estro

Estro is an herbal tincture containing plant-derived phytoestrogens, such as black cohosh, which are widely used in Europe as a safe alternative to synthetic estrogen. Phytoestrogens have been researched for their ability to support the body during PMS without many of the side effects associated with estrogen-replacement therapies. Contains the therapeutic-grade essential oil of clary sage *(Salvia sclarea)*, which contains natural sclareol, a plant-based estrogen. Start with one dropper two to three times daily. Increase as needed to as much as three droppers daily. Estro may take as long as four weeks to reach maximum effectiveness.

Contents:

Extracts of:

Black cohosh—approved by the German Commission E for combating PMS symptoms. Its constituents have been found to mimic those of estrogen.

Blue cohosh—the main ingredient brewed in a tea used by Native American women to relieve menstrual and labor cramping, now recommended by modern herbalists to induce menstruation and as uterine stimulant and antispasmodic.

Royal jelly—a secretion produced by the worker bee upon which all bee larvae feed during the first three days of life. Because queen larvae continue to feed on this substance (and live thirty to forty times longer), various herbalists claim that royal jelly is especially effective in halting or controlling the aging process, nourishing the skin, and erasing facial blemishes and wrinkles.

Essential Oils of:

Fennel *(Foeniculum vulgare)*—is antiseptic and stimulating to the circulatory and respiratory systems.

Lavender *(Lavandula angustifolia)*—is calming, relaxing, and balancing, both physically and emotionally.

Clary sage *(Salvia sclarea)*—is a source of natural estrogen.

Exodus

Exodus is the ultimate supercharged antioxidant containing a biblical blend of essential oils and other nutritional herbs to provide important support for the immune system.

Contents:

Uncaria tomentosa (Cat's Claw, Una de Gato) contains alkaloids such as mitraphylline that may fortify the immune system. Julian Whittaker, M.D., discusses this herb in an article entitled, "Take Una de Gato for All-around Immunity."

Amino acid complex of alanine, cystine, arginine, glycine, lycine, threonine, and thorine is used as the building block of the enzymes, proteins, and cells of our natural defenses.

Yucca has been used for its blood-cleansing properties.

Echinacea is one of the best-studied immune boosters. Extensive research indicates that it increases the number and activity of white blood cells involved with immunity and boosts the activity of T-cells and natural interferon.

Vitamin A is a powerful antioxidant that supports the eyes, hair, and skin.

Grapeseed extract is one of the strongest-known antioxidants.

Ionic minerals contain a specially balanced formula with trace minerals from boron to zinc. (See MINERAL ESSENCE)

Pantothenic acid supports adrenal function and the formation of antibodies, aids in vitamin utilization, and helps convert fats, carbohydrates, and proteins into energy.

Essential Oils:

Frankincense *(Boswellia carteri)* was well known for its healing properties during the time of Christ. It has antitumoral and immune-stimulating properties.

Hyssop *(Hyssopus officinalis)* has been used for thousands of years for its anti-inflammatory, anti-infectious, and antiparasitic properties. It helps discharge toxins and mucus, and regulates lipid metabolism.

133

Bay laurel (*Laurus nobilis*) contains antiseptic and antimicrobial properties.

Spikenard (*Nardostachys jatamansi*) is highly regarded in India as a medicinal herb.

Myrrh (*Commiphora myrrha*) is anti-infectious and supports the immune system.

Companion Products: ComforTone, Essential Manna, ImmuTune, Radex, Power Meal, Super C, and VitaGreen.

Companion Oil Blends: Exodus II, ImmuPower, Purification, and Thieves.

Suggested Use: Take three capsules, two to three times daily.

FemiGen

This is a formula with herbs and amino acids, to help balance the reproductive system from the developmental years all the way through menopause. FemiGen acts as a natural estrogen and helps balance the hormones.

Contents:

Damiana has been described as a blood purifier, an expectorant, and is used as a diuretic.

Epimedium has been used to help detoxify kidneys and help eliminate lower back pain and frequent urination.

Dong quai has estrogenic qualities and increases blood flow to the reproductive organs of the female system. It has also been used as a menstrual balancer.

Muira puama (potency wood) has been used for treatment of frigidity, menstrual cramps, impotency, and PMS.

Wild yam root contains compounds that are similar in structure to steroids. It is good for muscle spasms and contains anti-inflammatory compounds.

Also includes: American ginseng, licorice root, black cohosh, cramp bark, squaw vine, magnesium, L-carnitine, dimethylglycine, L-phenylalanine, L-cystine, L-cysteine, and L-trytophan.

Essential Oils:

Clary sage (*Salvia sclarea*) has been used for regulating cells and balancing hormones.

Fennel (*Foeniculum vulgare*) has hormone-like activity that helps balance hormones.

Sage (*Salvia officinalis*) helps alleviate premenopause symptoms, such as depression.

Ylang Ylang (*Cananga odorata*) has been used for sexual disabilities, lack of desire, and relaxation.

Suggested Use: Take two capsules with breakfast and two capsules with lunch. A maintenance dose of two capsules may be taken three times a day for ten days before a period.

Companion Products: AuraLight, Dragon Time Massage Oil, and Femalin.

Companion Oils: Dragon Time, Mister, PanAway, Peace & Calming, and Relieve It.

Femalin

Femalin is an essential tincture formulated to help protect the female reproductive system. Store in a cool place, out of sunlight. Take one dropper (approximately 25 drops) three to six times daily in distilled water as a dietary supplement. Keep in a cool place and avoid direct sunlight for longer life.

Contents:

Extracts of:

Goldenseal root—a Native American medicinal plant used for gastric and urinary disorders.

Blessed thistle—a popular folk remedy used by European monks to aid digestion and circulation.

Cayenne—traditionally used to aid digestion, it possesses fibrinolytic activity (able to break down blood clots).

Cramp Bark—used traditionally to combat endometriosis, osteoporosis, uterine cysts, and irregular menstruation. Also used as a labor tonic and to remedy cramping of the stomach, intestines, and uterus, from which its name is derived.

False unicorn—medicinal use is based in Native American tradition, especially in the regulation of menstruation, and to prevent miscarriages.

Ginger root—especially useful in calming nausea and stimulating appetite. It also alleviates motion sickness.

Red raspberry—especially helpful to women, this herb nourishes the reproductive organs, helping to strengthen and prepare the body for childbirth. It is also an effective remedy for digestive ailments and upset stomach.

Squaw vine—traditionally used for PMS symptoms: anxiety, edema, fibrocystic disease of the breast, postpartum depression, pregnancy, sore nipples (with olive oil and beeswax), and varicose veins.

Uva ursi—a mild diuretic, astringent, and urinary tract infection remedy.

Royal jelly—a secretion produced by the worker bee upon which all bee larvae feed during the first three days of life. Because queen larvae continue to feed on this substance (and live thirty to forty times longer), various herbalists claim that royal jelly is especially effective in halting or controlling the aging process, nourishing the skin, and erasing facial blemishes and wrinkles.

Essential Oils of:

Rosemary (*Rosmarinus officinalis*)—has been researched for its antiseptic and antimicrobial properties. It may be beneficial for the skin. It helps overcome mental fatigue.

Fennel (*Foeniculum vulgare*)—antiseptic and stimulating to the circulatory and respiratory systems.

Melaleuca (*Melaleuca alternifolia*)—highly regarded as an antimicrobial and antiseptic essential oil. Pure melaleuca has high levels of terpinenol, which is the key active constituent.

Clary sage (*Salvia sclarea*)—is a source of natural estrogen.

Bergamot (*Citrus bergamia*)—has been used in the Middle East for hundreds of years for skin conditions associated with an oily complexion.

Goji Berry Tea

Goji berry is the colloquial name for the wolfberry, which is grown in China. This delicious, nourishing tea, is made from the Chinese wolfberry, which has been used by the Chinese for centuries to strengthen the liver and reduce the effects of arthritis and other degenerative diseases. Several ingredients from other cultures enhance the immune-building effects of the wolfberry and provide tremendous nourishment to the body. Research at the Beijing Nutrition Research Institute and State Scientific and Technology Commission of China found that those who drank the tea and ate the berries did not experience liver disease, hepatitis, or other degenerative problems and lived 20-30 years longer than the average person in China.

Contents:

Chinese wolfberry (*Lycium barbarum*) has been prized in China to protect the body from degenerative disease by strengthening the body's defense mechanism, working as an antioxidant, and promoting longevity.

Cat's claw (*Uncaria tomentosa*) has been used to fight and prevent degenerative disease.

Nopal, harvested from a native cactus, is a traditional herb used in Mexico. It was tested and found to reduce cholesterol, burn fat, and support the pancreas.

Purple lapacho (also known as Pau D'arco in Brazil and Taheebo in Argentina) is reported to help support the body by cleansing the lymphatic system and building blood cells.

Panax ginseng has been used for thousands of years in the Orient to extend life and invigorate the body.

Essential Oils:

Lemon (*Citrus limon*) has been used to cleanse the lymphatic system and promote well being.

Peppermint (*Mentha piperita*) helps reduce candida, fever, and cools the body.

Spearmint (*Mentha spicata*) is antiparasitic and anti-infectious. Its hormone-like properties help bring about a sense of balance and well being.

135

Companion Products: ComforTone, Exodus, ImmuneTune, and Power Meal.

Companion Oil Blends: Exodus II, ImmuPower, Purification, Release, Thieves, and Valor.

Suggested Use: Bring one cup of purified or distilled water to the boiling point. Remove from heat and add one tea bag. Steep 15-30 minutes for desired taste. Add Stevia or honey as a nutritional supplement.

HRT

HRT tincture combines concentrated extracts of some of the best-studied herbs for supporting normal heart function, including hawthorn berry, garlic, and cayenne. Hawthorn berry's role in supporting the heart has been gaining increasing notice among both authors and physicians. According to Varro Tyler, Ph.D., one of the most highly esteemed herbalists in the U.S., "Studies are urgently needed for [an herb] as potentially valuable as this one." Take one to three droppers three times daily in distilled water or as desired.

Contents:

Extracts of:

Hawthorn berries—used since the time of Dioscorides in the first century A.D., they are one of the best studied herbs to support the heart, protecting against heart muscle weakness, angina, and mild arrhythmia. J. L. Rodale published an entire book on the subject, *The Hawthorn Berry for the Heart.*

Garlic—was shown by Louis Pasteur to have antibacterial properties in 1858. Albert Schweitzer used garlic to treat amoebic dysentery. Later researchers found that garlic can protect against heart disease and cancer. Garlic juice halts the growth of more than 60 types of fungi and 20 types of bacteria.

Lobelia—is a mild sedative and is helpful for allergies, coughs, colds, and headaches. Evaluated to be one of the most valuable herbs, due its dual properties of stimulation and relaxation.

Cayenne—traditionally an aid to digestion, this red pepper also possesses fibrinolytic activity (able to break down blood clots).

Royal jelly—a viscous, milky white secretion produced by the worker bee upon which future queens are continually nourished. Royal jelly's chemistry has been extensively studied and contains all the essential amino acids, unsaturated fats, natural sugars, minerals, and the vitamins B5 and B6. Tests have shown that royal jelly can have an effect on the adrenal cortex, stimulating the adrenal glands to produce a positive reaction on increased metabolism and enhanced energy.

Essential Oils of:

Lemon (*Citrus limon*)—has antiseptic-like properties and contains compounds that have been studied for their effects on immune function.

Rosewood (*Aniba rosaeodora*)—is soothing and nourishing to the skin. It has been researched at Weber State University for its inhibition rate against gram positive and gram negative bacterial growth.

Ylang ylang (*Cananga odorata*)—is traditionally used to support heart function and circulation.

Cypress (*Cupressus sempervirens*)—one of the oils most used for the circulatory system.

I.C.P.

I.C.P. Multiple Fiber Beverage is a unique source of fiber and bulk for the diet, which helps speed the transit time of waste matter through the intestinal tract. The psyllium, oat bran, flax, and rice bran are specifically balanced to eliminate allergy symptoms that many people experience when taking psyllium alone. Essential oils enhance the flavor and may help dispel gas and pain. This formula is unsurpassed as an aid in enhancing normal bowel function.

Contents:

Psyllium seed powder expands when mixed with water and is smooth and filling, not abrasive, to the intestinal walls.

Apple pectin slows absorption of food after meals, removes unwanted metals and toxins, is valuable against the effects of radiation therapy, and helps lower cholesterol.

Aloe vera extract is a natural laxative and lubricant that relaxes the colon.

Rice bran is an outstanding source of soluble and semisoluble fiber.

Oat bran binds up fat so it does not enter the blood stream.

cumin helps digestion and is an antioxidant.

Guar gum has been used in expanding and cleansing the colon.

Flax seed is an excellent cleanser for intestinal walls and the digestive system. It is also a lubricant, an antioxidant, and is very harmonious with essential oils.

Yucca helps break up obstructions in the digestive system and contains enzymes for digestion.

Fennel seed stimulates the gastrointestinal mucous membrane, which in turn stimulates the pancreas to secrete digestive enzymes to dissolve undigested proteins. It is antiparasitic.

Pepsin is an enzyme to aid digestion.

Essential Oils:

Fennel (*Foeniculum vulgare*) has been used to help reduce symptoms associated with menopause, help with gas, and is antibacterial and antiparasitical.

Tarragon (*Artemisia dracunculus*) has been shown to be anti-infectious, antispasmodic, and antiviral.

Ginger (*Zingiber officinale*) improves digestion and helps combat parasites.

Lemongrass (*Cymbopogon flexuosus*) is antifungal and promotes digestion.

Rosemary (*Rosmarinus officinalis*) reduces indigestion and helps regulate cholesterol.

Anise (*Pimpinella anisum*) helps flatulence, colon spasms, and indigestion.

Suggested Use: Take five times a week for maintenance (1/2 cup water, 1/2 cup apple juice, and one heaping teaspoon of I.C.P.). Take more often for cleansing (start with one heaping teaspoon, two to three times a day with carrot or other vegetable juices. Increase to three teaspoons, three times a day). I.C.P. dilutes better in warm water. Drink immediately as this product tends to thicken quickly when added to liquid.

For best results, take ComforTone first, then I.C.P., morning and night. I.C.P. absorbs toxins and can build and improve the wave-like movement of the intestinal walls.

Frequency: Approximately 56 MHz.

Companion Products: ComforTone, JuvaTone, Megazyme, and ParaFree (capsules or liquid).

Companion Oil Blends: Di-Tone, JuvaFlex, Purification, and Thieves.

ImmuGel

ImmuGel is a unique blend of naturally-occurring liquid amino acids, trace minerals, and herbal extracts with essential oils. This blend creates one of nature's most powerful antioxidant and antimicrobial formulas. It destroys fungi and bacteria, thereby boosting the immune defenses. This formula is used for general maintenance, and use should be increased during times of fatigue, depression, or to help prevent illness. It is also used as a support in eliminating candida.

Contents:

Deionized water helps cleanse and purify the body's tissues and organs.

Hydrolyzed protein (contains amino acids including alanine, arginine, aspartic acid, glutamic acid, glycine, histidine, hydroxyproline, leucine and isoleucine, lycine, methionine, phenylalanine).

Methylcellulose has been used by parasitologists to slow down single-cell organisms, such as amoebae, flagellates, etc.

German chamomile extract contains elements that are antibacterial and antifungal.

Trace minerals help restore electrolyte balance in the cells.

Essential Oils:

Cinnamon bark (*Cinnamomum verum*) is antifungal, antibacterial, and antiviral.

Clove (*Syzygium aromaticum*) is anti-infectious, antiviral, antifungal, antiparasitic, and has been used in European hospitals for viral hepatitis, bronchitis, flu, sinusitis, and cholera.

Rosemary (*Rosmarinus officinalis*) supports the heart and helps moderate hypertension.

Lemon (*Citrus limon*) promotes leukocyte formation and increases lymphatic (immune) function.

Thyme (*Thymus vulgaris*) is one of the strongest antibacterial, antifungal, and antiviral essential oils.

Oregano (*Origanum compactum*) has been used for infections, pneumonia, and dysentery.

Suggested Use: Take half to one teaspoon, three times daily. May be taken with water.

Companion Products: Exodus, ImmuneTune, JuvaTone, and Super C.

Companion Oil Blends: Exodus II, ImmuPower, JuvaFlex, Purification, Release, Thieves, and Valor.

ImmuneTune

ImmuneTune is a super antioxidant complex that supports the immune system and fights free radicals. The curcuminoid blend in this product has been found to be 60 percent stronger in antioxidant activity than pine bark or grape seed extract. However, synergy is the key to obtaining maximum effect. Through combining curcuminoids with grapeseed extract, the antioxidant power is almost doubled.

Contents:

Curcuminoids (from curcumin and turmeric) are potent antioxidants and immune supporters.

Grapeseed extract is one of the strongest antioxidants.

Magnesium is needed for normal muscle contractions and heart rhythm. High intake can reduce high blood pressure, fight arteriosclerosis, and improve insulin action.

Potassium citrate is needed for prevention of cancer, heart disease, strokes, and high blood pressure.

Calcium pantothenate may serve as protection against high blood pressure and colon cancer.

Alpha lipoic acid is found in many foods. It has produced great results in the prevention and treatment of diabetes, cataracts, heart disease, liver ailments, cancer, and kidney stones.

Chromium improves insulin sensitivity and blood sugar metabolism.

Selenium has been extensively researched for its anticancer and antioxidant properties.

Echinacea increases the white blood cells and stimulates the immune system.

Yucca is an excellent antioxidant that supports the liver and gall bladder.

Essential Oils:

Orange (*Citrus sinensis*) is excellent for flatulence, circulation, and fluid reduction.

Pine (*Pinus mariana*) is used for respiratory infection and bronchitis.

Fir (*Abies alba*) has also been used for different types of respiratory infections and bronchitis.

Cistus (*Cistus ladanifer*) has been used to improve immune function.

Ravensara (*Ravensara aromatica*), known as the "oil that heals," may help activity in the immune system.

Lemon (*Citrus limon*) promotes leukocyte formation and increases immune function.

Companion Products: Exodus, ImmuGel, ParaFree (capsules or liquid), or Super C.

Companion Oil Blends: Envision, Exodus II, ImmuPower, Release, and Thieves.

Suggested Use: For slow metabolism, take two to three capsules daily. For fast metabolism, take three to six capsules daily. It is best taken on an empty stomach. For stomach sensitivity, take with meals.

Frequency: Approximately 108 MHz.

JuvaTone

JuvaTone is a special herbal complex designed to support the liver. The liver is one of the most important organs of the body. It purifies the blood and is a key to converting carbohydrates to energy. An overtaxed liver may affect our energy, digestion, and skin. Fats and bile within the liver can easily become oversaturated with oil-soluble toxins, synthetic chemicals, and heavy metals. As toxins build, the liver becomes taxed and stressed, resulting in aggravating skin conditions, rashes, fatigue, headaches, muscle pain, digestive disturbances, pallor, dizziness, irritability, mood swings, and mental confusion. The liver also plays a major role in helping the body detoxify. The final products of digestion are transported through the portal vein from the colon to the liver to be cleansed.

Contents:

Choline bitartrate has been used in the treatment of many liver disorders, including elevated cholesterol levels, viral hepatitis, and cirrhosis.

Inositol helps the liver rid itself of fat and bile.

Dl-methionine is one of the most powerful antioxidants in the body, and especially important to protect the liver.

Oregon grape root contains berberine, which has been studied as a liver protectant and for its effects against hepatitis.

Dandelion root is used for disturbances in bile flow and liver disorders.

Other Ingredients: Alfalfa sprouts, echinacea root, parsley, sodium, and copper in herbal extracts.

Essential Oils:

Geranium (*Pelargonium graveolens*) has been used for centuries as a liver cleanser and to regenerate tissue and nerves.

German chamomile (*Matricaria recutita*) improves bile flow from the liver.

Rosemary (*Rosmarinus officinalis*) supports the liver and combats cirrhosis.

Lemon (*Citrus limon*) promotes leukocyte formation and increases lymphatic (immune) function.

Blue tansy (*Tanacetum annuum*) is anti-inflammatory and is used for hypertension and arthritis.

Myrtle (*Myrtus communis*) helps break up mucus and stimulate the thyroid.

Companion Products: ComforTone, I.C.P., Megazyme, ParaFree (capsules or liquid), and Power Meal.

Companion Oil Blends: Di-Tone, Forgiveness, JuvaFlex, Release, Surrender, and Thieves.

Suggested Use: For slow metabolism, take two tablets, three times daily. Increase as needed up to four tablets, four times daily. For fast metabolism, take three tablets, three times daily and increase to four tablets, four times daily or as needed. Best taken between meals. Tablets may be chewed, broken, or swallowed whole. For maximum results, use with ComforTone.

Frequency: Approximately 140 MHz.

K & B

K & B tincture contains extracts of herbs that support kidney and bladder function. Take one to three droppers, three times daily in distilled water or as desired.

Contents:

Extracts of:

Juniper berries—long used by Greek, Arabic, and Native American peoples as a kidney stimulant to encourage cleansing and increased filtration.

Parsley—commonly used to purify the urinary tract.

Uva Ursi—a mild diuretic, astringent, and urinary tract infection remedy.

Dandelion root—traditionally used for a host of disorders, including anemia, cirrhosis, colitis, constipation, cystitis, dermatitis, digestive complaints, edema, gallbladder disorders, liver disorders.

Roman chamomile—increases bile flow and liver function.

Royal jelly—a viscous, milky white secretion produced by worker bees upon which future queens are continually nourished. Through extensive study, royal jelly has been found to contain all the essential amino acids, unsaturated fats, natural sugars, minerals, and vitamins B5 and B6. Tests have shown that royal jelly can stimulae the adrenal glands to increase metabolism and enhance energy.

Clove (*Syzygium aromaticum*)—one of the most antimicrobial and antiseptic essential oils.

Juniper (*Juniperus osteosperma* and/or *J. scopulorum*)—a strong diuretic.

Sage (*Salvia officinalis*)—strengthens the vital centers and supports metabolism.

Fennel (*Foeniculum vulgare*) is antiseptic to the digestive tract. Supports digestion.

Geranium (*Pelargonium graveolens*)—opens the bile duct.

Roman chamomile (*Chamaemelum nobile*)—promotes the flow of bile to and from the liver, a key aspect of cleansing and detoxification.

Master Formula HIS/HERS and CHILDREN'S

The Master Formula vitamins are high-quality multivitamin, mineral, and amino acid supplements, manufactured using a special 16-stage Synergistic Suspension Isolation, which separates the antagonistic vitamins and herbs from the synergistic ones so they do not become abrasive and destroy each other's effectiveness. Master Formula contains the amino acid L-phenylalanine, enabling the body to recognize this supplement as a food, allowing for a faster conversion and assimilation.

Contents:

Vitamin A and beta carotene are powerful antioxidants that support the eyes, hair, and skin.

Vitamin D is beneficial for the absorption of calcium, and may prevent liver and kidney dysfunctions.

Vitamin E protects the heart and blood and combats free-radical oxidative damage.

Vitamin C supports immune function and blood vessel integrity, and combats free-radical damage associated with premature aging. It has been used to treat cataracts, glaucoma, high blood pressure, periodontal disease, eczema, gingivitis, and infections.

Folic acid plays an important role in cardiovascular health. Helps prevent neural tube defects.

Thiamin (vitamin B1) is essential for energy production, carbohydrate metabolism, and nerve cell function.

Riboflavin (vitamin B2) is crucial in the production of cellular energy, helps regenerate the liver, and helps prevent migraine headaches and some esophageal cancers.

Niacin is essential for turning carbohydrates into energy. It lowers cholesterol and helps regulate blood sugar. At least 4.4 mg is needed for every 1,000 calories consumed to avoid pellagra.

Vitamin B6 supports immune function and protects the heart and blood vessels. It inhibits skin cancer growth and helps prevent kidney stones and PMS symptoms. Vitamin B6 requires folic acid and magnesium to maximize its effects.

Vitamin B12 is critical for red blood cell formation and proper immune and nerve function.

Biotin helps convert fats and amino acids into energy. It promotes healthy nails and hair and combats yeast and fungus overgrowth.

Pantothenic acid is needed for the prevention of depression and tinnitus.

Choline bitartrate has been used in the treatment of many liver disorders, including elevated cholesterol levels, Alzheimer's disease, viral hepatitis, and cirrhosis.

Calcium is used primarily for the treatment of many conditions associated with osteoporosis, such as bone loss. It is also helpful for elevated blood pressure.

Iodine (kelp) helps prevent goiters, reduced thyroid hormones, and estrogen imbalance.

Iron is needed to prevent anemia, fatigue, hemorrhoids, and peptic ulcers.

Magnesium is crucial for proper enzyme function and is needed for normal muscle contractions and heart rhythm. High intake can reduce high blood pressure, fight arteriosclerosis, and improve insulin action.

Copper is necessary for proper red blood cell and immune function.

Zinc is crucial for proper immune function and is needed for proper action of many hormones, including insulin and growth hormone. It helps improve wound healing.

Potassium supports cellular fluid balance and healthy muscle, nerve, heart, and adrenal function. It reduces high blood pressure and balances water distribution.

Manganese is needed for blood sugar control, energy metabolism, and proper thyroid function. It is also good for antioxidant activity.

Chromium improves insulin sensitivity and blood sugar metabolism.

Selenium has been extensively researched for its anticancer and antioxidant properties.

Silicon is required for proper functioning of an enzyme that is essential for the formation of collagen in bone, cartilage, and other connective tissues.

In a base of betaine HCl, citrus bioflavonoids, L-cysteine, histidine, tyrosine, lysine, arginine, PABA (para amino benzoic acid), molybdenum, and amino acid complex.

Master Formula CHILDREN'S

A special chewable multivitamin formulated for children in the early growth years and for adult maintenance in late years. It is made with Chinese wolfberry *(Lycium barbarum)* and grain proteins for added immune support, with beta carotene, vitamin C, amino acids, and stevia.

Essential Oils:

Lime *(Citrus aurantiifolia)* is anti-inflammatory, antispasmotic, and supports cardiovascular function.

Mandarin *(Citrus reticulata)* is antifungal, antispasmotic, and promotes digestion.

Orange *(Citrus sinensis)* has been used as an anticoagulant to reduce flatulence and to stimulate circulation.

Companion Products: Body Balance, Essential Manna, Mineral Essence, Power Meal, and Wolfberry Power Bars.

Companion Oil Blends: Gentle Baby, Harmony, Joy, Peace & Calming, and White Angelica.

Suggested Use: Chew three tablets daily with breakfast as a dietary supplement.

Master Formula HERS

Master Formula HERS is formulated to specifically help the special nutritional needs of women.

Companion Supplements: AuraLight, Be-Fit, Estro, FemiGen, and VitaGreen.

Companion Oil Blends: Abundance, Dragon Time, Harmony, Joy, Magnify Your Purpose, and Mister.

Suggested Use: For slow metabolism: take three to six tablets daily. For fast metabolism: take six to eight tablets daily. Take 1/2 the amount before breakfast and 1/2 before dinner. Best taken before meals.

Free of allergens. Contains no artificial flavors, preservatives, sugar, cornstarch, corn, wheat, yeast or soy products.

Frequency: Approximately 88 MHz.

Master Formula HIS

Master Formula HIS is formulated especially for men.

Companion Supplements: Be-Fit, Essential Manna, Mineral Essence, ProGen, Power Meal, Sulfurzyme, VitaGreen, and Wolfberry Power Bars.

Companion Oil Blends: Envision, Magnify Your Purpose, Mister, and Sacred Mountain.

Suggested Use: Take three tablets with breakfast and three with lunch (take before meals).

Frequency: Approximately 86 MHz.

Megazyme

A high-quality enzyme complex that may improve and aid digestion and the elimination of toxic waste from the body. Megazyme was formulated to help supply enzymes to those who have difficulty digesting or assimilating food. Megazyme helps reestablish proper enzyme balance in the digestive system and throughout the body and helps improve intestinal flora. It may also help retard the aging process. Flavor enhanced with essential oils.

Contents:

Pancrelipase is an enzyme used to help digest foods.

Trypsin is an animal product that has amino acid precursor action, carbohydrate conversion, and assimilation.

Carrot powder has the second highest concentration of natural enzymes in vegetables.

Alfalfa sprouts help improve electrolyte balance for digestion.

Pancreatin is an enzyme complex that has been studied for the treatment of cancer.

Papain is a vegetable enzyme and carbohydrate digester.

Bromelain is a natural enzyme and carbohydrate digester.

Betaine HCl helps with the digestion of protein.

cumin assists with the digestion of protein.

Essential Oils:

Tarragon (*Artemisia dracunculus*) is antiviral, antibacterial, and anti-inflammatory.

Peppermint (*Mentha piperita*) has been used for indigestion, ulcers, and gastro-intestinal disorders.

Anise (*Pimpinella anisum*) is excellent in helping alleviate flatulence (gas) and congestion.

Fennel (*Foeniculum vulgare*) has been used for centuries for proper digestion.

Clove (*Syzygium aromaticum*) is beneficial for its antibacterial, antiviral, antifungal, anti-infectious, and antiparasitic properties.

Suggested Use: Take two or three tablets, three times daily or as needed. Take Megazyme with meals, especially protein meals, after 3 p.m., as it will help lessen the burden on the digestive system. Megazyme also helps with digestive functions in the liver.

Companion Products: ComforTone, JuvaTone, Mineral Essence, Mint Condition, Royaldophilus, and Power Meal.

Companion Oil Blends: Di-Tone, Harmony, and JuvaFlex.

Frequency: Approximately 83 MHz.

Mineral Essence

A balanced organic, ionic mineral complex with more than 60 different minerals. Without minerals, vitamins cannot be properly assimilated or absorbed by the body. Mineral Essence has a natural electrolyte balance, which enhances bioavailability, provides antimicrobial protection, and significantly improves oxygenation to the cell, helping to prevent disease and premature aging. Minerals are also necessary for proper immune and metabolism functions.

Mineral essence also includes essential oils to enhance their bioavailability. To demonstrate this, a group of volunteers consumed a teaspoon of liquid trace minerals without any essential oils. Each volunteer experienced diarrhea within 24 hours. Following a washout period of several days, the same volunteers were given double the dosage of the same liquid trace minerals blended with essential oils. None experienced any diarrhea.

In the July 1996 issue of the *Young Living Essential Edge,* an article entitled "Sunburn Relief" contained the following information: "Dr. Alex Schauss, a prominent mineral researcher, has discovered that burns are painful because certain trace minerals are depleted from the skin and surrounding tissue. If the trace minerals are replenished to the affected area, then the pain will subside almost immediately. . . . We have had many who have topically applied Mineral Essence directly on the sunburn or burn and received instant pain relief as the healing process began. . . ."

Contents:

Purified water is needed to dilute the minerals for liquifying this blend.

Honey is a an emulsifier and natural sweetener.

Royal Jelly is a very rich source of proteins and amino acids. It has been traditionally known to prolong youthfulness and improve skin beauty, increase energy, and reduce anxiety, sleepless-ness, moodiness, memory loss, and support the immune system.

Trace minerals include beryllium, bismuth, boron, bromine, calcium, carbon, cesium, chloride, chromium, copper, gallium, germanium, gold, hafnium, indium, iodine, iron, lithium, lutecium, manganese, magnesium, molybdenum, nickel, niobium, nitrogen, oxygen, phosphorus, potassium, rubidium, scandium, selenium, silicon, silver, sodium, strontium, sulfur, tanta-lum, thallium, tin, titanium, tungsten, vanadium, yttrium, zinc, and zirconium.

Essential Oils:

Lemon (*Citrus limon*) promotes leukocyte formation and increases lymphatic (immune) function.

Cinnamon bark (*Cinnamomum verum*) is anti-infectious, antibacterial, antiviral, antifungal, antiparasitic and anticoagulant.

Peppermint (*Mentha piperita*) is anti-infectious, antibacterial, antifungal, and used for pancreatic complaints, sinusitis, laryngitis, and hypotension.

Companion Products: Master Formula HIS/HERS and CHILDREN'S, Royal Essence, Sulfurzyme, VitaGreen, and Wolfberry Power Bars.

Companion Oil Blends: Citrus Fresh, Envision, Gathering, Harmony, and Valor.

Mint Condition

Mint Condition is a vegetarian digestive enzyme complex that combines select herbs with essential oils. It may help soothe irritated digestive systems and reduce inflammation, ulcers, colitis, irritable bowel syndrome, bloating, gas, and acid indigestion. It works well with Megazyme and Di-Tone. Use Megazyme before meals and Mint Condition after meals.

Contents:

Fennel seed powder has been researched for regulation of intestinal flora and as a digestive aid.

Papaya fruit powder is a source of natural fruit enzymes and fiber.

Apple pectin is a source of fiber that may help prevent high cholesterol and cancer and aid digestion.

Peppermint has many beneficial constituents that stimulate the production of digestive fluids. It also has anti-inflammatory and anti-ulcer properties.

Ginger root powder has been used to treat indi-gestion, flatulence, diarrhea, and stomachache.

Spearmint is used for many digestive disorders and as a remedy for flatulence (gas).

Trace minerals are needed for proper electro-lyte balance, and all functions in the body are dependent on these. They are essential for proper digestion and elimination.

Essential Oils:

Peppermint (*Mentha piperita*) has been used for indigestion, ulcers, and gastro-intestinal disorders for centuries. Recent clinical studies have shown it to reduce the intestinal spasms.

Spearmint (*Mentha spicata*) improves digestion.

Ginger (*Zingiber officinale*) improves digestion and combats constipation.

Tarragon (*Artemisia dracunculus*) is antipar-asitic, antispasmotic, and antiviral.

Companion Products: ComforTone, JuvaTone, Megazyme, Mineral Essence, Royaldophilus, and Power Meal.

Companion Oil Blends: Di-Tone, Harmony, and JuvaFlex.

ParaFree

An advanced blend of some of the strongest essential oils that have been studied for their antiparasitic properties.

Base Oils:

Sesame seed and olive oil.

Essential Oils:

Cumin (*Cuminum Cyminum*) has been shown to be antiparasitic and antiviral. It supports immune function.

Anise (*Pimpinella anisum*) is antiparasitic and promotes digestion and protein breakdown.

Fennel (*Foeniculum vulgare*) is antiseptic and antiparasitic and improves digestive and pancreatic functions.

Bay laurel (*Laurus nobilis*) is antiseptic, antibacterial, antiparasitic, and antiviral. It is also a diuretic, fungicidal, and digestive aid.

Vetiver (*Vetiveria officinalis*) is antiseptic, anti-inflammatory, and immune-supporting.

Nutmeg (*Myristica fragrans*) supports adrenal glands, is antibacterial and anti-inflammatory, and stimulates immune function. It has also been used to reduce diarrhea.

Melaleuca (*Melaleuca alternifolia*) is antifungal, antiparasitic, and antibacterial.

Idaho tansy (*Tanacetum vulgare*) is one of the most potent worm-expelling essential oils.

Clove (*Sygygium aromaticum*) has potent antiparasitic, antibacterial, and antifungal properties.

Thyme (*Thymus vulgaris*) among the most antiseptic of all of the essential oils.

Companion Products: ComforTone, I.C.P., JuvaTone, Megazyme, Rehemogen, and VitaGreen.

Companion Oil Blends: Di-Tone, JuvaFlex, Purification, Release, and Thieves.

Suggested Use: Take two to four droppers, three times daily for 21 consecutive days for liquid.

Take two to five gelcaps, two to three times a day for 21 consecutive days out of each month for gelcaps.

Repeat for three cycles or as needed. Use ParaFree with ComforTone and I.C.P. for cleansing. The I.C.P. will help break up plaque along the intestinal walls.

Note: Use in moderation during pregnancy, possibly two capsules daily. If diarrhea occurs, discontinue. A good parasite cleanse is recommended before conception. Consult your health care provider before starting a cleansing program.

For additional information, review the book, *Essential Oil Safety—A Guide for Health Care Professionals* by Robert Tisserand and Tony Balacs.

ProGen

ProGen is an all-vegetable and herbal support for the prostate and male glandular system. Saw palmetto is one of the most widely used herbs to combat the prostate enlargement that affects most men over 45. *Pygeum africanum* has been used for years to prevent prostate atrophy and malfunction.

Contents:

Seronoa serrulata (saw palmetto) has been used to help reduce enlarged prostate and relieve the inflammation and pain of benign prostatic hypertrophy.

Dioscorea villosa is another name for wild yam and is antispasmodic and helps supports the reproductive organs.

Pygeum africanum is used to prevent prostate atrophy and malfunction.

L-glutathione is a sulfur-bearing liver antioxidant.

Dl-methylglycine is excellent for heart muscle and tissue support.

L-carnitine supports the heart and helps convert calories into energy. It has been used to help lower cholesterol and improve memory.

Siberian ginseng is used for invigoration or concentration in times of fatigue.

Zinc is important for prostate health. It also may help restore sexual potency.

Essential Oils:

Yarrow (*Achillea millefolium*) is supportive to the prostate and nerves.

Sage (*Salvia officinalis*) has estrogen-like properties and may help balance hormones.

Myrtle (*Myrtus communis*) helps prevent candida and helps prevent an inflamed prostate.

Myrrh (*Commiphora myrrha*) has hormone-like properties and is anti-inflammatory.

Peppermint (*Mentha piperita*) helps decongest the prostate and urinary tract.

Fennel (*Foeniculum vulgare*) has estrogen-like properties and helps balance the hormones.

Lavender (*Lavandula angustifolia*) is calming and balancing.

Companion Products: Be-Fit, Exodus, Goji Berry Tea, Master Formula HIS, Protec, Power Meal, Sulfurzyme, or VitaGreen.

Companion Oil Blends: Exodus, Live with Passion, Magnify Your Purpose, Mister, or Valor.

Radex

Radex is an antioxidant complex that helps prevent the build-up of free radicals from air pollution and radiation while detoxifying, cleansing, and building the systems of the body.

Contents:

Vitamin E (d alpha tocopherol acid succinate) quenches free-radical damage that can contribute to premature aging. It also affords protection against cardiovascular diseases, diabetes, and menopausal conditions, and is beneficial for acne, allergies, and wound healing.

Vitamin C (ascorbic acid) helps the body to manufacture collagen for connective tissue, cartilage, tendons, etc., and is used for proper immune function. It is also an antioxidant.

Pantothenic acid supports adrenal function and the formation of antibodies, aids in vitamin utilization, and helps convert fats, carbohydrates, and proteins into energy.

Selenium has been extensively researched for its anticancer and antioxidant properties.

Wheat germ extract supports the body's ability to regenerate cells and tissue.

cumin helps digest protein and is an excellent antioxidant.

Essential Oils:

Melaleuca (*Melaleuca quinquenervia*) is anti-infectious and antibacterial.

Melaleuca (*Melaleuca alternifolia*) protects the body against radioactive materials and is anti-infectious and antibacterial.

Thyme (*Thymus vulgaris*) is one of the strongest antibacterial, antifungal, and antiviral essential oils.

Clove (*Syzygium aromaticum*) is antibacterial, antifungal, and antiviral.

Chamomile mixta (*Chamaemelum mixtum*) is a hybrid that supports skin and tissues.

Suggested Use: Take two tablets in the morning and two tablets in the evening.

Frequency: Approximately 89 MHz.

Rehemogen

Rehemogen tincture contains herbs that were used by Chief Sundance and the Native Americans as a blood cleanser and builder. **How to use:** Mix one to three droppers, three times daily in distilled water or as desired.

Contents:

Extracts of:

Red clover blossom—used to treat asthma, bronchitis, skin ailments, ulcers, and arthritis. Used in some cultures to prevent recurrence of cancer. Its combined properties act as a diuretic, sedative, and helps calm coughing.

Chaparral—used by Native American healers as a tonic for cancer, snake bite, infection, arthritis, and tuberculosis treatments.

Licorice root—traditionally used to defeat a host of degenerative ailments, including arthritis, asthma, bronchial ailments, cancer, catarrh, circulatory dysfunction, colitis, dyspepsia, irritable bowel syndrome, liver disorders, rheumatism, stress, and vertigo

Oregon grape root—contains berberine, a powerful liver protectant.

Sarsaparilla—contains saponins, steroid-like molecules that neutralize endotoxins, poisons secreted by fungi and bacteria in the human body that contribute to many kinds of disease.

Cascara sagrada—used to support the liver, pancreas, gallbladder, and stomach.

Burdock root—eaten as a vegetable in Japan, this root has been used to treat ulcers and arthritis, cleanse the blood, and cure skin diseases.

Essential Oils of:

Rosemary (*Rosmarinus officinalis*)—researched for its antiseptic and antimicrobial properties. It may be beneficial for the skin. It helps overcome mental fatigue.

Thyme (*Thymus vulgaris*)—one of the most antimicrobial and antiseptic essential oils.

Melaleuca (*Melaleuca alternifolia*)—highly regarded as an antimicrobial and antiseptic essential oil.

Roman chamomile (*Chamaemelum nobile*)—promotes the flow of bile to and from the liver, a key aspect of cleansing and detoxification.

Also contains: Buckthorn bark, stillingia, and prickly ash bark.

Royaldophilus

Royaldophilus is an outstanding source of *Lactobacillus acidophilus* and *bifidus* cultures required for optimum health. Derived from whole milk, these friendly bacteria are our first-line defense against disease and fungus overgrowth in the gastrointestinal system.

Excessive use of antibiotics and other drugs, chlorinated water, and processed foods reduces the number of friendly bacteria in our intestines, which can lead to systemic yeast infection (candida). Currently in the U.S., about 70 percent of females and 30 percent of males suffer from some form of candida overgrowth.

Acidophilus may remain potent for several weeks without refrigeration; however, it is recommended that it be refrigerated before opening the bottle and kept refrigerated at less than 40 degrees. It is unwise to freeze acidophilus as this may affect its potency.

Acidophilus works with the enzymes to digest our food. It also aids the growth of intestinal flora. When we have a good enzyme base, acidophilus will complement enzyme production. It is extremely important for acidophilus to implant on the intestinal wall for the returning of intestinal flora. *Acidophilus lactobacillus bifidus* derived from milk is the only form recognized and accepted by the human body. The whole milk acidophilus used in Royaldophilus provides greater culture and inhibits allergy reaction.

Plantain reduces digestive problems and is very soothing to irritable bowel problems where intestinal flora is absent. This formula has proven to be superior to all forms of acidophilus.

Contents:

Lactobacillus and *bifidus* cultures contain the best natural digestive aid, acidophilus, which has many benefits, including correcting lactose intolerance, eliminating bad breath and acne, reducing cholesterol, inhibiting candida, and preventing yeast infection.

Plantain has been used for bleeding of the lungs and stomach, consumption, and dysentery.

Companion Products: ComforTone, I.C.P., Megazyme, and VitaGreen.

Companion Oil Blends: Di-Tone, Forgiveness, JuvaFlex, Harmony, Release, and Thieves.

Royal Essence

Royal Essence promotes high energy.

Contents:

Yerba mate was a household cure for the Guarani people who used it to boost immunity, cleanse and detoxify the blood, tone the nervous system, combat fatigue, reduce stress, and stimulate the mind.

Stevia leaf extract supports pancreas function.

Aloe vera is is a natural laxative and lubricant, and helps relax the colon.

Trace minerals help restore electrolyte balance in the cells.

Royal jelly a viscous, milky white secretion produced by the worker bee upon which future queens are continually nourished. Royal jelly's chemistry has been extensively studied and contains all the essential amino acids, unsaturated fats, natural sugars, minerals, and vitamins.

Siberian ginseng strengthens the adrenal glands, enhances immune function, normalizes blood pressure, improves mental alertness, and promotes hormonal balance.

Fennel seed stimulates the gastrointestinal mucous membrane, which in turn stimulates the pancreas to secrete digestive enzymes to dissolve undigested proteins. It is antiparasitic.

Peppermint extract helps the digestion process and absorption.

Bee pollen is high in protein and low in fat and sodium. It contains many minerals and vitamins. including potassium, calcium, magnesium, zinc, manganese, copper, and B vitamins.

Also contains water, piper dilatatum, fo-ti extract, black walnut, licorice root, gentian extract, comfrey root extract, fennel seed extract, peppermint extract, bayberry extract, myrrh extract, bee pollen, saffron extract, eucalyptus globulus extract, lemongrass extract, cayenne extract.

Essential Oils:

Rosemary (*Rosmarinus officinalis*) helps fight candida and balance the endocrine system.

Nutmeg (*Myristica fragrans*) helps support the adrenal glands for increased energy.

Melaleuca alternifolia highly regarded as an antimicrobial and antiseptic essential oil. Pure melaleuca has high levels of terpinenol, which is the key active constituent.

Clove (*Syzygium aromaticum*) is anti-infectious, antiviral, antifungal, antiparasitic, and has been used in European hospitals for viral hepatitis, bronchitis, flu, sinusitis, and cholera.

Black pepper (*Piper nigrum)* is a stimulating, energizing essential oil that has been studied for its effects on cellular oxygenation.

Power Meal

Power Meal is a complete vegetarian protein drink mix powder containing Chinese wolfberry and rice protein with a large spectrum of antioxidant herbs, vitamins, enzymes, and minerals. Whether used as a meal alternative or snack, Power Meal can serve as an excellent weight management tool. Free of fats and synthetic ingredients, Power Meal provides most of the building blocks the body requires for regeneration and maintenance.

The protein-rich formula of Power Meal, when combined with exercise and proper nutrition, can help the body build lean muscle tissue, which is the foundation of a lean physique and an important element in weight management. Because muscle burns 22 times as many calories as fat, the addition of muscle tissue can significantly accelerate metabolism and contribute to a more slender body. Because muscle tissue weighs more than fat tissue, the addition of muscle mass to the body may not always be accompanied by weight loss, even though body fat may have dropped substantially.

Contents:

Chinese wolfberry (*Lycium barbarum*) has 18 amino acids, 21 trace minerals, beta carotene, and vitamins B1, B2, B6, and E. It is an excellent whole food and has many functions in the body.

Rice protein concentrate is high in branched chain amino acids required for building muscles.

Siberian ginseng root strengthens the adrenal glands, enhances immune function, normalizes blood pressure, improves mental alertness, and promotes hormonal balance.

Stevia leaf extract supports pancreas function.

Ginkgo biloba extract increases energy, improves memory and is excellent for cerebral circulation, oxygenation, and blood flow.

Bee pollen is high in protein and low in fat and sodium. It contains many minerals and vitamins. including potassium, calcium, magnesium, zinc, manganese, copper, and B vitamins.

Guar gum promotes healthy colon function.

Calcium carbonate is needed for healthy bones, teeth, and joints.

Lecithin (food for the brain) is excellent for liver disorders and helps to balance cholesterol.

Choline bitartrate has been used in the treatment of many liver disorders (including elevated cholesterol levels), Alzheimer's disease, viral hepatitis, and cirrhosis.

Silicon is required for skin, ligaments, bones, and tendons.

Magnesium is also crucial for proper enzyme function, muscle contractions, and heart rhythm. High intake can reduce high blood pressure, fight arteriosclerosis, and improve insulin action.

Potassium is important for proper muscle and nerve cell function.

MSM supports healthy hair, skin, liver, and immune function.

Inositol helps the liver rid itself of fat and bile.

Betaine HCl promotes protein digestion.

Amylase promotes fat digestion.

Kelp contains iodine, which is necessary to prevent goiters.

PABA (para amino benzoic acid) assists healthy bacteria in producing folic acid and helps form red blood cells.

L-carnitine helps convert fatty acids into energy.

Zinc is crucial for proper immune function and is needed for proper action of many hormones, including insulin and growth hormone. It helps improve wound healing.

Boron promotes the absorption and utilization of calcium.

Betatene is a mixed-carotenoid complex containing lycopene, lutein, zeaxanthin, and alpha carotene.

Copper is necessary for proper red blood cell and immune function.

Manganese citrate is an antioxidant that regulates blood sugar levels and increases cellular energy.

Vitamin E protects the heart and blood and combats free-radical oxidative damage.

Vitamin B3 is essential for turning carbohydrates into energy. It lowers cholesterol and helps regulate blood sugar.

Pantothenic acid supports antibody formation, aids in vitamin utilization, and helps convert fats, carbohydrates, and proteins into energy

Vitamin D3 stimulates the absorption of calcium and exerts many anticancerous properties, especially against breast and colon cancer.

Vitamin B6 supports immune function and protects the heart and blood vessels. It inhibits skin cancer growth and helps prevent kidney stones and PMS symptoms. Vitamin B6 requires folic acid and magnesium to maximize its effects.

Selenium has been extensively researched for its anticancer and antioxidant properties.

Riboflavin has shown to be crucial in the production of energy and is involved in regenerating glutathione and may help prevent certain esophageal cancers.

Thiamine HCl functions as part of an enzyme essential for energy production, carbohydrate metabolism, and nerve cell function.

Chromium improves insulin sensitivity and blood sugar metabolism.

Folic acid plays an important role in cardiovascular health and helps prevent neural tube defects.

Biotin helps convert fats and amino acids into energy. It promotes healthy nails and hair and combats yeast and fungus overgrowth.

Vitamin B12 is critical for red blood cell formation and proper immune and nerve function.

Also includes: Vanilla, Fructose, and Maltodextrin

Essential Oils:

Grapefruit (*Citrus paradisi*) has been used for disinfection and cellulite elimination.

Orange (*Citrus sinensis)* is anti-inflammatory, antispasmodic, and anticoagulant.

Lemon (*Citrus limon*) promotes leukocyte formation and increases immune function.

Cypress (*Cupressus sempervirens*) helps improve circulation and improve lymph flow.

Anise (*Pimpinella anisum*) promotes digestion and helps eliminate parasites.

Fennel (*Foeniculum vulgare*) is antiparasitic, antimicrobial, antispasmodic, helps regulate intestinal flora, is a digestive aid, and increases gastric secretions.

Nutmeg (*Myristica fragrans*) helps support the adrenal glands for increased energy.

Companion Products: Be-Fit, ComforTone, Essential Manna, I.C.P., Master Formula HERS/HIS, Megazyme, Thyromin, VitaGreen, and Wolfberry Power Bars.

Companion Oil Blends: Abundance, Citrus Fresh, EndoFlex, Envision, Live with Passion, and Magnify Your Purpose.

Stevia Extract

Stevia extract is a super-sweet, low-calorie dietary supplement that helps regulate blood sugar and supports the pancreas. It is valuable for anyone with diabetes and hypoglycemia.

It is a wonderful aid to weight loss and weight management because it contains no calories. In addition, research indicates that it significantly increases glucose tolerance and inhibits glucose absorption. People who ingest stevia daily often report a decrease in their desire for sweets and fatty foods. It may also improve digestion and gastrointestinal function, soothe upset stomachs, and help speed recovery from minor illnesses.

Stevia also inhibits the growth of some bacteria and infectious organisms, including those that cause tooth decay and gum disease. Many individuals using stevia have reported a lower incidence of colds and flu. Many who have used stevia as a mouthwash have experienced a significant decrease in gum disease.

When topically applied, stevia softens the skin and smooths out wrinkles while healing various skin blemishes, acne, seborrhea, dermatitis, and eczema. When used on cuts and wounds, stevia promotes rapid healing without scarring.

Contents:

Stevia leaf extract—intensely sweet with a mild licorice-like aftertaste.

Companion Products: AuraLight, Megazyme, Mineral Essence, Thyromin, and VitaGreen.

Companion Oil Blends: JuvaFlex and Thieves.

Suggested Use: As a dietary supplement and for skin care.

Stevia Select

Stevia Select is the powdered form of a popular South American food supplement combined with fructooligosaccharides that may balance blood sugar levels and support a healthy pancreas. This product is an excellent supplement for diabetics.

Contents:

Fructooligosaccharides (FOS) are one of the best-documented natural nutrients for promoting the growth the *lactobacilli* and bifidobacteria that are the linchpin of sound health. FOS has also been clinically studied for its ability to increase magnesium and calcium absorption, lower blood glucose, cholesterol, and LDL levels, and to inhibit production of the reductase enzymes that can contribute to cancer. Because FOS may increase magnesium absorption, it may also lead to lowered blood pressure and better cardiovascular health.

In addition, FOS also has another benefit: It has a naturally sweet taste.

Stevia leaf extract is an all-natural supplement. *(See Stevia for further nutritional information.)*

Companion Products: Megazyme, Mineral Essence, Power Meal, Stevia, Thyromin, and VitaGreen.

Companion Oil Blends: JuvaFlex and Thieves.

Sulfurzyme

Sulfurzyme is a unique combination of methyl-sulfonylmethane (MSM), the protein-building compound found in breast milk, fresh fruits and vegetables, and Chinese wolfberry (*Lycium barbarum*). Together, they create a new concept in balancing the immune system and supporting almost every major function of the body. Of particular importance is the ability of MSM to equalize water pressure inside of the cells—a considerable benefit for those plagued with bursitis, arthritis, and tendonitis.

Chinese wolfberry is contained in this product to supply the necessary nutrients for the proper assimilation and metabolism of sulfur.

Contents:

Methylsulfonylmethane (MSM)—a natural form of sulfur found in all living organisms, combats rheumatism, asthma, bursitis, and tendonitis, as well as autoimmune diseases, like arthritis, lupus, scleroderma, and allergies. One of the best sources of nutritional sulfur, MSM is critical to proper skin health, hair and nail growth, and liver function. MSM is the subject of a bestselling book, *The Miracle of MSM, The Natural Solution for Pain*, authored by UCLA neuropsychiatrist Ronald Lawrence M.D., Ph.D., and Stanley Jacob, M.D.

Chinese wolfberry (*Lycium barbarum*) contains minerals and coenzymes to support sulfur metabolism.

Companion Products: Arthro Plus, ArthroTune, ComforTone, I.C.P., Master HIS/HERS and CHILDREN'S, Megazyme, Ortho Ease and Ortho Sport massage oils, Power Meal and Ultra Young.

Companion Oil Blends: En-R-Gee, Envision, Magnify Your Purpose, PanAway, and Valor.

Super B

Super B is a comprehensive source of the B vitamins essential for good health, including, thiamine (vitamin B1), riboflavin (vitamin B2), niacin (vitamin B3), pyridoxine (vitamin B6), vitamin B12, biotin, folic acid, and PABA. It also includes minerals that aid the assimilation and metabolism of B vitamins.

B vitamins are particularly important during times of stress when reserves are depleted. Although research has shown that megadoses of B vitamins are not healthy, it has been known that the diets of many Americans do not provide the recommended amount of B vitamins that is essential for normal functions of immune response.

When many B vitamins are combined at once in the stomach, it can cause a fermentation resulting in stomach upset. To avoid this, Super B uses a synergistic suspension isolation process to isolate the various vitamins so they are released at different times.

Contents:

Folic acid is important in lowering homocysteine levels and protecting the heart and blood vessels. It also helps prevent osteoporosis, candidiasis, epilepsy, gout, and periodontal disease.

Thiamin (vitamin B1) is essential for energy production, carbohydrate metabolism, and nerve cell function.

Riboflavin (vitamin B2) is crucial in the production of cellular energy, helps regenerate the liver-protecting antioxidant glutathione, and may help prevent migraine headaches and some esophageal cancers.

Niacin is essential for turning carbohydrates into energy. It lowers cholesterol and helps regulate blood sugar. At least 4.4 mg is needed for every 1,000 calories consumed to avoid pellagra.

Vitamin B6 supports immune function and protects the heart and blood vessels. It inhibits skin cancer growth and helps prevent kidney stones and PMS symptoms. Vitamin B6 requires folic acid and magnesium to maximize its effects.

Vitamin B12 helps prevent deterioration of mental functioning, neurological damage, and a number of psychological disturbances. Vegetarians often lack adequate B12, since this nutrient is not found in non-animal products.

Biotin helps convert fats and amino acids into energy. It promotes healthy nails and hair and combats yeast and fungus overgrowth.

Magnesium is crucial for proper enzyme function and is needed for normal muscle contractions and heart rhythm. High intake can reduce high blood pressure, fight arteriosclerosis, and improve insulin action.

PABA (para amino benzoic acid) assists healthy bacteria in producing folic acid. It also helps the bones form red blood cells.

Zinc is crucial for proper immune function and is needed for proper action of many hormones, including insulin and growth hormone. It helps improve wound healing.

Selenium has been extensively researched for its anticancer and antioxidant properties.

Suggested Use: Take one-half to one tablet daily, preferably with a meal and not on an empty stomach.

Note: If taken on an empty stomach, one may experience a niacin flush, which may last up to an hour.

Frequency: Approximately 63 MHz.

Super C

Research has shown that physical stress, alcohol, smoking, and using certain medications may lower the blood levels of this essential vitamin. When citrus fruits are not readily available, diets may not contain enough vitamin C. Super C is properly balanced with rutin, biotin, bioflavonoids, and trace minerals to work synergistically, balancing the electrolytes and increasing the absorption rate of vitamin C. Without bioflavonoids, vitamin C has a hard time getting inside cells; and without proper electrolyte balance and trace minerals, it will not stay there for long.

Contents:

Vitamin C helps the body manufacture collagen for connective tissue, cartilage, tendons, etc., and is used for proper immune function, as well as an antioxidant.

Citrus bioflavonoids are anti-inflammatory, antiallergic, antiviral, and anticarcinogenic. They have been used to prevent heart disease.

Rutin helps prevent capillary fragility, easy bruising, swelling, and nosebleeds.

Calcium carbonate is needed for healthy bones, teeth, and joints.

Zinc is crucial for proper immune function and is needed for proper action of many hormones, including insulin and growth hormone. It helps improve wound healing.

Potassium is required for proper electrolyte balance and to prevent high blood pressure.

Essential Oils:

Orange (*Citrus sinensis*) helps reduce fluid retention.

Tangerine (*Citrus reticulata)* is an anticoagulant and helps decongest the lymphatic system.

Lemon (*Citrus limon*) promotes leukocyte formation and increases lymphatic function.

Grapefruit (*Citrus paradisi*) has been used for disinfection and cellulite elimination.

Lemongrass (*Cymbopogon flexuosus*) is antiparasitic, antifungal, and promotes digestion.

Companion Products: Exodus, ImmuGel, ImmuneTune, Rehemogen, and VitaGreen.

Companion Oil Blends: Citrus Fresh, Exodus II, ImmuPower, Motivation, Thieves, or Valor.

Suggested Use: For reinforcing immune strength, two tablets daily. For maintenance, one tablet daily. Best taken before meals.

Frequency: Approximately 80 MHz.

Super Cal

Formulated with calcium, potassium, and magnesium citrate (which is easier for the body to utilize) specifically for proper electrolyte balance, hormonal balance, and muscle and bone development.

Contents:

Calcium supports healthy bones and teeth and helps prevent kidney stones.

Magnesium works with calcium to build strong bones. It is also crucial for proper enzyme function, muscle contractions, and heart rhythm. High intake can reduce high blood pressure, fight arteriosclerosis, and improve insulin action.

Potassium is crucial for proper cellular fluid balance. It plays a role in reducing high blood pressure, increasing insulin sensitivity, and improving bone density.

Boron helps with the absorption and utilization of calcium.

Essential Oils:

Birch (*Betula alleghaniensis*) assists with bone, joint, and muscle pain.

Marjoram (*Origanum majorana*) supports muscles and nerves.

Lemongrass (*Cymbopogon flexuosus*) is used for ligament support.

Myrtle (*Myrtus communis*) has been researched for its effects in soothing the respiratory system.

Companion Products: Arthro Plus, ArthroTune, Megazyme, Ortho Sport and Ortho Ease massage oils, Power Meal, and Sulfurzyme.

Companion Oil Blends: Grounding, Harmony, PanAway, and Valor.

Suggested Use: Take one to two capsules before each meal.

Frequency: Approximately 78 MHz.

Thyromin

This product was developed to nourish the thyroid, balance metabolism, and reduce fatigue. It contains a combination of specially selected glandular nutrients, herbs, amino acids, minerals, and essential oils. All of the oils are therapeutic-grade quality and are perfectly balanced to bring about the most beneficial and nutritional support to the thyroid.

Contents:

Vitamin E is a potent antioxidant that protects against cardiovascular disease, diabetes, and menopausal conditions.

Iodine (kelp) is a key component of the T3 and T4 thyroid hormones that are pivotal for increasing energy levels and metabolism.

Potassium supports healthy thyroid function.

CoQ10 is used by cells in the body to convert food to energy. Heart cells require more CoQ10 to maintain muscle strength because of their higher demand for energy. CoQ10 helps in the prevention of heart disease and cancer and may help protect against blood cholesterol.

L-cysteine is an amino acid that supports proper liver function and healthy hair.

L-cystine is an amino acid that supports healthy liver function and hair.

In a base of: Irish moss and adrenal and pituitary extracts.

Essential Oils:

Peppermint (*Mentha piperita*) supports digestion and pancreatic function.

Spearmint (*Mentha spicata*) has hormone-like properties that support the thyroid.

Myrtle (*Myrtus communis*) may help increase thyroid function.

Myrrh (*Commiphora myrrha*) has hormone-like properties and is anti-inflammatory.

Companion Products: FemiGen, JuvaTone, Megazyme, Mineral Essence, Ultra Young, and VitaGreen.

Companion Oil Blends: Clarity, En-R-Gee, EndoFlex, JuvaFlex, and Magnify Your Purpose.

Suggested Use: Take one to two capsules daily, immediately before going to sleep.

Frequency: Approximately 52 MHz.

Ultra Young

Ultra Young is a revolutionary spray supplement that supports healthy pituitary and growth hormone secretion. It contains *Vicia faba*, which contains L-dopa. In 1976 a National Institute of Aging study found that administration of L-dopa to patients over 60 years of age resulted in a dramatic increase in growth hormone levels. A study conducted by Dr. George Cotzias showed that mice, fed small doses of L-dopa, lived twice as long as the control group not receiving L-dopa.

Contents:

Vicia faba major contains unusually high concentrations of L-dopa, an amino acid that has been shown in several studies to restore the sensitivity of the hypothalamus, which can lead to dramatic increases in both GHRH and GH levels.

Chinese wolfberry (*Lycium barbarum*) is rich in polysaccharides, which have potent immune-stimulating effects. These polysaccharides appear to be highly effective in raising levels of immunoglobulin A (IgA), an immune protein that steadily declines with age.

L-arginine is an amino acid that helps increase natural growth hormone production.

L-glutamine is an amino acid that has been researched for its hGH-promoting effects.

Zinc complex plays a pivotal part in maintaining optimal pituitary function.

GABA (Gamma-aminobutyric acid) is a nutrient that can amplify growth hormone production.

Vitamin B3 provides nutritional support for the hypothalamus and pituitary.

Vitamin B6 supports glandular and cognitive function.

Vitamin E protects the heart and blood and combats free-radical oxidative damage.

Selenium has been extensively researched for its anticancer and antioxidant properties.

Stevia is a super sweet supplement.

Contains therapeutic-grade essential oils of:

Sandalwood (*Santalum album*) is high in sesquiterpenes, which stimulate the hypothalamus and pituitary glands.

Fleabane *(Conyza canadensis)* overcomes retarded puberty, according to Dr. Daniel Penoël.

Companion Products: A.D.&E., Be-Fit, Essential Manna, JuvaTone, Mineral Essence, Power Meal, Sulfurzyme, Vitagreen, and Wolfberry Power Bars.

Companion Oil Blends: Abundance, En-R-Gee, EndoFlex, Envision, Joy, JuvaFlex, Live with Passion, Magnify Your Purpose, Release, and Valor.

Suggested Use: Spray Ultra Young directly inside cheeks and on the roof of the mouth. Avoid swallowing for one to two minutes. Spray upon waking, between meals, and just before retiring. Avoid spraying on the tongue because this reduces its effectiveness. It is best used one to two hours before or after meals, with no snacking in between because high blood sugar levels also reduce its effectiveness.

Ultra Young +

Contains the same ingredients as Ultra Young but with the addition of DHEA, a precursor to many important hormones.

VitaGreen

This supplement is a high protein, high-energy chlorophyll formula that invigorates and revitalizes the body. It contains ingredients that help cleanse the blood and support the immune, thyroid, and digestive systems.

Contents:

Spirulina is a source of chlorophyll, a magnesium-rich pigment that has been linked to improved energy and metabolism.

Barley grass juice concentrate is an antioxidant that is rich in minerals.

Bee pollen is high in protein and low in fat and sodium. It is loaded with vitamins and minerals, including potassium, calcium, magnesium, zinc, manganese, copper, and B vitamins.

Panax ginseng boosts energy and reduces stress. It also has the unique ability to stimulate lymphocyte formation (an essential part of the immune system).

L-arginine is an amino acid that promotes circulation in the small capillaries of our tissues, allowing greater nutrient absorption and cellular metabolism.

L-cystine is an amino acid that supports healthy liver function and hair.

L-tyrosine supports the formation of neurotransmitters, such as dopamine and serotonin.

Choline bitartrate has been used in the treatment of Alzheimer's disease and many liver disorders, including elevated cholesterol levels, viral hepatitis, and cirrhosis.

Kelp contains iodine that helps prevent goiters, thyroid hormonal imbalance, and estrogen imbalance.

Essential Oils:

Melissa (*Melissa officinalis*) is anti-inflammatory and energizing.

Lemon (*Citrus limon*) helps dissolve cholesterol and increase lymphatic (immune) function.

Lemongrass (*Cymbopogon flexuosus*) is antiparasitic, antifungal, and promotes digestion.

Rosemary (*Rosmarinus officinalis*) helps fight candida and balance the endocrine system.

Companion Products: AuraLight, Be-Fit, Juva-Tone, Royal Essence, Power Meal, Sulfurzyme, Thyromin, and Wolfberry Power Bars.

Companion Oil Blends: Abundance, Awaken, En-R-Gee, Envision, JuvaFlex, Live with Passion, Magnify Your Purpose, Motivation, Release, and Valor.

Suggested Use: Take three capsules, three times daily.

Frequency: Approximately 76 MHz.

Experience has shown that before putting oils in VitaGreen, there was 42 percent blood absorption in 24 hours. After adding essential oils to VitaGreen, blood absorption increased to 64 percent in 30 minutes and 86 percent in an hour. The conclusion was that the cells were now receiving nutrients that they had previously not been able to assimilate.

Wolfberry Power Bar (Peanut or Almond)

Wolfberry Power Bars are rich in the essential amino acids and minerals for building muscle and supporting immunity. These power bars combine Chinese wolfberries (over 15 percent protein) with amaranth (over 16 percent protein). Amaranth is rich in L-lysine, an essential amino acid lacking in traditional cereal grains, such as wheat and oats. The Power Bars also include dried cranberries and essential oils of orange and cinnamon. These essential oils are high in phenylpropanes and may activate the amino acid conversion of L-leucine in the body. L-leucine is converted into HMB, a powerful muscle builder.

Contents:

Rice protein concentrate is high in branched chain amino acids (valine, leucine, and isoleucine), which are crucial for muscle building.

Chinese wolfberry (*Lycium barbarum*) has been used for many years to help combat cancer and improve the immune system.

Honey is an emulsifier and natural sweetener.

Puffed amaranth is a South American grain rich in the amino acid L-lysine. Many traditional cereals, such as wheat and corn, lack sufficient amounts of L-lysine for optimum health.

Coconut is added for flavoring.

Cranberries have been proven effective for treatment of urinary tract infections in a number of clinical trials. Its action may be due to an antibacterial compound, hippuric acid, as well as other compounds that reduce the ability of bacteria to adhere to the lining of the bladder and urethra.

Soy protein is a complete source of amino acids, the building blocks of muscles and immunity. The FDA recently recognized soy's ability to combat cardiovascular disease and protect the heart.

Contains therapeutic-grade essential oils of:

Orange (*Citrus sinensis*) helps reduce fluid retention.

Cinnamon (*Cinnamomum verum*) is anti-infectious, antibacterial, antiviral, antifungal, antiparasitic, anticoagulant, and is used for all types of infections. It is used in the Wolfberry Power Bars as a natural preservative.

Companion Products: Be-Fit, ComforTone, Essential Manna, I.C.P., Master Formula HERS/HIS and CHILDREN'S, Megazyme, Thyromin, and VitaGreen.

Companion Oil Blends: Abundance, Citrus Fresh, EndoFlex, Envision, Live with Passion, and Magnify Your Purpose.

CHAPTER 10

Oral Hygiene

Antibacterial and Antiseptic

Essential oils are ideal for use in oral care products because they are both antiseptic and non-toxic—a rare combination. Jean Valnet, M.D., who used essential oils for decades in his clinical practice emphasized this: "Essential oils are especially valuable as antiseptics because their aggression toward microbial germs is matched by their total harmlessness toward tissue."

Dentarome, Dentarome Plus, and Fresh Essence Mouthwash use therapeutic-grade essential oils at the heart of their formulas. These oils include peppermint, birch, eucalyptus, thyme and a proprietary blend of therapeutic-grade essential oils, including clove, lemon, cinnamon, and rosemary. This blend was tested at Weber State University and found to dramatically inhibit the growth of many types of bacteria (both gram negative and gram positive), including *Micrococcus luteus* and *Staphylococcus aureus*. Even more remarkably, this blend exhibited a 99.96 percent kill rate against tough gram negative bacteria, like *Pseudomonas aeruginosa*. These bacteria, because of their thicker cell walls, tend to be far more resistant to antiseptics.

Dentarome Toothpaste

Dentarome is formulated with pure, natural ingredients, such as vegetable glycerine, sodium bicarbonate, ionic minerals, and steviocide (a natural, intensely-sweet extract from a tropical plant native to South America). In addition, Dentarome uses an exclusive formula of uniquely antiseptic and anti-microbial therapeutic-grade essential oils to combat plaque-causing microorganisms. Dentarome leaves the mouth fresh, fragrant, and clean.

Dentarome was tested at Weber State University and found to have potent antimicrobial properties against a wide range of oral microbes, including *Streptococcus oralis*, *Streptoccus pneumoniae,* and *Candida albicans.*

Dentarome Plus includes a higher concentration of thymol and eugenol for extra antiseptic action. Thymol is derived from thyme oil *(Thymus vulgaris)* and eugenol is derived from clove oil *(Syzygium aromaticum).*

Fresh Essence Mouthwash

Free from dyes, alcohol, preservatives, and other synthetic ingredients, Fresh Essence uses medicinal-grade essential oils, such as thyme, eucalyptus, birch, peppermint, and Thieves. These oils contain natural compounds clinically proven to kill the bacteria that can cause bad breath, plaque, and gum diseases, such as gingivitis. By using the entire essential oil rather than isolated active ingredients, Fresh Essence gains significant advantages in safety and antiseptic power. The complete oils of eucalyptus and thyme exhibit far stronger antimicrobial power than their active constituents alone. These whole oils are also safer because they contain a natural balance of elements that makes them nondamaging to human tissue.

Fresh Essence is also formulated with a patented liposome technology (using soy-derived lecithin) that binds the essential oils to the mucus membrane inside the mouth. This enables the essential oils to remain in the mouth longer so that they can provide long-lasting, germ-killing and breath-freshening effects.

Benefits of Liposomes in Fresh Essence

Controlled-release liposomes are a key ingredient in Fresh Essence Mouthwash. These liposomes adhere to either tooth enamel or mucus membranes in the mouth. The two primary benefits of using liposome technology are:

1. **Controlled release of active ingredients**

2. **Ingredient protection**

The controlled-release aspect of liposome technology is enhanced through the use of a patented "liposome anchoring" system. Liposomes

155

Comparing Toothpastes

	Dentarome & Dentarome Plus	Common Brand
Active Ingredients	Thieves*	Sodium Fluoride
	Thymol	Sodium Monofluorophosphate
	Eugenol	
	Birch oil	
Foaming Agent	None	Sodium Laurel Sulfate (SLS) **
Tooth Health Agent	Ionic Minerals	Pentasodium triphosphate
	Birch Oil	Tetrasodium pyrophosphate
Moisturizer	Vegetable Glycerine	Glycerine, sorbitol
Sweetener	Steviocide	Sodium saccharin
Coloring	None	Titanium Dioxide FD&C Blue #1
Cleansing Agent	Baking Soda	Abrasive Silica Synthetic Glycerine
Flavoring	Peppermint Oil	Artificial Sources Natural Sources
Thickener	Xanthum Gum	Xanthum Gum, Cellulose Gum

* A proprietary blend of clove, lemon, cinnamon, Eucalyptus radiata, rosemary.
** Also known as sodium laureth sulfate.

Comparing Mouthwashes

	Fresh Essence Mouthwash	Common Brand
Active Ingredients	Thieves*	Thymol
	Thyme oil	1,8 cineol
	Eucalyptus oil	Menthol
	Birch oil	Methyl Salicylate
	Peppermint oil	
Base	Water	Alcohol, SD Alcohol
Sweetener	Steviocide	Sodium saccharin
	Sorbitol	
Coloring	None	D&C Yellow #10
		FD&C Green #3
		FD&C Blue #1
		FD&C Yellow #5
Flavoring	Peppermint	Artificial Sources
Preservatives	None	Benzoic Acid
		Polysorbate 80
Dispersant	Natural Lecithin	Poloxamer 403
		Sodium Hydroxide (Lye)
		Synthetic Glycerine

*A proprietary blend of clove, lemon, cinnamon, eucalyptus radiata, rosemary.

that adhere to dental enamel can be used to improve dental health, because they contain active materials to prevent plaque formation, treat periodontal disease, and prevent dental caries. These active materials can be released slowly, enhancing their benefits.

The ability of dental liposomes to slowly release their therapeutic cargo is demonstrated in Fig. 1. A saliva-coated tooth is dipped into a solution containing dental liposomes. The liposomes contain a test material. The tooth is sequentially washed with 1.0 ml. of buffer 30 times. The test material is removed slowly with the washes. Even after 30 washes, some active material is retained on the tooth.

Slow Release Systems for Oral Soft Tissues

Liposomal systems that adhere to mucus membranes are designed to slowly release beneficial chemicals in the mouth, nose, and other tissues coated with mucin. This is useful in the slow release of flavors. For example, a breath lozenge containing menthol that is contained in a mucin-binding system can provide extended oral freshness longer than a standard menthol lozenge (Fig. 2).

In another experiment, two thymol-based mouthwashes were compared side by side. The first was a standard commercial product with no liposome-based delivery; the second used a liposomal delivery system. The results of the experiment are illustrated in Fig. 3. The level of thymol measured in saliva over a period of five minutes was measured. With the commercial product, thymol levels dropped off quickly, whereas with the liposome-based mouthwash, there was a significantly higher level of thymol in each saliva sample.

Liposomal Binding to Teeth

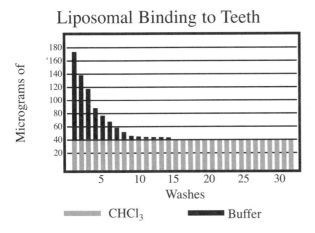

Figure 1. A saliva-coated human tooth was dipped in a solution of dental liposomes and rinsed repeatedly with 1.0 ml of water.

Controlled Release
Retention of thymol in the mouth

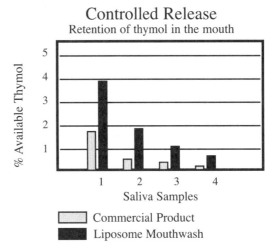

Figure 3. The retention of thymol was measured over a period of five minutes in various saliva samples. The level of thymol remaining in the saliva dropped off rapidly following usage of the commercial product. However, following usage of the liposome-based mouthwash, there was a significantly higher level of thymol in each saliva sample analyzed.

Comparison of Coolness
Retention of menthol flavor in the mouth

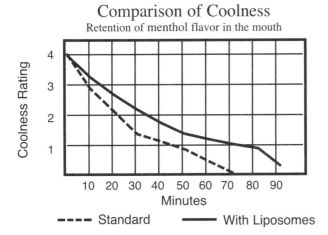

Figure 2. Lozenges made with mucin-binding system to release menthol flavor slowly are compared to control menthol lozenges. Timing began when the lozenge was completely dissolved in the mouth.

CHAPTER 11

Massage Oils

Massage and therapeutic touch have been part of both physical and emotional healing. When essential oils are combined with massage, the benefits are numerous. Massage improves circulation, lymphatic drainage, and aids in the elimination of tissue wastes. The oils bring peace and tranquility as well as keen mental awareness. Massage opens and increases the flow of energy, balancing the entire nervous system and helping to release physical and emotional disharmony. The unrefined carrier vegetable oils are rich in fat-soluble nutrients and essential fatty acids, easily absorbed through the skin and used in the body.

Cel-Lite Magic Massage Oil

Cel-Lite Magic combines vegetable oils and vitamin E with essential oils that tone and nourish the skin. Orange *(Citrus sinensis)* and grapefruit *(Citrus paradisi)* oils are beneficial in improving skin texture. Massage on location.

Contents:

Grapeseed Oil—light-textured and odorless, it is nourishing to the skin and is an excellent carrier for essential oils.

Olive Oil—a moisturizing agent in many organic cosmetics that will not clog pores.

Wheatgerm Oil—a rich and lush oil high in lecithin, vitamin E, and B vitamins.

Sweet Almond Oil—this nourishing oil is well suited for massage, aiding in a smooth application while reducing friction.

Vitamin E—protects skin and cell membranes against oxidative damage.

Cedarwood *(Cedrus atlantica)*—historically is recognized for its calming, purifying properties and is used to benefit the skin and tissues near the surface of the skin.

Cypress *(Cupressus sempervirens)*—one of the oils most used for the circulatory system. It is also antimicrobial.

Juniper *(Juniperus osteosperma* and/or *J. scopulorum)*—may work as a detoxifier and cleanser, as well as being beneficial for the skin.

Grapefruit *(Citrus paradisi)*—works as a mild disinfectant. Like many cold-pressed citrus oils, it has unique fat-dissolving characteristics.

Clary Sage *(Salvia sclarea)*—supports the cells and hormones. It contains natural estriol, a phytoestrogen.

Pepper *(Piper nigrum)*—a stimulating, energizing essential oil that has been studied for its effects on cellular oxygenation. It has been used for soothing deep tissue muscle aches.

Honeysuckle Fragrance Oil—adds the wonderful fragrance of honeysuckle to this massage oil.

Desert Breeze Massage Oil

Desert Breeze is a relaxing blend of oils designed to soothe muscles and promote calming and tension relief. Makes an excellent all-purpose massage oil.

Contents:

Grapeseed Oil—light-textured and odorless, it is nourishing to the skin and is an excellent carrier for essential oils.

Sweet Almond Oil—reduces friction and promotes smooth application during massage.

Olive Oil—a moisturizing agent in many organic cosmetics that will not clog pores.

Wheatgerm Oil—is a rich and lush oil high in lecithin, vitamin E, and B vitamins.

Vitamin E—protects skin and cell membranes against oxidative damage.

Bergamot *(Citrus bergamia)*—used in the Middle East for hundreds of years for skin conditions associated with an oily complexion. It soothes insect bites and may serve as an insect repellent.

Blue Tansy (*Tanacetum annuum*)—contains azulene, responsible for the rich blue color of the oil. Its extremely powerful anti-inflammatory properties make it perfectly suited to treat sprains, carpal tunnel syndrome, and sports injuries and to balance the emotions after traumatic emotional experiences.

German Chamomile (*Matricaria recutita*)—contains azulene, a powerful anti-inflammatory compound.

Roman Chamomile (*Chamaemelum nobile*)—may help calm and relieve restlessness and tension. Its anti-infectious properties benefit cuts, scrapes, and bruises. It is used extensively in Europe for the skin.

Lavender (*Lavandula angustifolia*)—is highly regarded for the skin. Excellent for burns and for cleansing cuts, bruises, and skin irritations. It is uniquely calming and relaxing.

Melissa (*Melissa officinalis*)—is antiviral and antimicrobial, yet gentle and delicate.

Rose (*Rosa damascena*)—is one of the oldest oils for treating skin conditions, including psoriasis and dermatitis. It has an exquisite fragrance that is both intoxicating and aphrodisiac-like. Daniel Penoël, M.D., used this oil for numerous skin conditions in his clinical practice.

Ylang ylang (*Cananga odorata*)—may be extremely effective in calming and bringing about a sense of relaxation.

Also includes **Joy** and **Valor** blends.

Dragon Time Massage Oil

Dragon Time combines essential oils that have been researched in Europe for their balancing effects on hormones. Can be used in massage or added to bathwater.

Contents:

Grapeseed Oil—light-textured and odorless, it is nourishing to the skin and is an excellent carrier for essential oils.

Sweet Almond Oil—this nourishing oil is well suited for massage, aiding in a smooth application while reducing friction.

Olive Oil—a moisturizing agent in many organic cosmetics that will not clog pores.

Wheatgerm Oil—a rich and lush oil high in lecithin, vitamin E, and B vitamins.

Vitamin E—protects skin and cell membranes against oxidative damage.

Clary Sage (*Salvia sclarea*)—supports the cells and hormones. It contains natural estriol, a phytoestrogen.

Fennel (*Foeniculum vulgare*)—antiseptic and stimulating to the circulatory and respiratory systems.

Lavender (*Lavandula angustifolia*)—is highly regarded for the skin. Excellent for burns and for cleansing cuts, bruises, and skin irritations. It is uniquely calming and relaxing.

Jasmine (*Jasminum officinale*)—beneficial for dry, oily, irritated, or sensitive skin. It can also be uplifting and stimulating in times of hopelessness and nervous exhaustion.

Sage (*Salvia officinalis*)—used in Europe for numerous skin conditions and recognized for its benefits of strengthening the vital centers and supporting metabolism. Containing sclareol, which stimulates the body to produce its own estrogen, sage may nutritionally support the body during PMS and menopause. Sage may also help in coping with despair and mental fatigue.

Ylang ylang (*Cananga odorata*)—may be extremely effective in calming and bringing about a sense of relaxation.

Massage Oil Base

The Massage Oil Base allows you the freedom to custom-blend your favorite oils to your personal specifications.

Contents:

Wheatgerm Oil—a rich and lush oil high in lecithin, vitamin E, and B vitamins.

Grapeseed Oil—light-textured and odorless, it is nourishing to the skin and is an excellent carrier for essential oils.

Sweet Almond Oil—reduces friction and promotes smooth application during massage.

Olive Oil—a moisturizing agent in many organic cosmetics that will not clog pores.

Vitamin E—also known as alpha-tocopherol, it protects skin and cell membranes against oxidative damage.

Ortho Ease Massage Oil

Ortho Ease is designed to soothe muscle aches, sports injuries, sprains, and minor swelling. It was created after extensive testing and has been used in European hospitals.

Contents:

Wheatgerm Oil—a rich and lush oil high in lecithin, vitamin E, and B vitamins.

Grapeseed Oil—light-textured and odorless, it is nourishing to the skin and is an excellent carrier for essential oils.

Sweet Almond Oil—reduces friction and promotes smooth application during massage.

Olive Oil—a moisturizing agent in many organic cosmetics that will not clog pores.

Vitamin E—protects skin and cell membranes against oxidative damage.

Birch (*Betula alleghaniensis*)—contains an active principle similar to cortisone and is beneficial for massage associated with bone, muscle, and joint discomfort.

Juniper (*Juniperus osteosperma* and/or *J. scopulorum*)—is stimulating to the nerves and beneficial for the skin. Works as a detoxifier and cleanser.

Marjoram (*Origanum majorana*)—used for soothing the muscles and the respiratory system. It also assists in calming the nerves. It is antimicrobial and antiseptic.

Red Thyme (*Thymus serpyllum*)—similar to *Thymus vulgaris*, this oil is powerfully antiviral, antimicrobial, and antibacterial. It is also rubefacient or warming to the skin.

Vetiver (*Vetiveria zizanioides*)—is well-known for its anti-inflammatory properties and traditionally used for arthritic symptoms. It is psychologically grounding, calming, and stabilizing.

Peppermint (*Mentha piperita*)—has been researched for its ability to block pain, counteract itching, and combat headaches (Gobel et al., 1996). Jean Valnet, M.D., studied peppermint's effect on the liver and respiratory systems. It is also antifungal and antibacterial.

Eucalyptus (*Eucalyptus ericifolia*)—is antibacterial and antifungal.

Lemongrass (*Cymbopogon flexuosus*)—has powerful antifungal properties that were documented in the journal *Phytotherapy Research*.

Ortho Sport Massage Oil

Ortho Sport is designed for soothing strained muscles and ligaments for both professional and amateur athletes. It is a stronger version of Ortho Ease, with a higher phenol content, which may produce a greater warming sensation.

Contents:

Wheatgerm Oil—a rich and lush oil high in lecithin, vitamin E, and B vitamins.

Grapeseed Oil—light-textured and odorless, it is nourishing to the skin and is an excellent carrier for essential oils.

Olive Oil—a moisturizing agent in many organic cosmetics that will not clog pores.

Sweet Almond Oil—reduces friction and promotes smooth application during massage.

Vitamin E—protects skin and cell membranes against oxidative damage.

Birch (*Betula alleghaniensis*)—contains an active principle similar to cortisone and is beneficial for massage associated with bone, muscle, and joint discomfort.

Oregano (*Origanum vulgare*)—one of the most powerful antimicrobial essential oils. Highly damaging to many kinds of viruses, oregano was shown in laboratory research conducted at Weber State University to have a 99 percent kill rate against *in vitro* colonies of *S. pneumoniae*, even when used in one percent concentration (Chao, 1998). (*S. pneumoniae* causes many kinds of lung and throat infections.)

Marjoram (*Origanum majorana*)—is used for soothing the muscles and the respiratory system. It also assists in calming the nerves. It is antimicrobial and antiseptic.

Red Thyme (*Thymus serpyllum*)—similar to *Thymus vulgaris*, this oil is powerfully antiviral, antimicrobial, and antibacterial. It is also rubefacient or warming to the skin.

Peppermint (*Mentha piperita*)—cooling and invigorating, it blocks the sensation of pain, counteracts itching, and combats headaches (Gobel et al., 1996). Antifungal and antibacterial.

Eucalyptus (*Eucalyptus globulus*)—is a powerful antimicrobial agent, rich in eucalyptol (a key ingredient in many antiseptic mouth rinses). Often used for the respiratory system, eucalyptus also repels insects.

Lemongrass (*Cymbopogon flexuosus*)—is a strong antifungal oil.

Vetiver (*Vetiveria zizanioides*)—is well-known for its anti-inflammatory properties and traditionally used for arthritic symptoms. It is psychologically grounding, calming, and stabilizing.

Elemi (*Canarium luzonicum*)—has been used in Europe for hundreds of years in salves for skin and was used in celebrated healing ointments, such as *baume paralytique*. Elemi belongs to the same botanical family as frankincense and myrrh. Antiseptic and antimicrobial, it is widely regarded today for soothing sore muscles, protecting skin, and stimulating nerves.

Protec

Protec is designed to be used in a night-long retention enema or douche. Suitable for both men and women. Use 1/2 to 1 ounce added to an enema or douche.

Contents:

Olive Oil—a moisturizing agent in many organic cosmetics that will not clog pores.

Grapeseed Oil—makes an excellent carrier for essential oils.

Sweet Almond Oil—this nourishing oil is well suited for massage, aiding in a smooth application while reducing friction.

Wheatgerm Oil—a rich and lush oil high in lecithin, vitamin E, and B vitamins.

Vitamin E—protects skin and cell membranes against oxidative damage.

Frankincense (*Boswellia carteri*)—is considered a holy anointing oil in the Middle East and has been used in religious ceremonies for thousands of years. It is stimulating and elevating to the mind and helps overcome stress and despair as well as supporting the immune system.

Myrrh (*Commiphora myrrha*)—is an antimicrobial oil referenced throughout the Old and New Testaments (*A bundle of myrrh is my well-beloved unto me*. Song of Solomon 1:13). Antibacterial, it is widely used in oral hygiene products.

Sage (*Salvia officinalis*)—is used in Europe for numerous types of skin conditions.

Cumin (*Cuminum cyminum*)—studied for its anticancer properties in "The Anticarcinogenic Effects of the Essential Oils from Cumin, Poppy, and Basil" (Aruna et al., 1996), it is rarer and more expensive than the commonly used white cumin. Antiseptic, calming, and a powerful support to the immune system, cumin seeds have been retrieved from the tombs of the pharoahs of Egypt.

Relaxation Massage Oil

Promotes relaxation and easing of tension.

Contents:

Grapeseed Oil—light-textured and odorless, it is nourishing to the skin and is an excellent carrier for essential oils.

Sweet Almond Oil—this nourishing oil is well suited for massage, aiding in a smooth application.

Wheatgerm Oil—a rich and lush-textured oil high in lecithin, vitamin E, and B vitamins.

Olive Oil—a moisturizing agent in many organic cosmetics that will not clog pores.

Vitamin E—protects skin and cell membranes against oxidative damage.

Tangerine (*Citrus reticulata*)—is soothing for anxiety and nervousness.

Rosewood (*Aniba rosaeodora*)—is soothing and nourishing to the skin. It has been researched at Weber State University for its inhibition rate against gram positive and gram negative bacterial growth.

Spearmint (*Mentha spicata*)—oil helps support the respiratory and nervous systems. Its hormone-like activity may help open and release emotional blocks and bring about a feeling of balance.

Peppermint (*Mentha piperita*)—cooling and invigorating, it blocks the sensation of pain, counteracts itching, and combats headaches (Gobel et al., 1996). Jean Valnet, M.D., studied peppermint's effect on the liver and respiratory systems. Antifungal and antibacterial.

Ylang ylang (*Cananga odorata*)—extremely effective in calming and bringing about a sense of relaxation.

Lavender (*Lavandula angustifolia*)—is highly regarded for the skin. Excellent for burns and for cleansing cuts, bruises, and skin irritations, it is uniquely calming and relaxing.

Sensation Massage Oil

Sensation leaves skin feeling silky and youthful.

Contents:

Grapeseed Oil—light-textured and odorless, it is nourishing to the skin and is an excellent carrier for essential oils.

Sweet Almond Oil—reduces friction and promotes smooth application during massage.

Wheatgerm Oil—a rich and lush-textured oil high in lecithin, vitamin E, and B vitamins.

Vitamin E—protects skin and cell membranes against oxidative damage.

Olive Oil—a moisturizing agent in many organic cosmetics that will not clog pores.

Rosewood (*Aniba rosaeodora*)—is soothing and nourishing to the skin. It has been researched at Weber State University for its inhibition rate against gram positive and gram negative bacterial growth.

Ylang ylang (*Cananga odorata*)—is extremely effective in calming and bringing about a sense of relaxation.

Jasmine (*Jasminum officinale*)—is beneficial for dry, oily, irritated, or sensitive skin. It can also be uplifting and stimulating in times of hopelessness and nervous exhaustion.

V-6 Mixing Oil

V-6 Mixing Oil is a mixture of nourishing, antioxidant vegetable oils that makes an ideal carrier for essential oils. It facilitates the penetration of essential oils into the skin.

Contents:

Olive Oil—a moisturizing agent in many organic cosmetics, the properties of olive oil also lend themselves to homeopathic applications.

Sesame Seed Oil—contains vitamins, minerals, amino acids, lecithin, and natural vegetable proteins that soothe skin conditions such as psoriasis and eczema.

Grapeseed Oil—light-textured and odorless, it is nourishing to the skin and is an excellent carrier for essential oils.

Sweet Almond Oil—this nourishing oil is well suited for massage, aiding in a smooth application while reducing friction.

Sunflower Seed Oil—compatible with the skin's natural oils and sebum, it is suitable to a variety of skin types.

Wheatgerm Oil—a rich and lush-textured oil high in lecithin, vitamin E, and B vitamins.

Vitamin E—protects skin and cell membranes against oxidative damage.

AromaSilk Skin and Hair Care

Skin Care Products

Use Facial Wash, Toner, and Moisturizer Creme together to promote younger and healthier-looking skin.

Orange Blossom Facial Wash

Ingredients: Deionized water, calendula extract, chamomile extract, rosebud extract, orange blossom extract, St. John's wort extract, algae, aloe vera gel, kelp extract, *Ginkgo biloba* extract, grapeseed extract, decyl polyglucose, MSM, wolfberry seed oil, essential oils of lavender, lemon, rosemary verbenon, and patchouly, multifruit acid complex, hydrolyzed wheat protein, citric acid, dimethyl lauramine oleate.

Instructions: For best results, use Orange Blossom Facial Wash twice daily. Follow up with Sandalwood Toner & Moisture Creme to promote younger and healthier looking skin.

Sandalwood Toner

Ingredients: Deionized water, MSM, glycerin, sorbitol, sodium PCA, allantoin, aloe vera gel, cucumber extract, chamomile extract, rosemary extract, echinacea extract, gotu kola extract, sodium hyaluronate, arnica extract, witch hazel extract, horse chestnut extract, wolfberry seed oil, essential oils of sandalwood, Roman chamomile, rosewood, and myrrh.

Instructions: Lightly mist face and neck with Sandalwood Toner. For best results follow up with Sandalwood Moisture Creme.

Sandalwood Moisturizer Creme

Ingredients: Deionized water, calendula extract, chamomile extract, rosebud extract, orange blossom extract, St. John's wort extract, aloe vera gel, kelp, *Ginkgo biloba* extract, grapeseed extract, caprylic/capric triglyceride, sorbitol, shea butter, goat's cream, glyceryl stearate, essential oils of myrrh, sandalwood, rosewood, lavender, and rosemary verbenon, wolfberry seed oil, rosehip seed oil, sodium PCA, algae extract, stearic acid, allantoin, lecithin, retinyl palmitate (vitamin A), tocopheryl acetate (vitamin E), ascorbic acid (vitamin C), locust bean gum, hydrolyzed wheat protein, sodium hyaluronate, tocopheryl linoleate.

Instructions: For best results, use Sandalwood Moisture Creme after cleansing and toning the face and neck to promote younger, healthier skin. Put small amount in hand, emulsify, and apply to face and neck using upward strokes.

Boswellia Wrinkle Creme

Ingredients: Deionized water, calendula extract, chamomile extract, rosebud extract, orange blossom extract, St. John's wort extract, aloe vera gel, kelp extract, *Ginkgo biloba* extract, grapeseed extract, ASC 111, goat's cream, glyceryl stearate, caprylic/capric triglyceride, shea butter, essential oils of frankincense, sandalwood, myrrh, geranium, and ylang ylang, wolfberry seed oil, stearic acid, stearyl alcohol, sodium PCA, sodium hyaluronate, allantoin, panthenol, retinyl palmitate (vitamin A), tocopheryl acetate (vitamin E).

Instructions: Boswellia Wrinkle Creme is a collagen builder. Used daily, it will help minimize and prevent wrinkles. Put small amount in hand, emulsify, and apply to face and neck using upward strokes.

Wolfberry Eye Creme

Eases eye puffiness and dark circles, and promotes skin tightening. Can be used before bed and in the morning.

Ingredients: Deionized water, aloe vera gel, caprylic/capric triglyceride, MSM, sorbitol, glycerin, glyceryl stearate, goat's cream, avocado oil, shea butter, kukui nut oil, rose hip seed oil, essential oils of lavender, rosewood, Roman chamomile, frankincense, and geranium, wolfberry seed oil, hydrocotyl extract, coneflower extract, sodium PCA, lecithin, dipalmitoyl hydroxyproline, phenoxyethanol, beta-sitosterol, linoleic acid, tocopherol, sodium ascorbate, mannitol, almond oil, jojoba oil, mango butter, sodium hyaluronate, comfrey extract, cucumber extract, green tea extract, tocopherol acetate, tocopherol palmitate (vitamin E), ascorbyl palmitate (vitamin A), ascorbic acid (vitamin C), citric acid, soy protein, wheat protein, allantoin, witch hazel extract, horse chestnut extract.

Instructions: Apply a tiny amount of Wolfberry Eye Creme under eye area and on the eyelid before bed. Repeat in morning if desired.

Satin Body Lotion

Nourishes and moisturizes skin. Contains herbal extracts, essential oils, and vitamin C.

Ingredients: Deionized water, MSM, glyceryl stearate, stearic acid, glycerin, goat's cream, sorbitol, wolfberry seed oil, essential oils of geranium, rosewood, ylang ylang, jasmine, sandalwood, peppermint, and Roman chamomile, tea tree oil, safflower oil, apricot oil, almond oil, jojoba oil, sesame oil, calendula extract, chamomile extract, orange blossom extract, St. John's wort extract, algae extract, aloe vera gel, *Ginkgo biloba* extract, grapeseed extract, tocopheryl acetate (vitamin E), retinyl palmitate (vitamin A), ascorbic acid (vitamin C), sodium hyaluronate.

Instructions: To moisturize the skin, promote healing, and leave the skin feeling soft, silky and smooth, apply Satin Body Lotion to hands, body, and feet. Also good for scars, burns, rashes, itching and sunburns.

Cinnamint Lip Balm

Is a natural lip balm enriched with essential oils and vitamins to soothe and prevent chapping.

Ingredients: Sweet almond oil, beeswax, MSM, hemp seed oil, sesame oil, orange wax, orange oil, tocopherol palmitate (vitamin E), ascorbyl palmitate (vitamin A), ascorbic acid (vitamin C), citric acid, wolfberry seed oil, essential oils of peppermint, spearmint, and cinnamon bark.

Instructions: To soften and moisturize lips, apply Cinnamint Lip Balm as often as needed.

LavaDerm Cooling Mist

This cooling mist is soothing to any burn from the slightest sunburn to the burn of a fire. Aloe vera has been a household remedy for years, and lavender made its re-entry into the therapeutic realm through healing the laboratory burn of Dr. Gattefossé. LavaDerm Cooling Mist will certainly become a must in every home.

How to use: Mist as often as needed to keep the skin cool and promote regeneration.

Ingredients: Re-structured water, aloe vera, and lavender essential oil.

Mint Facial Scrub

Eliminates layers of dead skin cells. Oatmeal and corn flour provide a mild abrasive texture that helps stimulate the pores, bringing oxygen to the surface. It is excellent for skin prone to acne. This scrub can be used as a drying face mask to draw impurities from the skin. If the texture is too abrasive, it can be mixed with the Orange Blossom Facial Wash.

How to use: Apply warm water to the face to moisten skin. Apply scrub directly to the face and gently massage in a gentle circular motion, creating a lather. Rinse thoroughly and gently pat dry. May also be mixed with Orange Blossom Facial Wash for a milder scrub. Mix 1/2 tsp. of both in palm of hand before applying. Use four or five times weekly, depending on need.

Ingredients: Floral water, corn flour, glycerin water, kaolin, almond meal, oatmeal, zinc oxide, vegetable oils, lecithin, magnesium silicate, chloro-phyllin-complex, and essential oils of laurelwood, lavender, melaleuca, palmarosa, peppermint, rosewood, and rosemary.

Rose Ointment

Is a skin ointment that protects and nourishes the skin and is outstanding when applied over essential oils to lock in their benefits. Note: Not recommended for burns initially, but is very helpful to maintain, protect, and keep the the scab soft.

How to use: Apply directly to skin.

Ingredients: Lecithin, lanolin, beeswax, mink oil, sesame seed oil, vitamin E oil, rose hip seed oil, and essential oils of carrot seed, melaleuca alternifolia, myrrh, palmarosa, patchouly, rose hip seed, rose, and rosewood.

Sensation Hand and Body Lotion

Is delightful to wear with its intoxicating blend of exotic essential oils. It leaves the skin soft and moist as it protects from harsh weather, chemicals, and dry air.

How to use: Dispense in hand and apply directly to skin.

Ingredients: Deionized water, cocoa butter, glyceryl stearate, cetyl alcohol, lanolin oil, floral water, vitamin E, and essential oils of rosewood, ylang ylang, and jasmine.

Hair Care Products

Lavender Volume Hair & Scalp Wash

Contains all natural ingredients for gently cleansing and volumizing fine hair. Horsetail and coltsfoot extract provide silica, and MSM provides sulfur to help build and strengthen hair. Fortified with vitamin complex, including panthenol, and vitamins A, C, and E. Contains essential oils for a beautiful fragrance.

Ingredients: Coconut oil, decyl polyglucose, MSM, vegetable protein (wheat, oat, soya), deionized water, rosemary extract, sage extract, nettles extract, coltsfoot extract, horsetail extract, fennel extract, essential oils of lavender, clary sage, lemon, and jasmine, aloe vera gel, retinyl palmitate (vitamin A), ascorbic acid (vitamin C), tocopheryl acetate (vitamin E), panthenol (vitamin B5), grapeseed extract, inositol, niacin.

Instructions: Wet hair thoroughly. Apply small amount of Lavender Volume Hair & Scalp Wash. Massage thoroughly into hair and scalp. Rinse well. Repeat if desired.

Lavender Volume Nourishing Rinse

Conditions and volumizes fine hair with MSM, amino acids, and a multi-vitamin complex. Essential oils enhance and provide vital components for healthy hair.

Ingredients: Natural vegetable fatty acid base, MSM, milk protein, phospholipids, amino acids cysteine and cysteine 8 methionine, glyco protein (glycogen and mucopolysaccharides), quinoa extract, rosemary extract, sage extract, horsetail extract, coltsfoot extract, hydrolyzed wheat protein, hydrolyzed soya protein, retinyl palmitate (vitamin A), ascorbic acid (vitamin C), tocopheryl acetate (vitamin E), panthenol (vitamin B5), grapeseed extract, essential oils of lavender, clary sage, lemon, and jasmine.

Instructions: Apply Lavender Volume Nourishing Rinse through the hair. Leave on hair for just a few seconds for light conditioning or for several minutes for deep conditioning. Rinse well.

Lavender Volume Sealer

Maintains volume and luster while it seals the hair shaft, preventing split ends and other damage.

Ingredients: Water, hyaluronic acid, panthenol sorbitol (vitamin B5), acetamide MEA, tocopherol, hydrolyzed soy protein, linoleic acid, arachidonic acid, jojoba oil, wheat germ oil, apple cider, balsamic vinegar, bee pollen extract, and essential oils of lavender, clary sage, lemon, and jasmine.

Instructions: Apply Lavender Volume Sealer evenly to towel-dried hair, leave in, then style.

Rosewood Moisturizing Hair & Scalp Wash

Contains natural ingredients to moisturize dry hair while gently cleansing. Contains herbal extracts, vitamins, and essential oils for nourishing the hair.

Ingredients: Coconut oil, decyl polyglucose, MSM, vegetable protein (wheat, oat, soya), deionized water, rosemary extract, sage extract, nettles extract, coltsfoot extract, horsetail extract, fennel extract, essential oils of bergamot, birch, geranium, sandalwood, clary sage, and rosewood, aloe vera gel, retinyl palmitate (vitamin A), ascorbic acid (vitamin C), tocopheryl acetate (vitamin E), panthenol (vitamin B5), grapeseed extract, inositol, and niacin.

Instructions: Wet hair thoroughly. Apply small amount of Rosewood Moisturizing Hair & Scalp Wash. Massage thoroughly into hair and scalp. Rinse well. Repeat if desired.

Rosewood Moisturizing Nourishing Rinse

Conditions and moisturizes dry hair with natural vegetable fatty acids, MSM, milk protein, vitamins, and essential oils.

Ingredients: Natural vegetable fatty acid base, MSM, milk protein, phospholipids, amino acids cysteine and cysteine 8 methionine, glyco protein (glycogen and mucopolysaccharides), quinoa extract, rosemary extract, sage extract, horsetail extract, coltsfoot extract, hydrolyzed wheat protein, hydrolyzed soya protein, retinyl palmitate (vitamin A), ascorbic acid (vitamin C), tocopheryl acetate (vitamin E), panthenol (vitamin B5), grapeseed extract, essential oils of bergamot, birch, geranium, sandalwood, clary sage, and rosewood.

Instructions: Apply Rosewood Moisturizing Nourishing Rinse to hair from roots to ends. Leave on hair for a few seconds for light conditioning or for several minutes for deep conditioning. Rinse well.

Rosewood Moisturizing Sealer

Seals the hair cuticle while maintaining moisture and volume in dry hair.

Ingredients: Water, hyaluronic acid, panthenol sorbitol (vitamin B5), acetamide MEA, tocopherol, hydrolyzed soy protein, linoleic acid, arachidonic acid, jojoba oil, wheat germ oil, apple cider, balsamic vinegar, bee pollen extract, and essential oils of bergamot, birch, geranium, sandalwood, clary sage, and rosewood.

Instructions: Apply Rosewood Moisturizing Sealer evenly to towel-dried hair, leave in, then style.

Lemon Sage Clarifying Hair & Scalp Wash

Removes buildup of styling products, leaving hair feeling naturally clean and healthy. Contains herbal extracts, vitamins, and essential oils to enhance the hair.

Ingredients: Coconut oil, decyl polyglucose, MSM, vegetable protein (wheat, oat, soya), deionized water, rosemary extract, sage extract, nettles extract, coltsfoot extract, horsetail extract, fennel extract, essential oils of lemon, lime, pine, geranium, Roman chamomile, ylang ylang, and sage, aloe vera gel, retinyl palmitate (vitamin A), ascorbic acid (vitamin C), tocopheryl acetate (vitamin E), panthenol (vitamin B5), grapeseed extract, inositol, and niacin.

Instructions: Wet hair thoroughly. Apply small amount of Lemon Sage Clarifying Hair & Scalp Wash. Massage thoroughly into hair and scalp. Rinse well. Repeat if desired.

Lemon Sage Clarifying Nourishing Rinse

Conditions hair of all types without building up on hair. Herbal extracts, vitamins, and essential oils work together to improve hair condition.

Ingredients: Natural vegetable fatty acid base, MSM, milk protein, phospholipids, amino acids cysteine and cysteine 8 methionine, glyco protein (glycogen and mucopolysaccharides), rosemary extract, sage extract, horsetail extract, coltsfoot extract, hydrolyzed wheat protein, hydrolyzed soya protein, retinyl palmitate (vitamin A), ascorbic acid (vitamin C), tocopheryl acetate (vitamin E), panthenol (vitamin B5), grapeseed extract, essential oils of lemon, lime, pine, geranium, Roman chamomile, ylang ylang, and sage.

Instructions: Apply Lemon Sage Clarifying Nourishing Rinse to hair from roots to ends. Leave on hair for just a few seconds for light conditioning or for several minutes for deep conditioning. Rinse well.

Lemon Sage Clarifying Sealer

Seals the hair shaft, protecting it from damage without adding buildup.

Ingredients: Water, hyaluronic acid, panthenol sorbitol (vitamin B5), acetamide MEA, tocopherol, hydrolyzed soy protein, linoleic acid, arachidonic acid, jojoba oil, wheat germ oil, apple cider, balsamic vinegar, bee pollen extract, and essential oils of lemon, lime, pine, geranium, Roman chamomile, ylang ylang, and sage.

Instructions: Apply Lemon Sage Clarifying Sealer evenly to towel-dried hair, leave in, then style.

CHAPTER 13

Bath and Shower Gels

Bath Gel Base

Bath Gel Base is a dispersing agent to help unlock the full effects of your aromatherapy bath. Contains natural botanical ingredients for cleansing the pores. You may add single essential oils or blends to create your own fragrance or a specific therapeutic action.

How to use: Add several drops of an essential oil single or blend (depending on the strength of the oil) to the Bath Gel Base. Shake before using.

Ingredients: Saponified oils of coconut and olive, vegetable gum extract, aloe vera, and rosemary extract.

Dragon Time Bath & Shower Gel

This bath and shower gel was blended for women's stressful time of the month. This custom-formulated blend of essential oils and vegetable oils is exceptionally balancing and uplifting, both physically and emotionally.

Ingredients: Saponified oils of coconut and olive, vegetable gum extract, aloe vera, rosemary extract, and the essential oils of bergamot, clary sage, geranium, jasmine, lemon, palmarosa, Roman chamomile, rosewood, lavender, blue tansy, mandarin, sage, fennel, marjoram, and ylang ylang.

Evening Peace Bath and Shower Gel

Evening Peace blends natural botanical ingredients with therapeutic-grade essential oils to relax tired, fatigued muscles and help dampen stress and tension.

Ingredients: Saponified oils of coconut and olive, vegetable gum extract, aloe vera, rosemary extract, and the essential oils of bergamot, Roman chamomile, clary sage, geranium, jasmine, lemon, palmarosa, rosewood, blue tansy, sandalwood, and ylang ylang.

Morning Start Bath & Shower Gel

Morning Start is an invigorating gel that combines uplifting, energizing essential oils to jumpstart your vigor and energy.

Ingredients: Saponified oils of coconut and olive, vegetable gum extract, aloe vera, rosemary extract, and the essential oils of lemongrass, rosemary, juniper and peppermint.

Sensation Bath & Shower Gel

Sensation contains an enchantingly fragrant mix of oils used by Cleopatra to enhance love and increase desire to be close to someone special.

Ingredients: Saponified oils of coconut and olive, vegetable gum extract, aloe vera, rosemary extract, and the essential oils of rosewood, ylang ylang, and jasmine.

CHAPTER 14

Vita Flex Technique

Vita Flex Technique means "vitality through the reflexes." It is a specialized form of hand and foot massage that is exceptionally effective in delivering the benefits of essential oils throughout the body. It is said to have originated in Tibet thousands of years ago, and perfected in modern times by Stanley Burroughs long before acupuncture was developed.

It is based on a complete network of reflex points that stimulate all the internal body systems. Oils are applied to contact points, and energy is released through electrical impulses created by contact between the fingertips and reflex points. This electrical charge follows the nerve pathways to a break in the electrical circuit caused by toxins, damaged tissues, or loss of oxygen. There are more than 1,400 Vita Flex points throughout the human body, encompassing the entire realm of body and mind, that are capable of releasing many kinds of tension, congestion, and imbalances.

In contrast to the steady stimulation of Reflexology, Vita Flex uses a rolling and releasing motion that involves placing all four fingers flat on the skin, rolling onto the fingertips, and continuing over onto the fingernail. Use medium pressure. Move ahead about half the width of the finger and repeat until the Vita Flex point, or area, is covered. Repeat this movement over the area three times.

Combine this technique with 1-2 drops of essential oil applied to those areas of the feet that correspond to the system of the body you wish to support (SEE DIAGRAM BELOW). The Vita Flex (VF) numbers correspond to locations on the feet and are noted on the foot chart. Rapid and extraordinary results are experienced when combining essential oils with Vita Flex stimulation, as it increases the effect of both. Vita Flex and Raindrop Technique are both demonstrated and explained on the "Science and Application" video available from Essential Science Publishing.

The following diagram shows the nervous system connection for the electrical points throughout the body.

Vita Flex Points

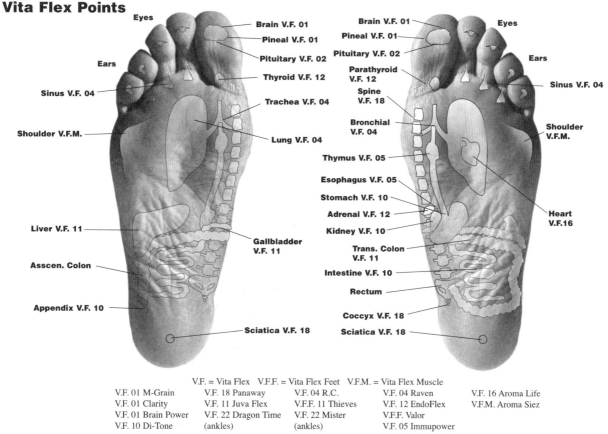

V.F. = Vita Flex		V.F.F. = Vita Flex Feet	V.F.M. = Vita Flex Muscle	
V.F. 01 M-Grain	V.F. 18 Panaway	V.F. 04 R.C.	V.F. 04 Raven	V.F. 16 Aroma Life
V.F. 01 Clarity	V.F. 11 Juva Flex	V.F.F. 11 Thieves	V.F. 12 EndoFlex	V.F.M. Aroma Siez
V.F. 01 Brain Power	V.F. 22 Dragon Time	V.F. 22 Mister	V.F.F. Valor	
V.F. 10 Di-Tone	(ankles)	(ankles)	V.F. 05 Immupower	

Nervous System Connection Points

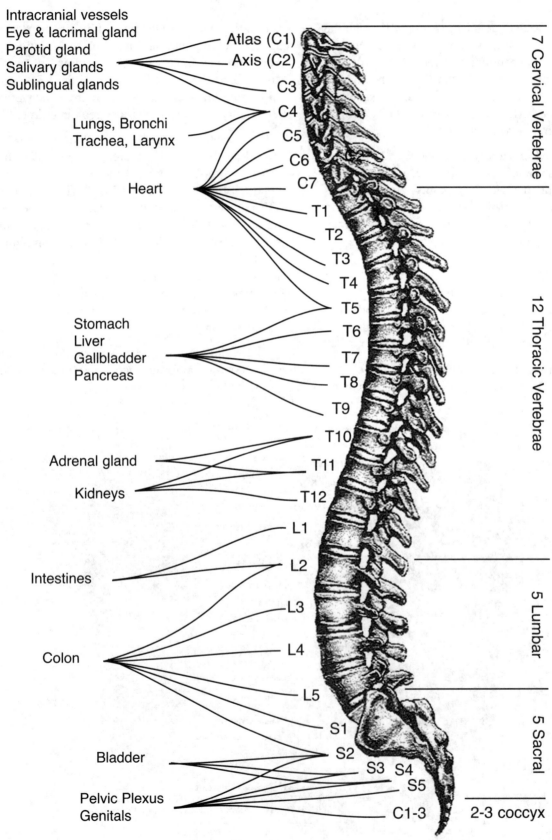

Intracranial vessels
Eye & lacrimal gland
Parotid gland
Salivary glands
Sublingual glands

Atlas (C1)
Axis (C2)
C3
C4

Lungs, Bronchi
Trachea, Larynx

C5
C6
C7

Heart

T1
T2
T3
T4
T5

Stomach
Liver
Gallbladder
Pancreas

T6
T7
T8
T9
T10

Adrenal gland

T11

Kidneys

T12

L1
L2

Intestines

L3
L4

Colon

L5
S1
S2

Bladder

S3 S4
S5

Pelvic Plexus
Genitals

C1-3

7 Cervical Vertebrae

12 Thoracic Vertebrae

5 Lumbar

5 Sacral

2-3 coccyx

CHAPTER 15

Raindrop Technique

Raindrop Technique is a powerful, non-invasive tool for helping to correct defects in the curvature of the spine. During the years that it has been practiced, it has resolved numerous cases of scoliosis and kyphosis and eliminated the need for back surgery for thousands of people.

Raindrop Technique originated from the research of D. Gary Young and a Lakota medicine man in the 1970s. It integrates Vita Flex and massage with essential oils to bring the body into structural and electrical alignment.

Raindrop Technique is based on the theory that many types of scoliosis and spinal misalignments are caused by viruses or bacteria that lie dormant along the spine. These pathogens create inflammation, which, in turn, contorts and disfigures the spinal column.

Raindrop Technique uses a sequence of highly antimicrobial essential oils designed to simultaneously reduce inflammation and kill the viral agents responsible for it. The principle oils used are: thyme (*Thymus vulgaris*), oregano (*Origanum compactum*), birch (*Betula alleghaniensis*), cypress (*Cupressus sempervirens*), peppermint (*Mentha piperita*), basil (*Ocimum basilicum*), and marjoram (*Origanum majorana*). The oils are dispensed like little drops of rain from a height of about six inches above the back and massaged along the vertebrae. Although the entire process takes about 45 minutes to complete, the oils will continue to work in the body for 5 to 7 days following treatment, with continued re-alignment taking place during this time.

The Raindrop Technique is not a cure-all or a magic bullet. A healthy body is the result of a well-rounded program of exercise and proper diet. Health is everything we do, say, hear, see, and eat. The Raindrop Technique is only one tool to help restore a balance in the body that will result in good health.

Healthy eating habits help prepare the body and skin to accept the oils better and more rapidly.

Although this therapy is explained as simply as possible, it is recommended that you contact Essential Science Publishing for a demonstration video on this remarkable technique. Viewing this video, combined with the outline presented here, will make this revolutionary technique relatively easy to understand and easy to put into practice.

It is recommended that the Raindrop Technique be performed in a quiet, semi-darkened area free of distractions. The temperature should be cool enough to prevent sweating, but warm enough to be comfortable as the receiver's back and legs will be exposed.

For this technique, you will need:

1. Each of the oils listed below

2. Massage table (preferably) or flat space to work on where the person doing the technique is not stressing their back. It also works using a chair. It is best to cover the table, bed, chair, etc. with a disposable sheet, towel, or blanket as several of the oils may stain certain surfaces.

3. Towels, two large and one hand towel. Use towels that can be stained or soiled. You will also need access to hot water.

4. Timer or watch

5. Tray or flat surface to place oils (and instructions) that are near the receiver.

Order in Which to Apply Essential Oils For Virus or Curvature (scoliosis)

STEP 1 — **Valor** is the most important oil used in this application, because it works on both physical and emotional levels, supporting the electrical and energy alignment of the body. The key to using this blend of oils is patience. Once the frequencies begin to balance in these areas, a structural alignment can occur.

STEP 2 — **Thyme** is documented to be highly antimicrobial. Thyme acts directly on the virus or bacteria. This essential oil easily penetrates the skin and travels throughout the body.

STEP 3 — **Oregano** has an antimicrobial action even more aggressive than thyme. It also has anti-inflammatory, antibacterial, and antiviral properties.

STEP 4 — **Basil** has antispasmodic activity that relaxes muscles. It is also anti-inflammatory and antimicrobial.

STEP 5 — **Birch** is anti-inflammatory and analgesic and relieves pain. It is excellent for bone since its primary constituent, methyl salicylate, has an analgesic effect.

STEP 6 — **Cypress** improves circulation and relieves spasms and swelling. Cypress also helps heal damaged tissue.

STEP 7 — **Marjoram** is antispasmotic and helps relax muscles.

STEP 8 — **Peppermint** has pain-killing properties. It is also antimicrobial, working synergistically with the other oils to enhance their activity. Peppermint also stimulates circulation and cools inflamed tissue.

STEP 9 — **Aroma Siez** is antispasmotic and helps relax and relieve sore or aching muscles.

STEP 10 — **Ortho Ease Massage Oil** is a blend of vegetable and essential oils with many properties such as being antioxidant, stimulating circulation, and alleviating sore muscles and joints. This blend has been reported to be beneficial for stress, muscle cramps, arthritic pain, and tension.

Ortho Ease also helps to seal in the essential oils, thereby, enhancing penetration. Ortho Ease is to be applied over the entire area after you have finished with the Raindrop Technique.

NOTE: For more information about each of these oils, you may refer to the single oils or oil blends section of this book.

V-6 Mixing Oil or any massage oil is required to dilute essential oils high in phenols that may produce an excess warming or reddening to the skin, a problem that occurs often with fair-skinned people. Following the application of thyme and oregano, it may be necessary to apply 5-10 drops of massage oil over areas with excess warming or reddening, especially the back of the neck or on the shoulders.

Preparation

• Remove all jewelry. This includes watches, pendants, rings, bracelets, earrings, etc.

• Wear clothing that is loose and comfortable. You may wish to remove your shoes for more ease and comfort.

• When administering this technique, you should have your fingernails clipped and filed down as short as possible. This will help you avoid unintentionally scratching the receiver.

• Put the oils into your non-dominant hand. Then use your dominant hand to rub them clockwise to stir the oils.

• You will need three medium-size towels, hot water, and a sheet or blanket to protect the modesty of the individual being treated.

NOTE: The facilitator may choose to apply Frankincense and/or White Angelica to themselves to deter any negative frequencies or energy coming from the receiver.

To begin:

• The receiver should lie face down on the massage table with the head slightly lower than the rest of the body, preferably resting in the face cradle.

• The facilitator should keep constant physical contact with the receiver to prevent feelings of insecurity or anxiousness.

• The receiver should lie as straight as possible with the hips flat on the table. The arms should be resting along the sides of the body.

Stage 1: Application of Valor. This procedure forms the foundation of everything that follows.

- Place 6 drops of Valor in each hand. Rub hands together.

- Apply Valor to the soles of the receiver's feet.

- Place your hands as flat as possible against the receiver's feet while holding the bottom of the foot. Hold the right foot with the right hand hold the left foot with the left hand. The facilitator may kneel or sit while holding the feet of the person receiving this technique.

- This step works best if there are two people to apply Valor. One to apply oils to the feet, the other to apply oils to the shoulders. However, if you are working by yourself, the application works well just holding the feet, which is the most important.

- Apply 3 drops on each shoulder: right hand placed on right shoulder and left hand placed on left shoulder. There must be as much hand to shoulder contact as possible.

- Let your mind be free and peaceful. Encourage the recipient to take deep breaths. Have them inhale and exhale deeply and slowly, allowing them to engage in their own healing. You may feel an energy flowing up through the patient into your body. The receiver may feel a little heat or tingling on the feet, or an energy working up through the legs to the back, even as high as the head. With some individuals, the giver may feel the hands become cold. Many times you may feel a pulsating feeling.

- Do not break physical contact with the individual. Hold your position for 5-10 minutes.

In most cases, you will see some realignment of the spine. The vertebrae can move under the skin with just this small amount of application. The results will depend largely on the frequency of the person holding the feet. If there are people present with negative attitudes, or if the person applying the oils lacks a high enough frequency to block out the negative interference, the results may be less than optimal. You should not apply the Raindrop Technique on another person if you are feeling angry, negative, or sick.

TIP: You may wish to put V-6 Mixing Oil or Massage Oil Base on the back of the receiver's neck at this point if the receiver's neck has a fold in the skin. This may prevent excessive burning as the oils tend to accumulate in this region of the spine the most.

Stage 2: Application of oregano and thyme.

- Hold the bottle six inches above the skin and evenly space 5-6 drops of each oil along the spine from bottom to top (sacrum to atlas).

- Apply one oil, layering it on along the spine. Apply the second oil the same way. It does not matter which oil is applied first.

- More is not better. If there is a burning sensation, apply a pure vegetable massage oil or blend, such as V-6 Mixing Oil or Massage Oil Base.

- With 4-inch brush-like strokes using the nail side of your fingertips, lightly feather up the spine. Repeat this action two more times, always starting at the sacrum (base of spine) and ending at the atlas (base of the skull).

- With **4-inch** brush-like strokes, flare your fingertips out to the sides of the back as your feather up the spine. The right hand will move to the right and the left hand to the left. Repeat motion two more times.

- Starting at the sacrum, stroke up **8 inches** before flaring out again. Repeat two more times.

- Starting at the sacrum, stroke up **12 inches** before flaring out again. Repeat two more times.

- Continue this step until your strokes feather up the full length of the spine up to the atlas. Flare your fingertips out over the shoulders when you reach the top. Repeat two more times.

- Repeat the feather stroking segments two times.

Stage 3: Application of basil, birch, cypress, marjoram, and peppermint.

- Apply 4-5 drops of basil along the sides of the spine. Layer it in by evenly spreading it with your fingertips.

- Repeat, using the other 4 oils in sequence.

- Starting on one side of the spine, gently massage the oils in along the muscles to the sides of the spine. **Do not work directly on the spine. Do not force it or apply direct pressure.** Start at the sacrum and use the fingertips of both hands placed side by side.

- In a circular clockwise motion, work up the side of the spine to the atlas, pushing or pulling the tissue in the direction you want the spine to move.

- After finishing one side of the spine, start on the other side. Repeat the feather stroking segments two more times.

- Using the index and middle finger of either hand, place the fingers so that they straddle the spine. Start at the coccyx (bottom of spine) and move to the top. Always work directionally toward the brain. With mild pressure and the fingers on either side of the spine, place one hand over the top of the fingers. Then, in a gentle sawing motion, rock the fingers of the hand on top back and forth while moving the fingers on both sides of the spine gently up the spine to the atlas. Repeat this procedure two more times.

- Beginning at the sacrum, with your thumbs on either side of the spine, you will use the Vita Flex technique working up the spine approximately a thumb's width apart with each move up to the atlas. With the thumbs on each side of the spine, nail side up and slightly angled out, rock the thumbs so they point upward with the joints slightly bent. Then, apply a mild pressure straight down. Continue to roll your thumbs slightly over onto the nails, and then release. Move your thumbs up about one-half thumb's width and apply the same technique. Do this all the way to the atlas. Repeat this step two more times.

Stage 4: Application of Aroma Siez.

- Apply 6-8 drops of Aroma Siez over each side of the back and rub into muscles on both sides of spine.

Stage 5: Back massage with massage oil.

- Apply 20-25 drops of Ortho Ease to each side of the spine, (not on the spine) into the muscle tissue of the back. Massage the oils in all over the back, using a gentle fingertip massage for a few minutes. After the oils have been massaged in, rest for five minutes. Then apply Ortho Ease over the entire back and legs.

Stage 6: Towel placement.

- Place a dry towel over the back. Then lay a hand towel (soaked in hot water, wrung out, and folded in thirds) along the entire length of the spine.

- Place another dry towel (folded in half) over the wet towel.

- Pay close attention to what the receiver is experiencing and ask how it is feeling, because the back can become very hot. The heat will generally build slowly and peak in 5-8 minutes before cooling down to the point where it feels pleasant. The greater the inflammation and viral infection along the spine, the hotter the area along the spine will become.

  Some will experience no heat, while others will find it mild and pleasant. Still others may find it uncomfortably hot. Pay attention to the receiver. Ask questions. If the heat becomes too uncomfortable, remove the towels and apply V-6 Mixing Oil or a massage oil on the back. Then massage it in. This will usually subside the heat within minutes.

  After placing the towels on the back, wait several minutes to gauge the individual's response. If the back does not become very hot, have the individual roll over onto his/her back. This usually creates more heat.

Stage 7: Leg massage with birch, basil, cypress, and peppermint.

- Apply 5-6 drops each of birch, basil, cypress, and peppermint along the inside shin bone of the lower legs. Start at the top of the knee and follow the shin bone down to the heel and sideways to the big toe on each foot. Apply one oil at a time, in order, massaging each oil in before applying the next oil.

• Place the fingers of one hand along the inside of the shinbone just below the knee. Using the Vita Flex Technique method, roll fingers around the leg down to the ankle and then along the foot up to the top of the big toe. Roll your fingers up and then over onto the nails of the fingers, applying slightly more pressure at the top of the roll and releasing as you roll the fingers over onto the nails. This is a time when the person on whom you are applying this technique to would appreciate short finger nails. Repeat this procedure twice on each leg (for a total of three times per leg).

Stage 8: Stretching the receiver's back.

• This next step works best with two people. With the receiver on his/her back, have your assistant hold each leg tightly, just above the ankles, while you cradle the individual's head under your right hand. Then place your left hand around the chin and gently pull to create slight tension. If you are working alone, hold the ankles and follow this step accordingly.

• Hold this traction for several minutes. Do not pull hard. The person holding the feet will act as the anchor, while you begin a mild rocking motion, repeatedly pulling and releasing. Continue the rocking motion for approximately 4-8 minutes. Then have the receiver roll back over onto their back.

Stage 9: Checking the results.

• With the receiver lying face down with his/her head snug in the head-cradle of the massage table, make sure the person is lying with their spine straight. Remove the towels and then check the spine. Corrections may or may not be visible. You may need to add another technique at a later time. Occasionally, results take several days to take effect.

SUMMARY:

This is the basic Raindrop Technique, although there are several variations. However, these are not easy to explain and require class instruction and demonstration. Every person is different, and what works for one may not work for another. Different body types respond to the applications in ways you may not expect. Learn to be sensitive to the person on whom you are working so that you can respond to his or her needs.

The question is often asked, "How long do the effects of this application last?" Again, each person responds differently. Generally speaking, the level of health and proper diet are key factors, as are exercise and attitude. The effects of one application may last four months for one person, but then for another it may be necessary to have the application repeated every week until the body begins to respond. The key is to retrain the body. In some cases, you will have to develop a new memory in the tissue in order for the body to stay where it should be. This may take a few weeks or even a full year.

Spinal alignment may have a completely different look when the individual is lying down, rather than sitting. There is more torque on the spine in a sitting or standing position, so these are the positions in which X-rays are usually taken. There may appear to be a total correction when the individual is lying down and then appear to be crooked when they are in a sitting position. This variance is normal and may be apparent until a total retraining of the tissue can occur. The object is to achieve straightening in all positions.

The Raindrop Technique is a powerful tool that not only can assist therapists but also helps everyone achieve a balance in the body.

Auricular Technique

Auricular aroma technique, the integration of essential oils with standard auricular technique, was developed by D. Gary Young after using essential oils in an acupuncture application in his clinic. He found that using essential oils in conjunction with acupuncture was extremely beneficial. He could localize and identify different functions and conditions that the body would respond to through direct acupuncture stimulation with essential oils than through acupuncture or oil application by themselves.

Acupuncture with essential oils seems to enhance benefits substantially. As Gary left his clinical practice and retired to researching, farming, and teaching, he could not continue the practice of acupuncture, so he started developing a technique that everyone could use. That technique is called auricular probe technique, using a small, pen-like instrument with a rounded end to apply the oils to the acupuncture meridians or Vita Flex points. This concept can be used in the emotional and physical

Physical Ear Chart

M - Mouth
E - Esophagus
CO - Cardiac Orifice
St - Stomach
SI - Small Intestine
LI - Large Intestine
Pr - Prostate
Bl - Bladder
Ur - Ureter
Kid - Kidney
Pan - Pancreas,
   Gall Bladder
Liv - Liver
Spl - Spleen
H - Heart
W - Windpipe,
   Trachea
Tri - Triple Warmer

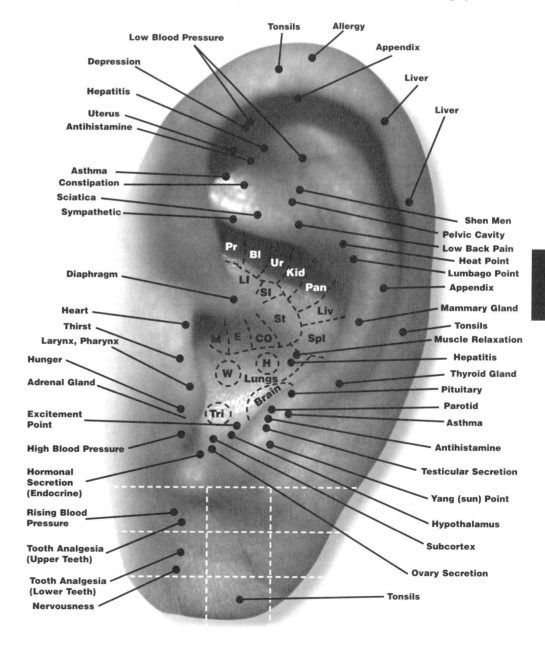

realm by applying oils to the acupressure points of the ears.

For working the spine and dealing with neurological problems that exist because of spinal cord injury, auricular probe technique was found to be extremely beneficial to deliver the oils to the exact location of the neurological damage.

Auricular probe technique is a program that Gary Young has been researching, developing, and teaching doctors about that has a tremendous value and will grow to be a well-known modality in the future.

Emotional Ear Chart

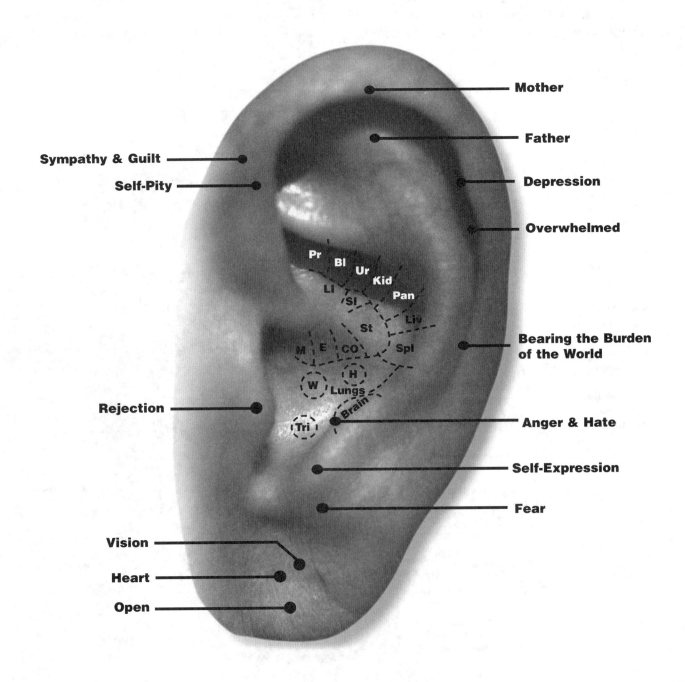

CHAPTER 17

Emotional Response with Essential Oils

Today, we live in a society of emotional turmoil. There is more focus on emotional behavior and psychological conditions of the body now than at any time in our history. Many doctors are recognizing the possibility that a number of diseases are caused by emotional problems that link back to infancy or even to problems that occurred during conception or while in the womb. These emotional problems may have compromised the immune system or genetic structuring, causing children to become allergic to something that the mother ingested while pregnant.

Essential oils play an important role in assisting people in getting beyond these emotional barriers. The aldehydes and esters of certain essential oils are very calming and sedating to the central nervous system (which consists of both the sympathetic and parasympathetic systems). These substances allow us to relax instead of letting anxiety build up in our body. Anxiety creates an acidic condition that activates the transcript enzyme that transcribes that emotion on the RNA template (RNA is the sister molecule of DNA) and stores it in the DNA. That emotion then becomes a predominant factor in our lives from that moment on.

When we have an emotional situation come up, instead of being overwhelmed by it, we can diffuse the oils, put them in our bath, or wear them as cologne. The oil molecules will absorb into the bloodstream from the nasal and buccal cavity to the limbic system. They will activate the amygdala (the memory center for fear and trauma) and sedate and relax the sympathetic/parasympathetic system. The oils help support the body in minimizing the acid that is created so that it does not create a reaction with the transcript enzyme.

Because essential oils affect the amygdala and pineal gland in the brain, they can help the mind and body by releasing emotional traumas and sharpening focus.

Essential oils provide assistance with staying centered in our goals. People have many distractions in today's fast-paced world. For example, if you are struggling to retain or remember informa-

tion, breathing the essential oils of peppermint, cardamom, or rosemary stimulate the brain and memory functions for better focus and concentration. Someone who is focusing on creating a business but finds other problems that interfere with that focus, could breathe the essential oils of galbanum, frankincense, sandalwood and melissa. These oils are extremely beneficial in enabling a person to bring his or her mind into a center of focus. The blend Gathering will also bring focus to people's minds. For emotional clearing and release, the essential oil blend Trauma Life is especially helpful.

Oils For Emotional Application

Abuse

Blends: SARA, Hope, Joy, Peace & Calming, Inner Child, Grounding, Trauma Life, Valor, Forgiveness, White Angelica.

Single Oils: Geranium, ylang ylang, sandalwood.

Agitation

Blends: Peace & Calming, Joy, Valor, Harmony, Forgiveness.

Single Oils: Bergamot, cedarwood, clary sage, frankincense, geranium, juniper, lavender, myrrh, marjoram, rosewood, rose, ylang ylang, sandalwood.

Anger

Blends: Release, Valor, Sacred Mountain, Joy, Harmony, Hope, Forgiveness, Present Time, Trauma Life, Surrender, Christmas Spirit, White Angelica.

Single Oils: Bergamot, cedarwood, Roman chamomile, frankincense, lavender, lemon, marjoram, myrrh, orange, rose, sandalwood, ylang ylang.

Anxiety

Blends: Valor, Hope, Peace & Calming, Present Time, Joy. Citrus Fresh, Surrender.

Single Oils: Orange, Roman chamomile, ylang ylang, lavender.

Apathy

Blends: Joy, Harmony, Valor, 3 Wise Men, Hope, White Angelica, Motivation, Passion.

Single Oils: Frankincense, geranium, marjoram, jasmine, orange, peppermint, rosewood, rose, sandalwood, thyme, ylang ylang.

Argumentative

Blends: Peace & Calming, Joy, Harmony, Hope, Valor, Acceptance, Humility, Surrender, Release.

Single Oils: Cedarwood, Roman chamomile, eucalyptus, frankincense, jasmine, orange, thyme, ylang ylang.

Boredom

Blends: Dream Catcher, Motivation, Valor, Awaken, Passion, Gathering, En-R-Gee.

Single Oils: Cedarwood, spruce, Roman chamomile, cypress, frankincense, juniper, lavender, fir, rosemary, sandalwood, thyme, ylang ylang, black pepper.

Concentration

Blends: Clarity, Awaken, Gathering, Dream Catcher, Magnify Your Purpose, Brain Power.

Single Oils: Cedarwood, cypress, eucalyptus, juniper, lavender, lemon, basil, helichrysum, myrrh, orange, peppermint, rosemary, sandalwood, ylang ylang.

Confusion

Blends: Clarity, Harmony, Valor, Present Time, Awaken, Brain Power, Gathering, Grounding.

Single Oils: Cedarwood, spruce, fir, cypress, peppermint, frankincense, geranium, ginger, juniper, marjoram, jasmine, rose, rosewood, rosemary, basil, sandalwood, thyme, ylang ylang.

Day Dreaming

Blends: Sacred Mountain, Gathering, Valor, Harmony, Present Time, Dream Catcher, 3 Wise Men, Magnify Your Purpose, Envision, Brain Power.

Single Oils: Eucalyptus, ginger, spruce, lavender, helichrysum, lemon, myrrh, peppermint, rosewood, rose, rosemary, sandalwood, thyme, ylang ylang.

Depression

Blends: Valor, Motivation, Passion, Hope, Joy, Brain Power, Present Time, Envision, Sacred Mountain, Harmony.

Single Oils: Frankincense, sandalwood, geranium, lavender, angelica, orange, grapefruit, ylang ylang.

Despair

Blends: Joy, Valor, Harmony, Hope, Gathering, Grounding, Forgiveness, Motivation.

Single Oils: Cedarwood, spruce, fir, clary sage, frankincense, lavender, geranium, lemon, orange, lemongrass, peppermint, spearmint, rosemary, sandalwood, thyme, ylang ylang.

Despondency

Blends: Peace & Calming, Inspiration, Harmony, Valor, Hope, Joy, Present Time, Gathering, Inner Child, Trauma Life, Envision.

Single Oils: Bergamot, clary sage, cypress, geranium, ginger, orange, rose, rosewood, sandalwood, ylang ylang.

Disappointment

Blends: Hope, Joy, Valor, Present Time, Harmony, Dream Catcher, Gathering, Magnify Your Purpose, Passion, Motivation.

Single Oils: Clary sage, eucalyptus, frankincense, geranium, ginger, juniper, lavender, spruce, fir, orange, thyme, ylang ylang.

Discouragement

Blends: Valor, Sacred Mountain, Hope, Joy Dream Catcher, Into the Future, Magnify Your Purpose, Envision.

Single Oils: Bergamot, cedarwood, frankincense, geranium, juniper, lavender, lemon, orange, spruce, rosewood, sandalwood.

Fear

Blends: Valor, Present Time, Hope, White Angelica, Trauma Life.

Single Oils: Bergamot, clary sage, Roman chamomile, cypress, geranium, juniper, marjoram, myrrh, spruce, fir, orange, sandalwood, rose, ylang ylang.

Forgetfulness

Blends: Clarity, Valor, Present Time, Gathering, 3 Wise Men, Dream Catcher, Acceptance, Brain Power.

Single Oils: Cedarwood, Roman chamomile, eucalyptus, frankincense, rosemary, basil, sandalwood, peppermint, thyme, ylang ylang.

Frustration

Blends: Valor, Hope, Present Time, Sacred Mountain, 3 Wise Men, Humility, Peace & Calming, Surrender, Passion.

Single Oils: Roman chamomile, clary sage, frankincense, ginger, juniper, lavender, lemon, orange, peppermint, thyme, ylang ylang, spruce.

Grief/Sorrow

Blends: Forgiveness, Valor, Joy, Hope, Present Time, White Angelica, Release, Trauma Life.

Single Oils: Bergamot, Roman chamomile, clary sage, eucalyptus, juniper, lavender.

Guilt

Blends: Valor, Release, Inspiration, Inner Child, Gathering, Harmony, Present Time, Magnify Your Purpose.

Single Oils: Roman chamomile, cypress, juniper, lemon, marjoram, geranium, frankincense, sandalwood, spruce, rose, thyme.

Irritability

Blends: Valor, Hope, Peace & Calming, Surrender, Forgiveness, Present Time, Inspiration.

Single Oils: All oils except eucalyptus, peppermint, black pepper.

Jealousy

Blends: Valor, Sacred Mountain, White Angelica, Joy, Harmony, Humility, Forgiveness, Valor, Surrender, Release.

Single Oils: Bergamot, eucalyptus, frankincense, lemon, marjoram, orange, rose, rosemary, thyme.

Mood Swings

Blends: Peace & Calming, Gathering, Valor, Dragon Time, Mister, Harmony, Joy, Present Time, Envision, Magnify Your Purpose, Brain Power.

Single Oils: Bergamot, clary sage, sage, geranium, juniper, fennel, lavender, peppermint, rose, jasmine, rosemary, lemon, sandalwood, spruce, yarrow, ylang ylang.

Obsessiveness

Blends: Sacred Mountain, Valor, Forgiveness, Acceptance, Humility, Inner Child, Present Time, Awaken, Motivation, Surrender, Passion.

Single Oils: Clary sage, cypress, geranium, lavender, marjoram, rose, sandalwood, ylang ylang, helichrysum.

Panic

Blends: Harmony, Valor, Gathering, White Angelica, Peace & Calming, Trauma Life, Awaken, Grounding.

Single Oils: Bergamot, Roman chamomile, frankincense, lavender, marjoram, birch, myrrh, rosemary, sandalwood, thyme, ylang ylang, spruce, fir.

Resentment

Blends: Forgiveness, Harmony, Humility, White Angelica, Surrender, Joy.

Single Oils: Jasmine, rose, Idaho tansy.

Restlessness

Blends: Peace & Calming, Sacred Mountain, Gathering, Valor, Harmony, Inspiration, Acceptance, Surrender.

Single Oils: Angelica, bergamot, cedarwood, basil, frankincense, geranium, lavender, orange, rose, rosewood, ylang ylang, spruce.

Shock

Blends: Clarity, Valor, Inspiration, Joy, Grounding, Trauma Life, Brain Power.

Single Oils: Helichrysum, basil, Roman chamomile, myrrh, ylang ylang, rosemary.

CHAPTER 18

Health Issues

Many of today's health concerns are caused by so-called modern conveniences. Increased use of sugars, artificial sweeteners, contaminated water, and even microwave ovens can all be harmful to health.

Sugars and Sweeteners

Nothing stresses the human body as much as refined sugar. Called a "skeletonized food" and a "castrated carbohydrate" by Edward Howell, Ph.D., and a "metabolic freeloader" by Ralph Golan, M.D., sugar actually drains the body of vitamins, minerals, and nutrients in the process of being burned for energy. Sugar also stresses the pancreas, forcing it to pump out a surge of unneeded digestive enzymes.

Sugars also undermine and downregulate immune response. One study measured the effects of 100 grams of sugar (sucrose) on neutrophils, a form of white blood cell that comprises a central part of immunity. Within one hour of ingestion, neutrophil activity dropped 50 percent and remained below normal for another four hours (Castleman, 1997).

Population studies have also linked sugar consumption with diabetes and heart disease. According to researcher John Yudkin, the reason sugar elevates the risk of heart disease is due to an automatic built-in safety switch inside the body. To protect itself from being immediately poisoned from excess sugar, the body converts it into fats, like triglycerides. So instead of killing you quickly, the body defends itself by clogging its arteries, thereby killing you on the installment plan.

The worst dangers, though, are not found in natural sugars but in the use of artificial sweeteners. Seventy-five percent of the adverse reactions reported to the U. S. Food and Drug Administration come from a single substance: the artificial sweetener aspartame.

Aspartame is marketed today as NutraSweet, Equal, Spoonful and Equal-Measure. With so many Americans on one diet or another, the market for aspartame is simply huge. And it matters not that aspartame users are suffering from symptoms ranging from headaches, numbness and seizures to joint pain, chronic fatigue syndrome, multiple sclerosis, and epilepsy.

This toxic artificial sweetener is made up of three chemicals: aspartic acid, phenylalanine and methanol. What these chemicals do in our bodies is anything but sweet.

Aspartame

A recent book by Dr. Russell L. Blaylock, professor of neurosurgery at the Medical University of Mississippi, *Excitotoxins: The Taste That Kills,* explains that aspartame is a neurotransmitter facilitating the transmission of information from one neuron to another. Aspartame allows too much calcium into brain cells, killing certain neurons, earning aspartame the name of "excitotoxin." With aspartame now in over 5,000 products such as instant breakfasts, breath mints, cereals, frozen desserts, "lite" gelatin desserts and even multivitamins, it is no surprise that there is a virtual epidemic of memory loss, Alzheimer's disease, and multiple sclerosis. In a move much like a telephone company selling your phone number to telephone solicitors and then charging you to block their calls, G. D. Searle (the Monsanto company that manufactures aspartame) is searching for a drug to combat memory loss caused by excitatory amino acid damage most often caused by aspartame.

Phenylalanine

The chemical phenylalanine, a by-product of aspartame metabolism, is an amino acid normally found in the brain. You may have heard of testing infants for phenylketonuria (PKU), a condition where phenylalanine cannot be metabolized, which can lead to death. It has been shown that excessive amounts of phenylalanine in the brain can cause serotonin levels to decrease. Have you ever concluded that half the people you know are on Prozac? Perhaps the flooding of American foods and soft drinks with aspartame is contributing to this need for drugs like Prozac and Zoloft.

But depression is not the most worrisome result of excessive phenylalanine levels in the brain. Dr. Blaylock writes that schizophrenia and susceptibility to seizures can occur as a result of these high levels. The Massachusetts Institute of Technology surveyed 80 people who suffered seizures following the ingestion of aspartame. The Community Nutrition Institute concluded that these cases met the FDA's own definition of an imminent hazard to the public health, but the FDA made no move to remove this dangerous product from the market.

Do you fly the friendly skies? You may be interested to know that both the Air Force's magazine, *Flying Safety,* and *Navy Physiology,* the Navy's publication, detailed warnings about pilots being more susceptible to seizures after consuming aspartame. The Aspartame Consumer Safety Network notes that 600 pilots have reported acute reactions to aspartame including grand mal seizures in the cockpit. Many other publications have warned about aspartame ingestion while flying, including a paper presented at the 57th Annual Meeting of the Aerospace Medical Association.

Methanol

Another by-product of aspartame is methanol. Free methanol results when aspartame is heated higher than 86 degrees F. If you cook a sugar-free pudding that contains aspartame, you are creating free methanol. If methanol were a criminal in a police lineup, it would wear a sign saying, "aka wood alcohol." For those desperate enough to drink it, wood alcohol can lead to blindness and even death. One quart of aspartame-sweetened beverage contains about 56 mg of methanol. The EPA states that methanol is "considered a cumulative poison due to the low rate of excretion once it is absorbed."

Methanol is truly criminal after it enters your body. It breaks down into formic acid and formaldehyde. Formaldehyde is a known carcinogen and can cause birth defects by interfering with DNA replication. Our Desert Storm troops were treated to free diet drinks that sat in the hot sun of Saudi Arabia. Many of the unusual symptoms found in Desert Storm veterans are similar to those of people chemically poisoned by formaldehyde.

The artificial sweetener aspartame would certainly not sell if people knew what kind of a toxic chemical stew they were ingesting.

Alternatives to Aspartame

Grade C Maple Syrup

Grade C maple syrup is the best sweetener and the most balanced sugar, since it contains a balance of positive and negative ions. It is processed in open kettles without formaldehyde. Other grades are processed in pressurized containers with formaldehyde added. Grade C Maple Syrup is also a low-glycemic index food, resulting in a slow, gradual rise in blood sugar levels.

Fructose

Fructose is a natural sweetener that has one of the lowest glycemic indexes of any food. A glycemic index measures the impact that a food has on blood sugar levels two to three hours after ingestion. The lower the glycemic level, the lower the rise in blood sugar levels.

With a glycemic index of only 20, fructose has one of the lowest of any food and many times lower than standard breads and processed grains. Fructose has a glycemic index that is only a third of that of glucose, a fourth of the glycemic index of white bread, and a fifth of the glycemic index for boiled potatoes.

Stevia

Known as *Stevia rebaudiana* by botanists and yerba dulce (honey leaf) by the Guarani Indians, stevia has been incorporated into many native medicines, beverages, and foods for centuries. The Guarani used stevia separately or combined with herbs like yerba mate and lapacho.

Fifteen times sweeter than sugar, stevia was introduced to the West in 1899, when M. S. Bertoni discovered natives using it as a sweetener and medicinal herb. With Japan's ban on the import of synthetic sweeteners in the 1960's, stevia began to be seriously researched by the Japanese National Institute of Health as a natural sugar substitute. In 1994, the U.S. Food and Drug Administration permitted the importation and use of stevia as a dietary supplement. However, its adoption by American consumers as a noncaloric sweetener has been very slow because the FDA does not currently permit stevia to be marketed as a food additive. This means that stevia cannot be sold as a sweetener (all sweeteners are classified as food additives by the FDA). Moreover, stevia faces fierce opposition by both the artificial sweetener (aspartame) and sugar industry in the U.S.

Stevia, however, is more than just a non-caloric sweetener. Several modern clinical studies have documented the ability of stevia to lower and balance blood sugar levels, support the pancreas and digestive system, protect the liver, and combat infectious microorganisms. (Oviedo et al., 1971; Suzuki et al., 1977; Ishit et al., 1986; Boeckh, 1986; Alvarez, 1986.)

Water

There is nothing more refreshing when you are hot and thirsty than clear, cold spring water. Water is not only refreshing but absolutely essential to life. The only nutrient more important to the body than water is oxygen.

Water is the crucial ingredient in our body's self-cleansing system. We are very aware of the body's normal elimination processes, but may not realize that unwanted substances are also eliminated through exhaled breath and perspiration, both of which also require water. Certainly our kidneys will not be able to cleanse efficiently if there is not enough water in our system to carry away waste.

Finding pure drinking water is becoming a challenge. Our increasingly polluted world has made it necessary for the Environmental Protection Agency to set water standards. The EPA screens for the presence of suspended solids, oil and grease, fecal coliform bacteria, chemicals and heavy metals. Unfortunately, the major source of pollution (65 percent in 1990) comes not from industrial sites, which can be regulated, but from storm-water run-off. Rainfall coming in contact with pollutants from agricultural and industrial operations absorbs these chemicals and transports them into lakes and rivers. Only 9 percent of water pollution came from actual industrial sites in 1990.

Municipal water should be avoided if possible. Most municipal waters have a high concentration of aluminum due to the use of aluminum hydroxide for water treatment. Moreover, the addition of chlorine results in the creation of cancer-causing chemicals when dissolved organic solids are chemically altered by chlorination. While there is a trend toward

replacing chlorination with peroxide treatment of water, it will be decades before peroxide is adopted as a standard.

We may turn to expensive bottled waters, but regulation in this industry is vague. Regardless of cost, the bottled water you buy may simply be tap water put through a filtration process. You may wish to invest in a water purifier for your home or drink distilled water to be sure you are getting pure water.

Distilled water washes out the system. With the help of essential oils and distilled water, the body can excrete petroleum residues, metals, inorganic minerals, and other toxins.

Essential oils, like lemon, also make outstanding water purifiers. One drop per glass is generally enough. Put the oil in a glass or container first, then run the water in. Since oils do not mix with water, this will distribute them through the water. Or put several drops in the out end of the carbon filter of a water purification system. This can drop nitrate levels by up to 3,000 ppm.

Since chlorine shuts down thyroid function, drink water that has the chlorine removed. You can either distill the water or let it stand unsealed (which allows the chlorine to evaporate over time). You can also add a drop of lemon or other oil. To obtain chlorine-free water for showering and bathing, get a shower head filter or aromatherapy shower head like the RainSpa. Avoid public swimming pools. While carbon filters are good for removing chlorine from water, the best water distillers have pre-flash or pre-boiling chambers, to flash off volatile gases, such as chlorine and petroleum products. The steam should rise at least 15 inches to balance the pH and fall 15 inches to oxygenate again.

One very popular water purification system is the ion exchange used in areas of the country with "hard" water or water with dissolved minerals. Water is passed through a filter exchanging charged particles (ions) in the water for charged particles in the filter. Most units use salt, with sodium and chloride ions exchanging for the contaminated ions in the water. Since the minerals are replaced with salt, at least one cold water tap needs to be left out of the system so that drinking water is not loaded with sodium.

The ideal amount of water to consume is half your body weight in ounces per day. That means if you weight 160 pounds, you should drink 80 ounces of water (or about ten, 8 ounce glasses per day. Avoid drinking any chlorinated water.

Microwave Ovens

Microwave ovens can be found in almost every home and restaurant because they are extremely convenient for thawing and heating food. Yet we are paying a great price for this convenience. In a study by Dr. Radwan Farag of Cairo University, it was discovered that just two seconds of microwave energy destroys all the enzymes in a food, thus increasing our enzyme deficiency and altering the frequency of the food. Heating proteins in the microwave for 10 minutes or more may create a new, harmful type of protein. You may decide that this is a high price to pay for convenience.

Also, microwave radiation has been known to leak and could disrupt the delicate balances in cellular growth. Our bodies are regulated by electrical frequencies and electromagnetic fields. It would be wise to avoid disrupting these frequencies.

And there is this to think about: the University of Minnesota warned that microwaving a baby's bottle can cause slight changes in the milk. In the case of a hip-surgery patient in Oklahoma, microwaving blood for a transfusion killed the patient. Warming blood for a transfusion is routine; unfortunately, using a microwave caused enough changes in the blood to be deadly.

For those who cannot give up convenience, please remember that plastic molecules could end up in your food if you microwave in plastic dishes or use plastic wrap to cover open dishes.

A research project with 20 volunteers was conducted in 1980 with microwave cooking. Ten volunteers in group A and 10 in group B fasted on liquids for 10 days. Then both groups were fed the same foods for another 10 days with only one exception: Group A foods were steamed, while group B foods were microwaved. After 10 days, stool samples were taken and analyzed. Group A stools appeared to be normally digested, while group B stools were of a plastic texture. Ultrasound scans showed adhesive food particles stuck to the stomach wall. In the stool sample, altered enzymes were found, as well as protein with altered molecular structure which could not be absorbed.

pH Balance

The Importance of Alkalinity to Health

The unfriendly bacteria and fungi that populate our intestinal tracts thrive in an acid environment and are responsible for secreting mycotoxins, which are the root cause of many debilitating human conditions. In fact, many researchers believe that most diseases can be linked to blood and intestinal acidity, which contributes to an acid-based yeast and fungus dominance.

The symptoms of excess internal acidity include:
• Fatigue / low energy
• Unexplained aches and pains
• Overweight conditions
• Low resistance to illness
• Allergies

• Unbalanced blood sugar
• Headaches
• Irritability / mood swings
• Indigestion
• Colitis / ulcers
• Diarrhea / constipation
• Urinary tract infections
• Rectal itch / vaginal itch

The ideal pH for the human body is between 7.4 and 7.6. Preserving this alkalinity (pH balance) is the bedrock on which sound health and strong bodies are built. When the blood loses its alkalinity and starts to become more acidic, the foundation of health is undermined. This creates an environment where we become vulnerable to disease and runaway yeast and fungus overgrowth.

The naturally-occurring yeast and fungi in the body thrive in an acidic environment. These same yeast and fungi are responsible for secreting a large number of poisons called mycotoxins, which are believed to be one of the root causes of many diseases and debilitating conditions.

When yeast and fungus decline in the body, so does their production of mycotoxins, the poisonous waste products and byproducts of their life cycles. There are numerous varieties of these mycotoxins, many of which are harmful to the body and must be neutralized by our immune systems. When our bodies are overwhelmed by large quantities of these toxins, our health becomes impaired, and we become susceptible to disease and illness.

Many cancers have been linked to mycotoxins. For example, the fungus *Aspergillus flavus*, which infests stored peanuts, not only generates cancer in laboratory animals but has been documented as the prime culprit in many liver cancers in humans.

By balancing the body's pH and creating a more alkaline environment, you can rein in the microbial overgrowth and choke off the production of disease-producing mycotoxins. With pH balance restored, the body can regain newfound vigor and health.

How to Restore Alkalinity

1. **Carefully monitor your diet.** Avoiding yeast- and fungus-promoting foods is a crucial factor in combating excess acidity and fungus overgrowth. Meats, sugars, dairy products, mushrooms, and pickled and malted products can be especially acidic. On the other hand, garlic is excellent for controlling fungi and yeast. Other high-alkaline, fungus-inhibiting foods include green and yellow vegetables, beans, and whole uncracked nuts. The natural ratio between alkaline and acid foods in the diet should be 4:1—four parts alkaline foods to one part acid. In his book, *the Yeast Syndrome*, Dr. Morton Walker outlines some antifungal diets.

   The pH of a raw food does not always determine its acidity or alkalinity in the digestive system. Some foods, like lemons, might be acidic in their natural state but when consumed and digested are converted into highly alkaline residues. Thus, the true determinant of a food's

pH is whether it is an alkaline-ash or acid-ash food. In this case, lemons are an alkaline-ash food.

2. **Avoid the use of antibiotics.** The overuse of antibiotics for incidental, minor, or cosmetic conditions not only increases the resistance of pathogenic microorganisms, but it kills the beneficial bacteria in your body, leaving the mycotoxin-generating yeast and fungi intact. This is why many women suffer outbreaks of yeast infections after antibiotic use.

3. **Use essential oils.** Many essential oils possess important antimicrobial, antibacterial and anti-fungal properties. French medical researchers in study after study have documented the healing properties of plant extracts and their ability to stimulate the immune system and inhibit bacterial growth.

   Essential oils work best when the body's blood and tissues are alkaline. When our systems become more acidic—due to improper diet or excessive levels of stress—essential oils lose some of their effects. So the best way to enhance the action of essential oils is to alkalize your body, and AlkaLime is a first-rate tool to accomplish this.

4. **Using alkaline salts.** AlkaLime is an outstanding source of alkaline salts that can help reduce internal acidity. An alkaline environment is hostile to fungi, which require acidity to survive and thrive. Lowered yeast and fungus populations translate into lower levels of body-damaging, disease-inducing mycotoxins.

5. **Lower stress.** Emotional and psychological tension can be especially damaging to bodily systems and act as a prime promoter of acid formation in the body. To properly appreciate how acidic stress can be, just think back to the last time you were seriously stressed-out and had to reach for an antacid tablet to soothe your heartburn or stomach discomfort.

   Some of the most common varieties of negative bacteria, yeast, and fungi that live in the intestines are inactive. However, when the body is weakened by illness, stress, and excess acidity caused by stress, these bacteria become active, damaging and assuming an invasive mycelic form.

Blends of essential oils high in sesquiterpenes, such as frankincense, myrrh, and sandalwood, can produce profound balancing and calming effects on emotions. They work by affecting the limbic system of our brain, the seat of our emotions.

6. **Boost friendly flora.** From three to four pounds of beneficial bacteria permanently reside in the intestines of the average adult. Not only are they the first line of defense against foreign invaders, but they are absolutely essential for health, energy, and optimum digestive efficiency. These intestinal houseguests not only control mucus and debris, but they produce B vitamins, vitamin K, and maintain the all-important pH balance of the body.

These friendly flora are also important in counteracting and opposing yeast and fungus overgrowth. When our natural cultures are compromised or disrupted by taking antibiotics or by poor dietary practices, yeast and fungus start growing unopposed and begin colonizing and invading larger swaths of our internal terrain, secreting ever-increasing volumes of poisonous mycotoxins.

Using an acidophilus or bifidus supplement, such as Royaldophilus, may be especially valuable in boosting levels of naturally occurring beneficial bacteria in the body and preventing fungal and yeast overgrowth. They also help the body maintain proper pH balance for nutrient digestion and absorption. Ideally, the lactobacillus acidiphilus and bifidobacterium bifidus cultures must be combined with plantain to promote implantation on the intestinal wall.

Research indicates a significant proportion of bacteria from many acidophilus supplements do not reach the lower intestine alive, or they arrive in such a weakened state that they are not of much benefit. This is why combining the acidophilus and bifidus cultures with plantain is so important because plantain helps these cultures adhere to the intestinal walls.

An even more effective means of fortifying the friendly flora in our intestines is by consumption of fructooligosaccharides (also known as FOS). FOS is one of the most powerful natural agents for feeding our friendly flora. FOS is made up of medium-chain sugars that cannot be used by pathogenic yeast and fungi. The end result is that FOS starves fungi while feeding the acidophilus and bifidus cultures that are our main defense against disease.

But FOS is far more than just an outstanding means of rebuilding and protecting the beneficial bacteria inside the body. Over a dozen clinical studies have documented the ability of fructooligosaccharides to prevent constipation, lower blood sugar and cholesterol levels, and even prevent cancer. (Hidaka et al., 1991; Briet et al., 1995); Bouhnik et al., 1996; Kawaguchi et al., 1993; Luo et al., 1996); Rochat et al., 1994; Tokunaga et al., 1993).

Stevia Select is a supersweet supplement that combines stevia with FOS.

Testing Your pH

You can easily test your pH at home by purchasing small litmus-paper strips at your drug store or pharmacy. To get the most accurate reading, expose the strip to a sample of your saliva immediately after awakening in the morning and before eating breakfast. Color changes on the litmus paper will determine pH; check the instructions of your kit for specific details on how to read the litmus paper.

Biofrequency and Disease

Frequency is a measurable rate of electrical energy that is constant between any two points. Every living thing has an electrical frequency.

- Robert O. Becker, M.D., documents the electrical frequency of the human body in his book, *The Body Electric*.

- A "frequency generator" was developed in the early 1920s by Royal Raymond Rife, M.D. He found that by using certain frequencies, he could destroy a cancer cell or virus. He found that these frequencies could prevent the development of disease, and others would destroy disease.

- Nikola Tesla said that if you could eliminate certain outside frequencies that interfered with our own electrical frequencies, we would have greater disease resistance.

- Bjorn Nordenstrom, a radiologist from Stockholm, Sweden, wrote the book *Biologically Closed Circuits*. He discovered in the 1980s that by putting an electrode inside a tumor and running a milliamp D.C. (Direct Current) through the electrode, he could dissolve the cancer tumor and stop its growth. He found electropositive and electronegative energy fields in the human body.

- Bruce Tainio of Tainio Technology in Cheney, Washington, developed new equipment to measure the biofrequency of humans and foods. He used this biofrequency monitor to determine the relationship between frequency and disease.

Measuring in megahertz, it was found that processed/canned food had a zero MHz frequency; fresh produce measured up to 15 MHz; dry herbs from 12-22 MHz; and fresh herbs from 20-27 MHz. Essential oils started at 52 MHz and went as high as 320 MHz, which is the frequency of rose oil. A healthy body typically has a frequency ranging from 62 to 78 MHz, while disease begins at 58 MHz.

Clinical research shows essential oils, having the highest frequency of any natural substance known to man, can create an environment in which microbes cannot live. Truly, the chemistry and frequencies of essential oils have the ability to help man maintain an optimal health frequency.

It is wonderful to discover that essential oil frequencies are several times greater than frequencies of herbs and foods.

For years, research has been conducted on the use of electrical energy to reverse disease. Scientists in the field of natural healing have believed there has to be a more natural way to increase the body's electrical frequency. This led to the research and subsequent discovery of electrical frequencies in essential oils.

Patients felt better emotionally when oils were diffused in their rooms. It seemed that, within seconds, these patients were more calm and less anxious with little exposure and inhalation. Certain oils acted within 1-3 minutes; others acted within seconds. It is fascinating to think that an oil applied to the bottom of the feet could travel to the head and take effect within one minute. The more results that have been seen, the more research has been initiated.

Unhealthy Substances Cause Frequency Changes

In one test, the frequency of two individuals – the first a 26 year. old male and the second a 24 year old male – was measured at 66 MHz each. The first individual held a cup of coffee (without drinking any), and his frequency dropped to 58 MHz in 3 seconds. He put the coffee down and inhaled an aroma of essential oils. Within 21 seconds, his frequency had returned to 66 MHz. The second individual took a sip of coffee and his frequency dropped to 52 MHz in the same 3 seconds.

However, no essential oils were used during the recovery time, and it took 3 days for his frequency to return to its initial 66 MHz.

One surprising aspect of this study measured the influence that thoughts have on the body's electrical frequency. Negative thoughts lowered the measured frequency by 12 MHz and positive thoughts raised the measured frequency by 10 MHz. It was also found that prayer and meditation increased the measured frequency levels by 15 MHz.

Health Programs with Essential Oils and Supplements

Cleansing and Digestion

The Risks of Internal Pollution

As we grow older, we risk suffering greater and greater buildup of chemical contamination in our bodies. As toxins accumulate, we are more likely to suffer the energy-robbing effects of poor health and degenerative changes. We feel sluggish, tired, and prone to illnesses.

This is why cleansing our bodies is so important. When we purge our systems of heavy metal contamination, undigested foods, and internal pollution, we relieve our organs and tissues of enormous stress.

Cleansing becomes especially important whenever we consume animal products, such as meats and dairy products. These foods are loaded with naturally-occurring, disease-related microbes. According to Robert O. Young, Ph.D., D.Sc., meats contain an average of 300,000 to 3 million microorganisms per gram, or roughly 336 million per serving. Cheese contains from 300,000 to 1 million microorganisms per gram; milk, 20,000. These animal products can be a major source of internal pollution. Clean plant food, on the other hand, contains only 10 microbes per gram.

Humans were built to be primarily plant-eaters, not meat-eaters. Our long intestinal tracts are similar to many plant-eating species and are specifically designed by nature to digest a high-fiber, high-roughage, plant-based diet. Its long length gives our enzymes a chance to unlock the nutrient value of our food. This contrasts markedly with the short intestines of flesh-eating animals, which are designed to quickly digest and pass through meats, without allowing them to putrefy, feed fungi, and create illness.

What happens when we consume meats and dairy products? Lacking fiber, such proteins move through our lengthy intestines very slowly and easily become trapped in the intestine's many nooks and crannies. Acting like toxic time bombs, putrefying pockets of undigested food gradually release their payload of heavy metals, chemicals, hormones, and toxins directly into the blood and tissues. Even worse, this undigested debris is fermented by our body's naturally-occurring yeast and fungi, polluting us with toxic by-products called mycotoxins. These mycotoxins have been linked to many diseases.

Who Needs Cleansing?

Everyone needs cleansing. All of us are stressed, to a lesser or greater degree, by an ever-mounting buildup of toxins, chemicals, bacteria, and parasites. A distinguished medical researcher, Kenneth Bock, M.D., states that humans are "walking toxic dumps." Why? Because of the industrial wastes, herbicides, pesticides, additives, and heavy metals we unknowingly absorb from our food, cosmetics, air, and water—even the mercury fillings in our teeth. Moreover, our place at the top of the food chain means that we are subjected to concentrated doses of potentially harmful chemicals from the meats and dairy products we consume.

According to a large 1990 survey by the Environmental Protection Agency, every single person tested showed some evidence of petro-chemical pollution in their tissues and fats. Some of the chemicals found included styrene (used in plastics), xylene (a solvent in paint and gasoline), benzene (a chemical found in gasoline), and toluene (another carcinogenic solvent).

Cleansing is also beneficial for degenerative diseases, allergies, Alzheimer's, arteriosclerosis, arthritis, asthma, bursitis, diabetes, cancer, hypertension, insomnia, multiple sclerosis (MS), and rheumatism, and of course infections, colds, and influenza, and often just sluggishness and general poor health. Cleansing allows the body to work towards fighting off the disease and not be encumbered or overloaded with the accumulation of toxins, mucous, and parasites that have built up over the years.

Understanding a Complete Cleansing

The ideal cleansing program should combine high water consumption with high-potency herbs, digestive enzymes, and therapeutic-grade essential oils. Essential oils have a special lipid-soluble makeup, which gives them a remarkable ability to penetrate cell membranes, break up undigested food, and oppose toxins. Essential oils also deliver oxygen, which has an unparalleled ability to inhibit the growth of many types of microbes. In fact, many essential oils have been studied for their unique antimicrobial, antifungal, and antiparasitic properties. Some oils, like rosemary, have demonstrated significant antiseptic activity, with documented research appearing in many scientific journals.

A cleansing program should target many different parts of the body (colon, intestine, stomach, liver, pancreas) and cover many different types of internal pollution, including waste buildup, heavy metals, parasites, fungi, and yeast.

When Should You Cleanse?

Cleansing your system should not be just a once- or twice-a-year event. It should be continuous.

Cleansing is especially important for anyone over 40. With age comes a greater buildup of debris in our bodies caused by a decreased production of the stomach acids and enzymes. Without proper enzyme production, we lack the ability to properly break down undigested proteins and other fermenting debris that obstruct our digestive system and impede the assimilation of nutrients.

To get the most out of any cleansing regimen, **drink plenty of distilled or purified water** (never chlorinated tap water) throughout the day. A good rule of thumb is to divide your body weight (in pounds) by half, then drink that number of ounces of water. For example, if you weigh 150 pounds, drink 75 ounces of water daily.

The Stanley Burroughs Master Cleanse

The Master Cleanse is not a fast, but a cleansing program. A true fast consists only of water, while the Master Cleanse incorporates a mixture of lemon juice, maple syrup, and cayenne pepper that is consumed throughout the day and is a source of calories, vitamins, and minerals.

The Master Cleanse is ideal for anyone who is not diabetic and can safely cleanse for at least three to seven days. The ideal duration of a cleanse can extend from one to three weeks. As with any program of caloric restriction, however, it is strongly recommended that you consult with your health care professional before undertaking any extended fast or cleanse.

Program:

Take juice of 1/2 fresh lemon (preferably organic)

Mix juice into 8 oz. of distilled water

Add 1-2 tablespoons of grade B maple syrup

Add 1/8 to 1/4 tsp. cayenne pepper (red)

Drink as many 8-10 oz. glasses as required according to your body weight per day. If you weigh 100 pounds then you would drink half your weight in ounces which would be 50 ounces or 5 glasses.

Grade B maple syrup is one of the most balanced of all sugars, containing a balance of positive and negative ions. Grade B does not enter the bloodstream as rapidly as honey or sugar which is better for people who react adversely to sugars, (becoming restless, sleepless, and energetic after consuming sugar), or may be borderline or pre-diabetic. Diabetics should substitute blackstrap molasses for the maple syrup, using up to 1/4 tablespoon.

Contrary to popular belief, lemon is not acidic in the body. It turns alkaline in the mouth. If an acid-like reaction is observed when using lemon with water, it is because of the minerals in the water. Distilled water will not react in this manner.

Cayenne pepper is a blood vessel dilator, thermal warmer, and provides vitamin A. People who have type O blood tend to have poor circulation. As a result, their body temperature may drop during a cleanse. Because cayenne is an herb known for its ability to warm and restore circulation, it may be taken internally and used topically (especially on the feet).

For the deepest cleanse, it is recommended that you cleanse for at least two to three weeks. Exercise enhances the cleansing action of the program.

During the middle and later phases of the cleanse, the body chemistry changes, and energy levels may begin to increase. One may experience minor discomforts, such as headaches, upset stomach, or low energy, as toxins and parasites are released from the body. These symptoms will be short-lived.

It is important to have a positive attitude during cleansing or fasting. If you are unaccustomed to the process, you can prepare yourself by fasting one day a week. Sunday, or your Sabbath day, is a wonderful day for this purpose. The biggest obstacle to successful cleansing is fear of failure and not knowing what to expect.

To fast for 24 hours, it is easier if you begin at noon of one day and finish at noon of the next day or from one dinner to the next.

Again, drink plenty of water.

As you begin to fast, you may experience some unpleasant side effects of cleansing, such as a headache, nausea, bloating, or irritability. These symptoms are part of the cleansing response and are often a result of toxins and waste matter being purged from the body which usually takes place within 12 to 36 hours. In any case, you may want to consult your health care professional.

You may have an unexpected emotional clearing. There are various essential oil blends designed to help control your emotions, and modulate and facilitate the emotional release. Herbs, like St. John's wort, kava, and hops extract, are excellent for managing stress and negative emotions. Ideally, these herbs should be taken using oral infusion therapy (sprayed into the inside of the mouth where they can be most efficiently delivered into the blood).

The first 2 to 4 days of the fast are often the most difficult, since you will be overcoming the powerful psychological need to eat. As your body is cleansed

of parasites and putrefying toxins, you will experience a sudden surge in energy and well being. Tapeworms, pinworms, and roundworms often start to appear in your stools (after 4 to 6 days), physical hunger will fade away. As the cleansing progresses, your mind will become sharper, your memory will improve, and your spirit will become more buoyant.

Remember: It is crucial to drink plenty of distilled water throughout the day, at least 8 to 10 eight ounce glasses. Water is crucial for not only flushing out toxins, but maintaining the metabolic machinery of your cells and tissues in proper working condition.

The Complete Cleanse

It is difficult to control internal pollution with a simple one-time fix or a single magic-bullet type solution. Complete cleansing requires a battery of different solutions all targeted at specific systems of the body. Cleansing the liver needs different herbs, oils and minerals than cleansing the colon which requires a different cleansing solution than the intestines.

Complete cleansing also requires a broad array of products that are effective against a wide variety of contaminants and microorganisms—not just one or two. Contaminants, like heavy metals, need a different set of tools to deactivate and purge them from the body than parasites do.

An important part of a complete cleansing program is essential oils. Highly antibacterial, antifungal, and antiviral, essential oils help dissolve and chelate toxic chemicals in the body. They also promote digestive function and enhance the intestinal contractions that are the cornerstone of waste elimination.

Tips

To aid the transition to vegetarianism and help re-program the system, take Body Balance three or four times per week. Also, for two weeks, take VitaGreen, then follow the master cleanse for another 30 days.

The Herbal Colon Cleanse: ComforTone

Some of the best natural laxatives include diatomaceous earth, buckthorn bark, licorice root, apple pectin, bentonite, and black current extract. These herbs are particularly effective in cleansing the colon (large intestine) and can help counteract bloating and constipation. Purging the colon of toxins and impurities is just as important as cleaning the small intestine. Waste products and gases that are held in the colon have a far higher concentration of toxic by-products than those in the small intestine. When these leach into the organs and tissues, they can wreak havoc in our bodies.

The essential oils of rosemary and tarragon are antimicrobial and combat fungal buildup in the colon. Peppermint oil promotes peristalsis, the wavelike motion of the intestines that moves waste matter out of the body.

Program:

Take two capsules every morning and two every night for two days.

Bowel movements should increase to 3-4 daily.

If elimination does not improve, then increase capsules to 3 each night and morning.

Keep increasing amount each day by one more capsule until you have achieved results.

If you feel cramping without results, you may have a dehydrated colon, spastic colon, loss of peristalsis, or a collapsed colon.

Drink 8 ounces. of aloe vera and/or prune juice daily, which will work as a lubricant.

You should drink half your body weight of water in fluid ounces daily. When cleansing, you need 20 percent more water. However, water is not a lubricant. It works to soften and flush. Clay-like stools indicate dehydration caused by not drinking enough.

When bowel movements occur 3 to 4 times per day, ComforTone has done its job. If you retain this regularity, after stopping ComforTone, you have taken enough. An ideal bowel movement is 1 movement for each meal consumed per day;

i.e.: 3 meals per day equal 3 bowel movements per day. When the movement slows to 1 or 2 per day or you begin to feel sluggish, begin again with ComforTone. You may completely reduce the amount to zero or you may find that you need 1-2 capsules daily for a few weeks until you feel that you do not need it any more.

Anyone, including pregnant women, should stop ComforTone if diarrhea occurs for 1 to 2 days Restart again with a smaller amount. Other than this, it is safe to take the supplement through the entire pregnancy.

ComforTone and JuvaTone should not be taken together as they might cause a release of too many toxins at the same time creating nausea, vomiting, dizziness or simple discomfort. They are best taken one hour apart to allow them to work separately within the body.

The Fiber Cleanse: I.C.P.

Coarsely ground grains rich in soluble and semi-soluble fiber are some of the best intestinal cleansers known. Psyllium powder and husks, rice bran, oat bran, and flax seed all help loosen and expel undigested and fermenting materials from the intestines that may block nutrient absorption and poison our internal environment.

Fibers act as a biochemical sponge for the body, absorbing impurities, gases, and toxins. They also speed up the flow of waste matter through the intestines, helping to minimize the exposure to harmful substances. The slower the "transit time," or movement of waste matter through the gastro-intestinal tract, the higher the incidence of disease.

Fiber satisfies the appetite by giving people a feeling of fullness without adding excessive calories. Fiber may also help balance blood sugar levels. It also helps maintain regularity as we grow older, preventing and overcoming constipation, diarrhea, and gas. Essential oils, such as fennel, tarragon, ginger, lemongrass, and rosemary, not only help dissolve and chelate toxins, but they also combat pathological microorganisms that reside in the intestines.

Program:

Take 1 tsp. morning and night for two or three days.

Increase to 2 tbs. morning and night while you cleanse and drink plenty of water.

Maintenance: 2 tbs., 3-4 time per week.

Mint Condition can be taken with ComforTone to soothe, help digestion, and relieve upset stomach.

Beta carotene, found in carrot juice and beet juice, also helps elimination.

Carrot seed oil detoxifies the liver, expels kidney stones, cleanses the bowel, and relieves flatulence.

To maintain a healthy colon, it is best to stay away from dairy products, cheeses, white sugar, and yeasts.

If ComforTone or I.C.P. produce heartburn, this indicates that the gut is not working properly. If the cleansing process reduces the intestinal flora, add the following to the program:

- Royaldophilus: 1 capsule, 2 to 3 times daily.

- Megazyme: 1-3 tablets per meal and up to 6 with heavy meat meals late in the day or at night.

- Yogurt: Take 1/2 hour before meals on an empty stomach.

These supplements provide the stomach with the friendly bacteria and enzymes necessary for good digestion, conversion, and assimilation. Master Formula HERS/HIS and CHILDREN'S, Royal Essence, and Mineral Essence provide trace minerals that the body requires to make enzymes.

When taken together, ComforTone and Megazyme have synergistic effects, so less of each is required to achieve similar benefits.

Colonics

Mix:
- 5 drops rosemary
- 5 drops basil
- 4 drops juniper

Add to colonic water and mix well.

The Enzyme Cleanse: Megazyme

Enzymes help break down foods and proteins that might otherwise ferment and putrefy in the gastrointestinal tract. Undigested foods tax our bodies, sap our energy, and spur the overgrowth of yeast, fungi, and parasites. Inadequate digestive enzyme activity has also been linked to chronic inflammations elsewhere in the body: fibromyalgia, herpes, inability to gain or lose weight, bad breath, body odor, skin rashes, and migraines. Enzymes like pancreatin and pancrelipase are very efficient in breaking down proteins. Vegetable enzymes from the unripe papaya and pineapple (papain and bromelain) provide enzyme support.

Digestive enzymes not only promote complete digestion but also help supply enzymes to people who have difficulty digesting and assimilating food. The older we get and the more food we consume, the more enzymes we need for complete digestion. Enzymes are essential in unlocking the vitamins, minerals, and amino acids from our food.

Enzymes help digest cooked and processed foods that lack the natural enzymes of fresh foods.

Program:

For maintenance: 2 or 3 tablets 3 times daily. They are best taken before meals.

Eating out: Carry tablets with you or take them when you return home. After a heavy meal at night and before going to bed, make sure to take plenty of tablets to help prevent fermenting.

A, B, and AB blood types: 2-4 tablets

O blood types: 3-6 or more tablets if you feel it necessary.

Cancer or other degenerative diseases:

Phase 1: Take 3 tablets 3 times daily. Increase by one tablet every day until you become nauseated or vomit. Then discontinue Megazyme for 24 to 36 hours.

Phase 2: Take 4 tablets 3 times daily. Increase daily by one tablet until you become nauseated or vomit. Rest again 24-36 hours.

Phase 3: Take 5 tablets 3 times daily. Increase daily by one tablet until you become nauseated or vomit. Rest again for 24-36 hours.

Phase 4: Start again with the amount that was being taken before nausea or vomiting occurred the third time. For example: If you were taking 30 tablets when you started to vomit, you would then start Phase 4 with 29 tablets spread out over each day. Continue with this amount for 6 weeks.

Phase 5: In the 7th week, start the enzyme saturation program again. This means that you begin Phase 1 and increase the amount by one each day until nausea or vomiting starts again. Repeat and continue for 6 weeks as previously described.

If your doctor determines that you are in remission, you can maintain with 20-30 tablets daily for one year, 6 days a week.

Maintenance: 6 Megazyme tablets, 2 times daily.

Caution: This is a rigorous program so you should consult with your doctor before starting and have your doctor monitor you.

The Liver Cleanse: JuvaTone and JuvaFlex

The liver is one of the most important organs in the body. It is pivotal for purifying the blood and plays a key role in converting carbohydrates to energy, as well as storing energy in the form of glycogen and fats. An overburdened liver can affect our energy, digestion, skin and blood.

Fats and bile within the liver can easily become saturated with toxic by-products, chemicals and heavy metals—many of which are oil-soluble. As these toxins accumulate, the liver becomes taxed and stressed. Skin conditions, rashes, fatigue, headaches, muscle aches, digestive disturbances, pallor, dizziness, irritability, mood swings and mental confusion can all become evident. Cleansing the liver can remove toxins and alleviate the problems caused by them.

Several dietary compounds have been shown to be helpful in cleansing the liver. The lipotropic agents, choline, inositol, and the powerful antioxidant, dl-methionine, have been researched for their ability to defat and remove toxic byproducts from the liver. Dl-Methionine is a sulfur-based amino acid that acts as an important liver-protecting antioxidant.

Oregon grape root is a source of berberine, a compound researched for its liver-protecting properties, as well as its ability to slow the liver damage and scarring (cirrhosis) associated with alcohol consumption and hepatitis B and C.

Essential oils can also be valuable in increasing the flow of bile from the liver. These oils include blue chamomile, carrot seed, and geranium. Carrot seed oil is well-regarded by herbalists for its role in liver cleansing.

Program:

Week 1: Take 3 tablets, 3 times daily for one week.

Week 2: Increase to 4 tablets, 3 times daily for one week.

Week 3: Increase to 5 tablets, 3 times daily for one week.

Week 4: Increase to 6 tablets, 3 times daily for 90 days.

Then decrease in the reverse order.

Rest for two weeks after the completed 120 day cycle.

Nausea or vomiting indicates a toxic liver. Stop and rest 2-3 days and then start again with 1/2 tablet per day. Gradually increase amount.

JuvaTone and ComforTone should not be taken together as they might cause a release of too many toxins at the same time creating nausea, vomiting, dizziness or discomfort. They are best taken an hour apart to allow them to work individually as the body needs.

JuvaFlex may be massaged over the liver once daily and may also be applied in a hot compress application (see compress). A compress may be applied once a week. JuvaFlex may also be applied on the bottom of the feet through the Vita Flex technique over the liver points.

The Parasite Cleanse: ParaFree

Almost everyone has parasites in one form or another. For the most part, they go entirely unnoticed until they begin to cause fatigue and unwellness.

Pure essential oils have some of the strongest antiparasitic properties known. Some of these oils include thyme, clove, anise, nutmeg, fennel, vetiver, wild tansy, cumin, melaleuca, and bay laurel.

Program:

The duration of this program depends on the individual.

Take 3-6 gelcaps, 2 times daily for one week. Rest for one week to allow the parasite eggs to hatch and become active.

Continue for a minimum of 3 weeks and then rest for 3 weeks. Repeat for 3 weeks.

The Heavy Metal Cleanse: Chelex Tincture

Heavy metals such as lead, mercury and cadmium can damage our bodies—even in microscopic amounts. They disrupt normal functions and can lead to allergic reactions, fatigue, headache, muscle pains, digestive disturbance, dizziness, depression and mental confusion.

Of even graver concern is their tendency to accumulate in the brain, kidneys, nerves, immune system, and fatty tissues. Some highly poisonous heavy metals, such as cadmium, can remain in the body for up to 30 years.

Herbs such as astragalus, garlic, sarsaparilla, and red clover have the ability to bind heavy metals so they can be expelled from the body. Essential oils also have a natural ability to dissolve insoluble heavy metal salts so that they can be eliminated.

Program:

Put 3-4 droppers in distilled water and drink 3-4 times daily for up to 120 days. Depending on type of mineral or chemical toxicity it may be necessary to follow this regimen for 1 1/2 years.

Maintenance: 1-2 droppers, 2 times daily, 5 days a week. The duration of this program depends on one's own knowledge of exposure and contamination.

Hair analysis may help in determining the duration of this program.

Blood Cleanse: Rehemogen Tincture

This tincture contains herbs that were traditionally used by Chief Sundance and the Native Americans for cleansing and purifying the blood. It builds red blood cells and is recommended for any blood disorder. It works as a strong companion with JuvaTone and Chelex.

Program:

Chelation with Chelex and JuvaTone: 2 droppers (50 drops) in water 2-3 times daily.

Blood disorders: Put 2-3 droppers (50-75 drops) in distilled water every 2-3 hours. JuvaTone with Rehemogen is invaluable.

Maintenance Cleansing

Our lifestyles should incorporate cleansing at all times. The extremity of the cleansing depends on the individual. You should always take ComforTone, Megazyme and I.C.P. at the same time.

Program:

ComforTone: 1 tsp. 5-6 days per week.

Megazyme: 3 tablets, 3 times daily to continue the digestion of toxic waste in your body from everyday metabolism.

Other Health Programs

Anti-Aging and Longevity

The Hunza Diet - Limited Caloric Intake

A people living in the remote Hunza Valley in Northern Pakistan are renowned for their longevity. The Hunzakuts (as they call themselves) routinely live past ages 100, 110 and even 120. They also share another remarkable trait: the near absence of degenerative disease.

It is known that the diet of the Hunza people is high in potassium and low in sodium. Apricots, barley, millet, and buckwheat are the main staples of their diet along with mineral-rich water with a pH of 8.5. But there is yet another unusual factor that may protect the health of the Hunza people and increase their longevity: their limited food intake.

Because the land provides just enough food to cover their basic caloric expenditures, the Hunzakuts rarely indulge in overeating. In fact, prior to the construction of the Korakoram Highway, they annually endured near-fasting conditions for several weeks each spring, a time when the previous year's food was depleted and the current year's harvests had not yet begun.

Restricted caloric intake can have powerful effects on longevity because it increases blood levels of growth hormone which is one of the most significant anti-aging hormones to be identified during the last two decades. Secreted by the pituitary gland, growth hormone production steadily declines with age. By age 70, the human body produces less than one-tenth of the growth hormone it did at age 20.

Clinical studies have repeatedly shown that growth hormone production is stimulated by low glucose levels. Because fasting depresses glucose levels, it leads to a surge in natural growth hormone production (Khansari et al., 1991).

Other studies have shown that the practice of caloric restriction (providing all necessary nutrients but limiting calorie intake) results in increased longevity and postponement of disease. Clive McCay at Cornell University showed that rats fed a diet low in calories but high in vitamins, minerals, and nutrients lived up to *twice as long* as rats fed on a regular diet (McCay et al., 1939). Ray Walford of the University of California in Los Angeles found that in studies on mice, the greater the reduction in calories, the longer the animal lived—as long as the vitamin and mineral content remained constant and the calories consumed did not drop below 40 percent of the normal (Walford et al., 1987).

Single oils: Frankincense, sandalwood, myrrh, cypress, and patchouly.

Blends: Brain Power, Di-Tone, EndoFlex, Clarity, Harmony, Live With Passion, and Valor.

Body massage weekly with the oils.

Supplements:

- Power Meal: 2 scoops, 2-3 times daily.

- Ultra Young: 3-4 sprays inside cheeks, 3-4 times daily.

- Be-Fit: 3-4 capsules, 2 times daily.

- Master Formula: 3-6 tablets, 2 times daily, depending on blood type.

- Goji Berry (wolfberry) Tea: 1-3 cups daily.

- Sulfurzyme: 1-2 tbs. daily. For some, 2 times weekly is sufficient.

- VitaGreen: O blood types: 6-12 capsules daily, A and AB blood types: 2-4 capsules daily.

- Super C: 1-3 capsules daily.

- A D & E: 1 dropper daily. Mix Power Meal, Body Balance, I.C.P., or any thicker liquid and drop in A.D.&E.. It will stay as a drop and will be easy to drink and not stick to sides of glass. Others simply drop into mouth and swallow.

- AlkaLime: 1 tsp. in water once daily or less (depending pH levels).

- Use AromaSilk Satin Body Lotion to hydrate the skin.

Also use Essential Manna, Thyromin, Immune-Tune, Royal Essence.

Babies and Children

Babies and children respond very well to oils and supplements. The only difference from adult use is smaller dosage.

Babies: Put 1-2 drops of oil in your hand and rub them together until the hands are practically dry. Then hold them over any particular area of the baby. This works very well without direct application.

Direct application: Mix 1-2 drops of an essential oil in V-6 Mixing oil or Massage Oil Base and apply to bottom of feet.

Children: Put 1-2 drops on bottom of feet or anywhere else on the body as long as the oil is diluted in V-6 Mixing oil, Massage Oil Base, or any vegetable or massage oil. The dilution is always the important factor in comfortability.

Balancing Body Frequency

Much of the cause of imbalance is in the endocrine glands, which create the electrical balance throughout the physical body.

Where the imbalance is due to allergy in sinuses, throat, or pituitary insufficiency, apply the complementary oil to the crown of the head, the forehead, and the thymus.

The blend Release stimulates harmony and balance by releasing memory trauma from liver cells, which store emotions of anger, hate, and frustration. Rub neat over liver, apply compress over liver, or massage Vita Flex points on feet and hands (see COMPRESSES).

Sandalwood oxygenates the pineal/pituitary gland, thus improving attitude and body balance. Rose has a frequency of 320 MHz, the highest of all oils. Its beautiful fragrance is aphrodisiac-like and almost intoxicating. The frequency of every cell is enhanced, bringing balance and harmony to the body. Rose is stimulating and elevating to the mind, creating a sense of well being.

Lavender is very good unless it is an oil that is disliked. Harmony will probably work in most situations. Inner Child is also excellent.

For overall body electrical imbalance, put a couple of drops of the complementary oil in each palm, have the person hold the right palm over the navel and the left palm over the thymus and take three slow, deep breaths. Place the dominant hand over the navel and the other hand over the thymus and rub clockwise three times. This works through the body's electrical circuitry by pulling the frequency in through the umbilicus, the thymus, and the olfactory to the limbic system in the brain to create electrical balance.

Apply Thieves on the bottom of the feet. Sage is good for balancing frequencies when disease lowers body frequency.

Harmony on the energy centers (or chakras) helps balance the body, enhancing the healing process and facilitating the release of stored emotions.

The energy points corresponding to the endocrine glands are:

- The crown (top) of the head (pineal)
- Forehead (pituitary)
- Neck (thyroid)
- Thymus
- Solar plexus (adrenal)
- Navel (pancreas)
- Groin (ovaries/gonads)

Other oils that can be used are frankincense, myrtle, Valor, 3 Wise Men, and Joy.

Blood Types and Food Supplements

In 1996, Dr. Peter J. D'Adamo's book, *Eat Right 4 Your Type*, presented the concept of separate diets for each of the four blood types.

People with blood type A and AB are natural vegetarians and have the easiest time converting to a vegetarian diet. However, these people also have a tendency for thyroid problems and tend to be overweight. For them, exercise that increases heart rate is necessary to have weight reduction.

People with type B blood are probably the most balanced in nutritional needs and can more easily be either vegetarians or meat-eaters.

People with type O blood need additional protein, possibly through meat consumption. They have a more difficult time converting to vegetarianism. These people can get all the protein they need if they consume the correct portions of seeds, nuts and grains. VitaGreen should be a mainstay for this group. These people often have digestive deficiencies. They eat more but assimilate less, have excess gas, get full quickly but are hungry sooner, and tend to weigh less.

People who have type O blood tend to have poor circulation and as a result tend to be cold when fasting. Cayenne pepper improves this situation. One can also put some cayenne in one's shoes and socks when they are worn. Cayenne becomes damp from foot perspiration creating warmth to the feet.

During fasting, O blood types may require more protein. During the first two weeks these people should take Body Balance twice a day and should also take VitaGreen three times per day. These supplements will provide the necessary proteins. After two weeks, the supplements should be ceased, because protein intake must be zero in order to effect DNA memory change. The body will convert its minimal protein requirements as needed.

Blood type is one of many variables to be considered in selecting what you eat and the supplements you take.

Building the Body

Nutritional supplements enhanced with essential oils can help support and balance body systems. The following products will nourish, strengthen and build your body.

Program:

Power Meal — The all-vegetarian protein drink with Chinese wolfberries.

Use 2 scoops (4 tbs.) in liquid 2-3 times per day. Mix in water, rice or soy milk. It can be mixed in orange or apple juice, but this may make it too sweet and lower the pH. It also may be mixed with cereal, fruits, deserts, and other foods.

Combine equal parts Power Meal and Body Balance for a high-powered protein blend.

Drink as needed.

Master Formula HERS/HIS — Premium multivitamin, mineral, and amino acid supplements.

O Blood Type: 8-10 tablets daily.

B Blood Type 6-8 tablets daily.

A Blood Type 4-6 tablets daily.

Megazyme — Enzyme function for mental clarity and physical activity.

O Blood Type: 4-8 tablets daily (depending on type of food eaten and time of day).

B Blood Type: 8-10 tablets daily.

A Blood Type: 10-12 tablets daily (A types tend to have more digestive needs).

Note: When eating heavy protein foods after 3:00 p.m., it is very helpful to take more Megazyme before going to bed.

Exodus — Supercharged antioxidant formula for immune supporting.

O Blood Type: 6-8 capsules daily.

B Blood Type: 6-7 capsules daily.

A Blood Type: 4-6 capsules daily.

VitaGreen — Protein-rich chlorophyll formula.

O Blood Type: 8-10 capsules daily.

B Blood Type: 6-8 capsules daily.

A Blood Type: 4-6 capsules daily.

Ultra Young — Supports healthy pituitary and growth hormone secretion.

Apply 3 sprays on the inside of the cheeks to maximize absorption. Avoid swallowing. Inhale the fragrance of the oils if possible.

Age 15-30: 3 sprays, 2 times daily (for immune support).

Age 30-45: 3 sprays, 2-3 times daily.

Age 45-65: 3 sprays, 4-6 times daily.

Juvenile Pituitary Retardation: 3 sprays, 3-6 times daily.

Spray 6 days a week for 3 weeks and rest for one week and then repeat.

ImmuneTune

O Blood Type: 6-8 capsules daily.

B Blood Type: 6 plus capsules daily.

A Blood Type: 4 plus capsules daily.

Super C

1 capsule daily for maintenance.

2 capsules daily for reinforcing immune strength.

Super Cal

2-6 capsules daily or as needed.

Mineral Essence

3-6 droppers (75 to 150 drops) in water 1-2 times daily.

Sulfurzyme

Start: 1-2 tsp daily for 1-2 days

Increase: 1-2 tbs 2 times daily for maximum results.

The Clock Diet

The Clock Diet was originated by Dr. Charlotte Holms who maintained a private practice even at 100 years of age in 1989. This diet was based on the fact that stomach acid and enzyme production (pepsin and hydrochloric acid) begins in the morning (about 6 a.m.) and tapers off during the afternoon (between 1:00 and 3:00 p.m.).

This diet mandates that we should schedule our consumption of animal and plant protein to coincide with the highest output of stomach acid and enzymes. Unless our body produces the enzymes to break down protein, high-protein foods will merely ferment in the stomach and lead to fungal and bacterial overgrowth, laying the groundwork, not only for indigestion, but also for disease.

Ideally, we should consume all of our high-protein foods once a day during the morning meal. These foods include grains, such as oats, cornmeal, millet, soy milk, and brown rice, and animal products, such as cheese, milk, and meats.

When the stomach's production of acid and enzymes drops during midafternoon, the best foods to eat consist of simple and complex carbohydrates such as fresh fruits and cooked and raw vegetables.

Avoid mixing protein and carbohydrates in the same afternoon or night meal.

Daily Maintenance

The human body has a daily need for nutrients to keep it in peak condition. The nutritional products listed below contain essential oils to help support normal digestive function and nutrient absorption.

Power Meal or Body Balance—Complete protein foods.

Combine or use individually: 1-2 scoops in water, rice milk, oat milk, or other liquid.

VitaGreen—Protein-rich chlorophyll formula very beneficial for vegetarians and O blood types.

O Blood Type: 8-10 capsules daily.

B Blood Type: 6-8 capsules daily.

A Blood Type: 4-6 capsules daily.

Master HIS/HERS—Gender-specific vitamin, mineral, and amino acid complexes.

O Blood Type: 8-10 tablets daily.

B Blood Type: 6-8 tablets daily.

A Blood Type: 4-6 tablets daily.

ComforTone—All natural colon cleanser.

Essential Manna—Whole food complex, a fiber- and mineral-rich snack.

Fasting

Fasting has been called nature's single-greatest healing therapy. Fasting is the avoidance of solid food with liquid intake varying from no liquids to just water to fresh juices. A fast can last 24 hours or several weeks. Fasting has long been a tradition in Judaism, Christianity and the Eastern religions. Religious fasting can involve purification, penitence or preparation for approaching God. An increasing number of doctors are recognizing that fasting can be physically healing while allowing us to focus our energy inward, bringing clarity and change.

Gabriel Cousens, M. D. writes that "fasting in a larger context, means to abstain from that which is toxic to mind, body and soul. A way to understand this is that fasting is the elimination of physical, emotional and mental toxins from our organs, rather than simply cutting down on or stopping food intake. Fasting for spiritual purposes usually involves some degree of removal of oneself from worldly responsibilities. It can mean complete silence and isolation during the fast which can be a great revival to those of us who have been putting our energy outward.

Fasting is generally safe but those with medical conditions should check with their health care professional.

Elson M. Haas, M. D. notes that fasting is a catalyst for change and an integral part of transformational medicine. He writes, "Fasting clearly improves motivation and creative energy; it also enhances health and vitality and lets many of the body systems rest."

An extremely important benefit of fasting is the elimination of toxins. By minimizing the work our digestive system must do, we allow it to repair itself and clean up stored toxins. In the beginning of a fast, the liver will convert stored glycogen to energy. As the fast continues, some proteins will be broken down unless juices provide calories.

The best way to convert to vegetarianism is by fasting. To be healthy, have energy, be free of sickness and disease, you must learn to discipline yourself and listen to the needs of your body.

Our bodies do not need meat to maintain good health, even though many of us have programmed ourselves through years of meat consumption to have the desire to eat meat. Our bodies can get all the protein required from a diet containing a wide variety of non-meat foods: beans, lentils, vegetables, whole grains, seeds, some cheeses, dairy products (preferably unpasteurized and natural colored), and occasionally eggs. However, you must be sure to eat enough protein to maintain a balanced, healthy body.

Exercise makes fasting work better, particularly if one is trying to lose weight.

Anyone fasting for more than three days should do so under supervision.

Never begin a shut-down fast unless you have been fasting regularly for at least two years. This type of a fast should always be done under supervision.

NOTE: Pregnant or lactating mothers should seek medical supervision before beginning a fast.

Fitness

Power Meal—2 scoops, 4-6 times daily in water or rice milk or as needed.

Be-Fit—2 capsules before working out and 2 capsules after working out.

Capsules may be increased or decreased as needed according to body weight and blood type.

VitaGreen—As desired, anywhere from 4-10 capsules daily.

Master HIS/HERS—As desired, anywhere from 4-8 capsules daily.

Fortifying the Immune System

The immune system is the most important body system. It must be strong and responsive in order to combat infectious diseases and counteract toxins. Some 40 percent of immune system function is found in the intestinal tract and is called *pirus patchet*. Another 40 percent is accounted for by the thymus gland, which produces immune-stimulating cells.

Dietary supplements containing essential oils provide nutritional support for normal immune system function. Many ingredients in these nutritional products are used to reinforce the body's natural defense system. Research has found that microorganisms do not develop resistance to essential oils as much as they do to many other products.

Exodus II—blended with oils referenced in the Old and New Testaments.

Massage 3-6 drops on bottom of feet, thymus, throat, or wherever desired.

Exodus—a strong immune builder.

Maintenance: 2-4 capsules daily; O blood types may increase amount.

For weaker system: Take 6-10 capsules, 3 times daily for 10 days and then reduce. Type A bloods may want to use less.

Sulfurzyme—contains MSM and Chinese Wolfberry.

> **Maintenance:** 1-2 tsp. daily in water or juice. May increase as needed.

> **Deficiencies:** Begin 1-2 tsp. daily and work up to 3-4 tbs. daily or more if desired.

ImmuneTune—has strong antioxidant, anti-inflammatory, and anti-tumoral properties. Helps maintain electrolyte and pH balance.

> **Maintenance:** 2-4 capsules daily.

Radex—contains herbs and essential oils that have been researched for their antioxidant properties and their effects on DNA-damaging free radicals. This blend also contains Super Oxide Dismutase, widely reported to be another powerful free-radical scavenger.

Super C—a special formula of ascorbic acid, scientifically balanced with rutin, bioflavonids, and trace minerals to balance electroytes and assist in the absorption of vitamin C. The essential oils of grapefruit, tangerine, lemon, and mandarin may increase the oxygen and bioflavonoid activity.

Thyromin—an herbal complex with amino acids, minerals, herbs, and essential oils to support to the thyroid. This gland regulates body metabolism and temperature and is important for immune function.

Immugel—a blend of liquid amino acids, ionic trace minerals and herbal extracts with essential oils. Amino acids are the building blocks of protein and form the enzymes used to support immune function.

Protec—a blend of essential and vegetable oils for the prostate, designed for a night-long retention enema.

Mineral Essence—a precisely balanced complex of essential oils and more than 60 trace minerals that are essential to a healthy immune system. It includes well-known antioxidants and immune-supporters such as zinc, selenium and magnesium.

Other Products for Supporting the Immune System

Single oils:

- Frankincense with ravensara, thyme, helichrysum, oregano, rosemary, chamomile, Idaho tansy, mountain savory, melissa, lavender, grapefruit, lemon, cinnamon, clove, cumin, cistus, melaleuca, myrrh, myrtle, rose, vetiver, or lemongrass.

Blends:

- Frankincense with Thieves, ImmuPower, Abundance, Acceptance, Humility, Raven, or 3 Wise Men.

Supplements:

Super B, Royal Essence, VitaGreen, Power Meal, ArthroTune, Goji Berry Tea, Rehemogen, Alka-Lime, Ultra Young, Cleansing Trio, JuvaTone, and Wolfberry Power Bar.

Other Steps for Maintaining a Healthy Immune System

1. Cleanse the colon and liver of toxins and accumulated waste that can sap energy and down-regulate immune response.

   — The Cleansing Trio is a complete cleansing solution.

2. Avoid excess fear, anxiety, and depression, which can undermine and compromise immune function. Continual daily use of essential oils is optimal to overcome stress (see STRESS).

3. Avoid physical and mental overexertion which can downregulate immune response. Essential oils, such as lavender, can have powerful relaxant effect on the mind and body, and thus stimulate immune function.

4. Maintain a healthy, balance diet. A diet high in minerals, such as magnesium, potassium, selenium, zinc, and folic acid play a crucial role in optimizing immune response.

   — Mineral Essence is rich in magnesium and trace minerals.

   — Essential Manna is rich in potassium, magnesium, selenium, zinc and numerous other nutrients.

— Super B is a good source of all B vitamins. Those with impaired immune systems often lack vitamin B5.

5. Avoid contaminated or chlorinated water.

   Chlorine inhibits thyroid function interfering with its uptake of iodine and the amino acid tyrosine and therefore slows down metabolism, circulation, and immune function.

   — Add 1 drop of lemon, peppermint, or spearmint to drinking water.

   — Use chlorine-free water for showering and bathing. The RainSpa shower head is specially designed to accept bath salts loaded with essential oils.

6. Stimulate the immune system using selected essential oils and supplements.

   — Grapefruit, lemon, lemongrass, and Raven promote leukocyte (white blood cell) formation.

   — ImmuneTune and Exodus (herbal complex) build and support the immune system. Exodus II (essential oil blend) is a companion to both supplements.

   — VitaGreen encourages healthy blood and boosts immune function.

7. Diffuse essential oils to reduce airborne pathogens and viruses that can overwhelm the immune system.

   — ImmuPower and Thieves

   NOTE: Do not diffuse Thieves more than 15 to 30 minutes at a time as the cinnamon may irritate the nasal passages. Also be sure that the room is well ventilated.

8. Inhalation of essential oils can increase immune function through their ability to stimulate the hypothalamus. According to studies conducted by Dr. Asawa of Japan and Dr. Richardson of England, inhalation of unadulterated essential oils increase blood flow to the brain by 15 percent and brain blood oxygen levels by 25 percent.

9. Eliminate parasites which compromise immune function by overloading the system (see PARASITES).

10. Use essential oils in massage applications or take as dietary supplements. Research from the Universities of Cairo, Geneva, and Paris indicate that essential oils are one of the highest known sources of antioxidants.

    — Thieves, Exodus II, mountain savory, abundance, ImmuPower.

    Dilute 1 or 2 drops in massage oil or V-6 Mixing Oil and massage on the thymus, bottom of feet, and throat. These oils can also be used as dietary supplements: Use 3 drops, four to six times daily for seven days. Repeat the cycle again, if needed, after four day rest.

11. Support the thyroid gland. The thyroid is crucial to regulating body metabolism, energy levels, and balancing immunity.

    — Thyromin strengthens the thyroid (see THYROID).

12. Use antioxidants.

    — Super C contains vitamin C and bioflavonoids and acts as a strong immune support.

    — Essential Manna contains an extremely wide variety of natural antioxidants.

    — Radex is power free-radical eliminator.

13. Reduce candida and fungal overgrowth in the body. These can seriously impair and overload immune function. Alkaline ash whole foods and FOS (fructoligosaccharides) can minimize fungal growth.

    — Stevia Select is a supersweet, noncaloric supplement containing FOS and stevioside.

    — Essential Manna is a whole food complex of alkaline-ash nutrients.

    (See BODY pH ACID/ALKALINE BALANCE)

14. Increase intake of antioxidants when exposed to radiation. If you know you have been exposed to radiation, feeling fatigued from it, or if you are flying with commercial airlines (because of the greater exposure to radiation due to the high altitude) an increased daily amount antioxidant supplements is needed. When flying, increase intake 10 days before the trip and continue this higher dosage for 10 days after the trip.

Guidelines for the Healthiest Diet

Breakfast is the most important meal of the day. Some people get up and work for an hour or two until they have a good appetite and the digestive system is awake. Then they have breakfast.

Eat breakfast between 6 and 7 a.m. Do not eat any fruit. The exception to this is strawberries with cereal or occasionally bananas. Yogurt is good since it supplies friendly bacteria. Cereals may be oatmeal, millet, wheat, barley, triticale, or a mixture of these, with coconut milk, rice milk, soy milk, whey powder, or goat milk. Since we do not have enough enzymes to handle multiple foods, it is best to not mix over 3 grains or different foods at a time. Bread should always be toasted; this changes it from a wet food to a dry food, making it more digestible.

Breakfast is the best meal of the day for eating proteins, such as beans and rice, or if you eat meat, then meats, eggs, fish, etc. Avoid meat after the noon meal; meat is best for breakfast. This will provide more energy and stamina in the afternoon because in the morning the enzymes are in place for meat digestion.

Our bodies cannot absorb vitamins and minerals without the presence of protein (protein powders suffice). This is particularly true for those who have had their gall bladder removed. Power Meal, Sulfurzyme, and Megazyme magnify the nutritional effects of vitamins vital to the production of amino acids that are responsible for protein synthesis.

Lunch should consist of carbohydrates and complex carbohydrates in the form of pasta, fruit, vegetable broth (not solid vegetables), or juices.

Dinner should be eaten as close to 3 p.m. as possible. It is better not to eat late at night. Both fruit and solid vegetables are fine for the evening meal.

If one must eat a large, heavy meal late in the day or evening, an extra portion of Megazyme is most beneficial. This will assist with digestion and assimilation of the heavy food, allowing restful sleep and a reduction of gas production.

Be patient. It may take 2 to 2 1/2 years of very diligent work to establish good digestive function. Listen to your body and modify the program as your body changes.

Hering's Four Laws of Healing

Constantine Hering, a German homeopath who emigrated to the United States in the 1830s, is considered the father of American homeopathy. He formulated four fundamental principles of healing:

1. Healing progresses from the deepest part of the organism—the mental and emotional levels and the vital organs—to the external parts, such as the skin and extremities.

2. As healing progresses, symptoms appear and disappear in the reverse of their original chronological order of appearance.

3. Healing progresses from the upper to the lower parts of the body. This means that head symptoms may clear before stomach symptoms. Deep toxins in the colon or liver will be released before the more surface areas.

4. The most recent illnesses will be the first to leave. This means that flu symptoms experienced a month ago will leave earlier in the healing than the bronchitis suffered two years before.

Hormone Balance: Men

ProGen

Helps feed and nourish the male reproductive system.

Maintenance: Take 2-3 capsules, 2 times daily

Aggressive deterioration: 6 capsules, 3 times daily.

Mister

Supports male reproductive system. May be taken as a dietary supplement: 3-10 drops under tongue, 2-3 times daily. Take 10-20 drops in water or in a capsule, 2 times daily. Use no more than 7 days and then rest 4 days. Massage on Vita Flex points and between scrotum and rectum.

Hormone Balance: Women

Estro Tincture

Estro is designed for women who are estrogen deficient. Numerous studies have researched the benefits of black cohosh for relieving PMS symptoms, without the side effects associated with synthetic estrogen. The German Commission E recommends black cohosh for premenstrual discomfort and ailments associated with menopause.

Estro is comforting for cramping and irregular bleeding. In these cases, FemiGen should accompany Estro to help give more balance to the estrogen.

To begin: Drink 2-3 droppers in water, 1-3 times daily.

FemiGen

FemiGen is a dietary supplement designed to strengthen the reproductive system, creating better hormonal balance and helping with night-time sweats.

For deficiencies, take 3-4 capsules, 2-3 times daily.

For maintenance, take 4-8 capsules, 2 times weekly.

Femalin

May help cervical lesions and cysts, ovarian cysts, and endometriosis.

Begin: 2-3 droppers in water, 3 times daily.

Increase if necessary: 3-4 droppers in water, 4 times daily or as necessary to alleviate cramping and irregular bleeding.

Douche: Mix 6 droppers in distilled water, 2-3 times daily.

Dragon Time

Massage 3-4 drops around inside and outside of ankles and over lower back for premenstrual problems, ovarian imbalance, cramping or irregular flow. Two to three drops of clary sage may also be added for extra strength.

Suppository: 20 drops in a capsule, insert at night for night retention.

Bath: Mix 30 drops in bath gel base for a relaxing and soothing bath.

Mister

Many women ages 40-plus have found that Mister helps in preventing hot flashes. May be used in bath, on Vita Flex points, rubbed on lower back and over lower abdomen. It is a good companion to Dragon Time.

Royaldophilus: Restores proper flora in bowels

If taking antibiotics or undergoing chemotherapy or radiation: Take 3 capsules, 3 times daily for one week after finishing with antibiotics or medical intervention.

Maintenance: Take 3 capsules, 3 times weekly.

Yogurt taken before lighter meals also helps provide friendly bacteria. The need for yogurt is sometimes indicated by an intolerance of dairy products.

CHAPTER 21

Veterinary Medicine

Veterinary Medicine

Essential oils have been used very successfully on many different kinds of animals from tiny kittens to 2,000-pound draft horses. Animals often respond to essential oils in similar ways as humans. Animals are not as sensitive to the phenol and sesquiterpene constituents so the oils can be applied "neat," or full strength. A determination must be made which oils are applicable to the situation. For long term treatments or health regimens, a few drops of oil can be applied 3-4 times daily.

General Guidelines:

For small animals: (cats and small dogs) Apply 3-4 drops per application.

For larger animals: (large dogs) Apply 6-7 drops per application.

For horses: Apply 15-20 drops per application.

Helpful Tips:

When treating animals for viral or bacterial infection, arthritis, or bone injury, use the same oil and protocol recommended for humans.

For open wounds or hard-to-reach areas, oils can be put in a spray bottle and sprayed directly on location.

After applying the oils locally, cover the open wound with Rose Ointment to seal the wound and protect it from further infection. It also prevents the essential oils from evaporating.

There is no right or wrong way to apply essential oils. Use common sense and good judgment as you experiment with different methods.

Take care not to get essential oils in the animal's eyes.

When treating animals with essential oils internally, make sure that the oils are pure and free of chemicals, solvents, and adulterants.

How to Apply Essential Oils:

For non-ungulate animals (not having hooves) such as dogs or cats, oils can be applied to paws for fast absorption.

For hoofed animals, apply oils on the spine or auricular points of the ears.

Apply on the gums, tongue, or underneath the top lip.

Sprinkle a few drops on the spine or flanks and massage them in.

Example of Application:

If you have a high-spirited, jittery horse that is tough to saddle, apply Peace & Calming and Valor on yourself. As you approach him, he will have a tendency to bow his head or flare his nostrils when he perceives the aroma. Kneel down or squat beside him and remain still so that the animal can become accustomed to the smell. As he breathes in the fragrances, he will become calmer and easier to manage.

Animal Treatment A to Z

Arthritis: (common in older animals and pure-breeds). Ortho Ease or PanAway (massage on location or put several drops in animal feed).

Use Raindrop-like application of PanAway, birch, pine, or spruce and massage the location. For larger animals use at least 2 times more oil than a normal Raindrop Technique would call for on humans.

For prevention: Put Power Meal and Sulfurzyme in feed or fodder. Small animals: 1/8 to 1/4 serving per day. Large animals: 2-4 servings per day.

Birthing: Gentle Baby.

Bleeding: Geranium, helichrysum.

Bones (pain, spurs—all animals): PanAway, birch, lemongrass, and spruce.

Bones (fractured or broken): Mix PanAway with 20-30 drops of birch and spruce. Cover the area. After 15 minutes rub in 10-15 more drops of birch and spruce. Cover with Ortho Sport Massage Oil.

Calming: Peace & Calming, Trauma Life, lavender (domestic animals respond very quickly to the smell).

Colds and flu: For small animals put 1-3 drops Exodus II, ImmuPower, or Di-Tone in feed or fodder. For large animals, use 10-20 drops.

Colic: For large animals (cows) put 10-20 drops of Di-Tone in feed or fodder. For small animals, use 1-3 drops.

Fleas and Other Parasites

> **Single oils:** Lemongrass, citronella, and peppermint.
>
> **Blends:** Di-Tone Add 1 or 2 drops of lemongrass to pet shampoo. Oils repel fleas and other external parasites. Wash blankets with oils added to the wash water. Place 1-2 drops of lemongrass on collar to eliminate fleas.
>
> For internal parasites, rub Di-Tone on the pads (bottom) of the feet. Many people have reported that they have seen the parasites eliminated from the animal.

Horses (To Calm): Add chamomile to feed.

Inflammation: Apply Ortho Ease, PanAway, pine, birch, or spruce on location. Put Sulfurzyme in feed.

Insect Repellent: Put 10 drops each of citronella, Purification, Eucalyptus globulus, and peppermint in 8 ounce spray bottle with water. Alternate formula: Put 2 drops pine, 2 drops Eucalyptus globulus, and 5-10 drops citronella in a spray bottle of water. Shake vigorously and spray over area. Floral waters, such as peppermint and Idaho tansy, can also be used.

Ligaments/tendons (torn or sprained): Apply lemongrass and lavender (equal parts) on location and cover area. For small animals or birds, dilute essential oils with V-6 Mixing Oil (2 parts mixing oil to 1 part essential oil).

Mineral deficiencies: Mineral Essence. (In one case, an animal stopped chewing on furniture once his mineral deficiency was met).

Mites (ear mites): Apply Purification and peppermint to a Q-Tip and swab the inside of the ear.

Nervous anxiety: Valor, Trauma Life, geranium, lavender, and valerian.

Pain: Helichrysum.

Saddle sores: Melrose and Rose Ointment.

Shiny coats: Rosemary and sandalwood.

Sinus problems: Diffuse Raven, R.C., pine, myrtle, and Eucalyptus radiata in animal's sleeping quarters or sprinkle on bed.

Skin Cancer: Frankincense, lavender, clove, and inula: Apply neat.

Strangle in horses: Mix 4 parts Exodus II and with 1 part Melrose.

Ticks: To remove ticks, apply 1 drop cinnamon or peppermint on cotton swab and swab on tick.

Trauma: Trauma Life, Valor, Peace & Calming, melissa, rosewood, lavender, valerian, and chamomile.

Tumors or cancers: Mix frankincense with lavender or clove and apply on area of tumor.

Worms and parasites: ParaFree and Di-Tone.

Wounds (open or abrasions): Melrose, helichrysum, and Rose Ointment.

CHAPTER 22

How to Use
The Personal Usage Reference

How Essential Oils Work

Essential oils can work through inhalation, ingestion, topical application, or through rectal implantation.

Topical application is one of the most effective means of using essential oils. According to researcher Jean Valnet, M.D., an essential oil that is directly applied to the skin can pass into the bloodstream and diffuse throughout the tissues in 20 minutes or less. More recent studies have also documented the ability of essential oils to penetrate the stratum corneum (the upper layer of skin) to reach the subdermal tissues and blood vessels beneath. (Huang et al., 1999; Ogiso et al., 1995)

Some of the compounds in essential oils that work synergistically to enhance permeation include alpha-pinene, beta-pinene, alpha-terpineol, 1,8-cineole and d-limonene.

Inhalation is an extremely effective means of therapeutically using and delivering an essential oil. The fragrance of an essential oil can have a direct influence on both the mind and body due to its ability to stimulate the brain's limbic system (a group of subcortical structures including the hypothalamus, the hippocampus, and the amygdala). This can produce powerful effects that can effect everything from emotional balance and energy levels to appetite control and heart function.

Some researchers believe that the inhalation of an essential oil can also enhance the body's electrical frequency, which can have a direct impact on disease. Disease and emotional trauma foster a negative frequency that may be disrupted or broken by essential oils. Oils with higher frequencies can elevate the entire frequency of the body whether topically or orally administered, thereby creating an internal environment that opposes the establishment of some disease conditions.

When to Mix Oils and Blends

The essential oils and blends that are listed for a specific condition can be used either separately or together. By combining a single oil with another recommended single oil or blend, a synergistic or additive effect is produced that results in stronger total effect than the sum of the actions produced by each oil or blend separately.

As a rule, when a list of oils or blends is recommended and does not list specific quantities, equal parts (usually 1-3 drops) of each oil should be used. For example, if the list reads, "Lavender with lemongrass, marjoram, or ginger," this means that 1 drop of lavender should be mixed with one drop of either lemongrass, marjoram, or ginger). This does not mean that lemongrass or marjoram cannot be also mixed. In fact, any four—or even all four—of these oils could be combined to produce a blend.

How to Convert Measurements

15 ml	= 1 tablespoon (1/2 fl. oz.)	= 250 drops
5 ml	= 1 teaspoon	= 85 drops
240 ml	= 1 cup	
30 ml	= 1 fluid ounce	
28 grams	= 1 ounce	

How to Choose an Essential Oil

The essential oils listed for a specific condition are not designed to be a comprehensive or complete list; they are merely a starting point. Other oils that are not listed can also be effective, so it may be necessary to experiment with different oils to pinpoint the most effective ones.

In addition, essential oils are not listed in any particular order. This is because an oil might be more compatible with one person's chemistry than another's. If results are not felt within several minutes, try another oil, blend, or combination.

How to Use Essential Oils

Essential oils should be used in moderation as they are extremely concentrated. In most cases, one or two drops is sufficient to produce significant effects. It is highly recommended that most essential oils be diluted in vegetable oil prior to either topical or internal application.

Many essential oils can be used as dietary supplements, and a list of these oils appears in Appendix C. All essential oils should be diluted prior to oral use, and no more than 1-2 drops should be consumed at one time (in a single serving) unless indicated otherwise. The best way to dilute essential oils for ingestion is to mix a drop in a teaspoon of honey or a cup of soy or rice milk.

Avoid Petrochemicals

Exercise caution when applying essential oils to skin that has been exposed to cosmetics, personal care products, or soaps and cleansers containing synthetic or petroleum-based chemicals. Essential oils may react with such chemicals and cause skin irritation, nausea, or headaches.

Consult Your Health Care Professional

Consult your health care professional about any serious disease or injury. Do not attempt to self-diagnose or prescribe any natural substances such as essential oils for health conditions that require professional attention.

Essential oils can also react with toxins built up in the body from chemicals in food, water, and work environment. If you experience a reaction to essential oils, temporarily discontinue their use and start an internal cleansing program (30 days using the Cleansing Trio) before resuming regular use of essential oils.

Tip on Safe Use:

- Skin-test the diluted essential oil on a small patch of skin. If any redness or irritation results, cleanse skin thoroughly and reapply. If skin irritation persists, discontinue use.

Start with Cleansing

You should always address the overall health improvement of the body when considering a specific health solution. While essential oils have powerful therapeutic effects, they are not, by themselves, a total solution. They must be accompanied by a program of internal cleansing, proper diet, and supplementation.

Step 1. Cleanse

Cleansing the colon and liver is the first and most important step to take when dealing with any disease condition. Many imbalances can be corrected by cleansing alone. Products that cleanse the body include: Cleansing Trio (Megazyme, ComforTone, and ICP), Chelex, ParaFree, JuvaTone, and JuvaFlex.

Step 2. Balance and Build

Once the body has been cleansed, various systems of the body can be balanced and nourished. This includes rebuilding and nourishing our beneficial intestinal flora, and remineralizing the blood and tissues. Products that build the body include: Mineral Essence, Essential Manna, Royaldophilus, Stevia Select, Master Formula vitamins, VitaGreen, Power Meal, and Super Cal.

Step 3. Support

Supporting the endocrine and immune system comprises the third phase. Products include: AuraLight, ImmuneTune, Exodus, Be-Fit, Wolfberry Bars, Goji Tea, Super C, Super B, Estro Tincture, Ultra Young.

NOTE: Infants or children under 8 should not undergo a colon and liver cleanse. Instead, use 3 drops of Di-Tone in a tsp. of V-6 Mixing Oil or Massage Oil Base, rub around the navel, and place warm hot packs over the stomach. Also apply on bottom of the feet.

Abscess (Skin)

(See ACNE or SKIN DISORDERS)

Absentmindedness

(See BRAIN DISORDERS)

Single Oils: Peppermint, cardamom, frankincense, sandalwood, rosemary, or basil.

Blends: Clarity, Brain Power, or M-Grain.

Supplements: Power Meal, Ultra Young, Sulfurzyme, VitaGreen, or Mineral Essence.

Abuse (mental and physical)

The trauma from mental and physical abuse can result in self-defeating behavior that can undermine success later in life. Through their powerful effect on the limbic system of the brain (the center or stored memories and emotions), essential oils can help release pent up trauma, emotions, or memories.

Single Oils: Geranium, sandalwood, or melissa.

Blends: SARA, Trauma Life, Release, Acceptance, Forgiveness, Surrender, Humility, Joy, White Angelica, Inner Child, Release, Harmony, Hope, Brain Power, Citrus Fresh, Christmas Spirit, or Valor.

Supplements: Power Meal, Super C, AuraLight, or Super B.

Sexual Abuse: Forgiveness, Trauma Life, SARA, Release, or Joy.

Spousal Abuse: Forgiveness, Trauma Life, Acceptance, Release, Valor, Joy, or Envision

Spiritual, Ritual, and Physical Abuse: Begin with Forgiveness, unless suicidal. It is most effective around the navel. Follow with Release over the Vita Flex points, on liver points of feet, and under the nose.

Parental, Spousal, Ritual, or Sexual Abuse: SARA over the area where abuse took place; then Forgiveness, Release, Joy, or Present Time.

Feelings of Revenge: 1-2 drops of Surrender on the sternum over the heart, 2-3 drops of Present Time on the thymus, and Forgiveness over navel.

Suicidal: 2 drops Hope on rim of ears, Melissa, Brain Power, or Present Time.

Protection/Balance: 1-2 drops of White Angelica on shoulders, Harmony over thymus and on energy chakras of the body.

Acid/Alkaline Balance

(See FUNGAL INFECTIONS)

Acidosis

(See ACIDOSIS AND ALKALOSIS)

Acidosis is a condition where the pH of the intestinal tract and the blood become excessively acidic. This can promote the growth pathogenic fungi like candida and exacerbate yeast infections. Eventually this can lead to many forms of chronic and degenerative diseases.

To raise pH, avoid acid-ash foods, overuse of antibiotics, and monitor the pH of the saliva (6.4-6.5), urine (5.5-5.6), and blood (7.3-7.6). (See APPENDIX B)

Single Oils: Peppermint or lemon.

Blends: Di-Tone.

Supplements: Royaldolphilus, Stevia Select, AlkaLime, Megazyme, Mint Condition, and VitaGreen.

Take Royaldophilus and Mint Condition with peppermint until acid level is balanced, then add Megazyme.

To reduce acid indigestion and prevent fermentation that can contribute to bad dreams and interrupted sleep: 1 tsp. AlkaLime in water before bedtime.

To raise pH, take 2-6 capsules of VitaGreen 3 times daily and take 1 tsp. AlkaLime in water one hour before or two hours after meals each day. For maintenance, take 1 tsp. AlkaLime once per week.

To stimulate enzymatic action in the digestive tract: Raw carrot juice, alfalfa, trace minerals, and papaya.

Acne

(See SKIN DISORDERS)

ADD

(See ATTENTION DEFICIT DISORDER)

How to Tap the Full Therapeutic Potential of Essential Oils

An outstanding way to tap the full therapeutic potential of essential oils is to combine them with bath salts and use them in the shower. The RainSpa aromatherapy shower head has a specially designed chamber that can be filled with essential oils and bath salts. As the water passes through the mixture, it disperses the essential oils into the spray, creating a fragrant, antiseptic spa.

Addictions

Many food and chemical dependencies, such as addictions to tobacco, caffeine, drugs, alcohol, and sugar may originate in the liver. Cleansing and detoxifying the liver is a crucial first step toward breaking free of these addictions. A colon and tissue cleanse is also important.

Using stevia, stevioside, or FOS can help reduce sugar cravings. Stevia is a supersweet noncaloric extract derived from an ancient South American herb, while FOS is a sweet-tasting natural sugar derived from chicory roots and Jerusalem artichokes that has no calories and important health benefits. (See APPENDIX G)

Trace mineral and mineral deficiencies can also play a part in some addictions. Magnesium, potassium, calcium, and zinc should all be included in the diet.

Blends: Harmony, Peace & Calming, or JuvaFlex.

Supplements: JuvaTone, Stevia, Essential Manna, Mineral Essence, Super Cal, Stevia Select, ComfortTone, Megazyme, I.C.P.

(See LIVER and SMOKING CESSATION)

Addison's Disease

(See ADRENAL GLAND IMBALANCE)

Adrenal Gland Imbalance

The adrenal glands consist of two sections: An inner part called the medulla produces stress hormones and an outer part called the cortex secretes critical hormones called glucocorticoids and aldosterone. Because of these hormones, the cortex has a far greater impact on overall health than the medulla does.

Why are aldosterone and glucocorticoids so important? Because they directly affect blood pressure and mineral content and help regulate the conversion of carbohydrates into energy.

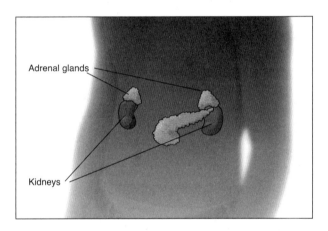

Adrenal glands

Kidneys

Addison's Disease

In cases like Addison's disease, adrenal cortex hormones are no longer produced or severely limited. This can lead to life-threatening fluid and mineral loss unless these hormones are replaced.

Because Addison's disease is an autoimmune disease in which the body's own immune cells destroy the adrenal glands, it may be treated with MSM. MSM is an important source of organic sulfur that has been shown to have extremely positive effects with many types of autoimmune diseases, including lupus, arthritis, and fibromyalgia.

If adrenal insufficiency is accompanied by a lack of thyroid hormone, condition is known as Schmidt's syndrome.

Symptoms:
- Severe fatigue
- Lightheadedness when standing
- Nausea
- Depression/irritability
- Craving salty foods
- Loss of appetite
- Muscle spasms
- Dark, tan-colored skin

Essential oils can play a part in correcting deficiencies in adrenal cortex function. Nutmeg, for example, has adrenal-like activity that raises energy levels.

Single Oils: Nutmeg

- Sage with nutmeg, clove, rosemary, or basil.

Blends: EndoFlex, Joy, or En-R-Gee.

Supplements: Thyromin, VitaGreen, Royal Essence, Super B, Master Formula, Mineral Essence.

Regimen:

- Thyromin: 1 immediately after awakening.

- Super B: 1 after meals. If you experience a niacin flush (skin becoming red and itchy for about 15 minutes), use only 1/2 of a tablet.

- Master Formula: 2-6 tablets, 3 times daily according to blood type and need.

Cushing's disease

Cushing's disease is the opposite of Addison's disease: It is characterized by the overproduction of adrenal cortex hormones. While these hormones are crucial to sound health in normal amounts, their unchecked overproduction can cause as much harm as their underproduction. This results in the following symptoms:

Slow wound healing
Low resistance to infection
Obesity
Acne
Moon-shaped face
Easily-bruised skin
Weak or wasted muscles
Osteoporosis

Although Cushing's disease can be caused by a malfunction in the pituitary, it is usually triggered by excessive use of immune-suppressing corticosteroid medications—such as those used for asthma and arthritis. Once these are discontinued, the disease will abate.

Single Oils: Lemon.

Blends: ImmuPower or Thieves.

Supplements: Exodus or ImmuneTune.

Supporting the Adrenal Glands

Add essential oils to 1 teaspoon of massage oil and apply as a hot compress over the adrenal glands (located on top of the kidneys).

- 3 drops clove
- 3 drops nutmeg
- 7 drops rosemary

Agent Orange Exposure

Blends: JuvaFlex and EndoFlex.

Rub JuvaFlex over liver area or apply in a hot compress. Apply 2-4 drops of EndoFlex over adrenal gland area.

Supplements: Radex, ImmuneTune, Cleansing Trio, JuvaTone, and Thyromin.

- Megazyme: 3 servings daily.

- ComforTone, I.C.P., and JuvaTone: 3 servings daily.

- ImmuneTune: 4 servings daily.

- Rub 3 drops EndoFlex on the thyroid (hollow at base-front of neck) and 3 drops over the kidneys 3 times daily. Also rub 3 drops on the thyroid and kidney Vita Flex points of the feet.

217

- After 90 days on the program, gradually reduce the above amounts but stay on the program for a full year.

- Add 1 cup Epsom salts and 4 ounces of 35 percent food-grade hydrogen peroxide to bath water once daily.

- Take a 30-minute bath with 6 cups of Epsom salts per tub of water. Drink 3 glasses of lemonade while bathing.

Agitation

Single Oils: Lavender, orange, and Roman chamomile.

Blends: Peace & Calming, Forgiveness, Surrender, and Joy.

Supplements: AuraLight, Super B, Super C, and Super Cal.

AIDS (Acquired Immune Deficiency Syndrome)

The AIDS virus attacks and infects immune cells critical to the function of normal immunity.

Essential oils such as lemon, cistus, thyme, lavender have immune building properties. Other oils like cumin (*Cuminum cyminum*) have an inhibitory effect. In May 1994, Dr. Radwan Farag of Cairo University demonstrated that cumin seed oil had an 88 to 92 percent inhibition effect against HIV, a precurser to the AIDS virus.

Single Oils: Cistus, Lemon, cumin.

Blends: Brain Power, Exodus, Valor, Thieves, and ImmuPower.

Regimen:

1. Exodus II: 6-8 drops on spine alternating days with Raindrop Technique.

2. Valor and Thieves: 4-6 drops on feet for 3 weeks.

3. ImmuPower: 6 drops in vegetable oil or honey

4. Raindrop Technique: 3 times weekly.

Supplements: Cleansing Trio, JuvaTone, Immu-Gel, Rehemogen, Thyromin, ImmuneTune, VitaGreen, Sulfurzyme, Exodus, Super B, Ultra Young, Goji Berry Tea.

Regimen:

1. Cleansing Trio for 120 days with JuvaTone.

2. ImmuGel: 1/2 tsp., 3 times daily. Hold in mouth for better absorption.

3. Thyromin: Start with 2 at night, 1 in morning.

4. ImmuneTune: 6-8 capsules daily.

5. VitaGreen: 6-10 capsules daily.

6. Sulfurzyme: 1 tablespoon.

7. Exodus: Up to 18 capsules daily.

8. Super B: 1 tablet daily with a meal.

9. Ultra Young: 3 sprays on inside of each cheek, 4-5 times daily.

10. Eat 5-6 mini-meals daily, primarily Power Meal (3 times daily) and fish for protein. Do not eat chicken for first 3-6 weeks to allow more energy for immune building.

11. Goji Berry Tea: 10-12 cups daily.

Alcoholism

(See ADDICTIONS)

Single Oils: Lavender, Roman chamomile, orange, helichrysum, elemi, and rosemary verbenon.

Blends: JuvaFlex, Forgiveness, Acceptance, Surrender, Motivation, and Joy.

Supplements: JuvaTone, Cleansing Trio, Thyromin, Power Meal, and Mineral Essence.

Alkalosis (see acidosis)

Alkalosis is a condition where the pH of the intestinal tract and the blood becomes excessively alkaline. While moderate alkalinity is essential for good health, excessive alkalinity can cause problems and result in fatigue, depression, irritability, and sickness.

The best solution is to lower, or acidify, the internal pH of the body. Rudolf Wiley, Ph.D., recommends several tactics to accomplish this in *Biobalance: The Acid/Alkaline Solution to the Food-Mood-Health Puzzle*.

Single Oils: Ginger, tarragon, and anise.

Blends: Di-Tone.

Supplements: Megazyme, Sulfurzyme, and Body Balance.

Allergies

Allergies can be triggered by food, pollen, dander, dust, and insect bites and can impact:

Respiration—wheezing, labored breathing

Mouth—swelling of the lips or tongue, itching lips

Digestive tract—diarrhea, vomiting, cramps

Skin—rashes, dermatitis

Nose—sneezing, congestion

Food Allergies

Food *allergies* are different from food *intolerances.* The former involve an immune system reaction, whereas the latter involves a gastrointestinal reaction (and is far more common). For example, peanuts often produce a lifelong allergy in adults due to peanut proteins being targeted by immune system antibodies as foreign invaders. In contrast, intolerance of pasteurized cow's milk that causes cramping and diarrhea is due to the inability to digest lactose (milk sugar) because of a lack of the enzyme lactase.

Food allergies are often associated with the consumption of peanuts, shellfish, tree nuts, wheat, cow's milk, eggs, and soy. Infants and children are far more susceptible to food allergies than adults, due to the immaturity of their immune and digestive systems.

A thorough intestinal cleansing is one of the best ways to combat most allergies. Start with the Cleansing Trio and JuvaTone.

Hay fever (allergic rhinitis)

Hay fever is an allergic reaction triggered by airborne allergens (pollen, animal hair, feathers, dust mites) that cause the release of histamines and subsequent inflammation of nasal passages and sinus-related areas. Allergies resemble asthma, which manifests in the chest and lungs.

Symptoms: Inflammation of the nasal passages, sinuses, and eyelids that causes sneezing, runny nose, watery, red, itchy eyes, and wheezing.

Single Oils: Lavender and Roman chamomile.

Blends: Harmony and Valor.

Supplements: Sulfurzyme, Power Meal, Megazyme, Royaldophilus, Mineral Essence, Master Formula, VitaGreen, Cleansing Trio, JuvaTone.

Alopecia Areata

Alopecia is an inflammatory hair-loss disease that is the second-leading cause of baldness in the U.S. A randomized, double-blind study at the Aberdeen Royal Infirmary in Scotland found that certain essential oils were extremely effective in combating this disease (Hay et al., 1998; Kalish, 1999).

Single Oils:

- Thyme (thymol chemotype), rosemary (cineol chemotype), lavender, and cedarwood.

Mix with carrier oils of jojoba and grapeseed. Massage into the scalp daily.

Aluminum Toxicity

Aluminum is a very toxic metal that can cause serious neurological damage in the human body—even in minute amounts. Aluminum has been implicated in Alzheimer's Disease.

People unwittingly ingest aluminum from their cookware, beverage cans, and antacids. Even deodorants have aluminum compounds. The first step toward reducing aluminum toxicity in the body is to avoid these types of aluminum-based products.

Single Oils: Helichrysum.

Blends: PanAway.

Supplements: Chelex, JuvaTone, Super Cal, and ComforTone.

Alzheimer's

(See NEUROLOGICAL DISEASE)

Analgesic

Single Oils: Elemi, birch, clove, peppermint, lavender, lemongrass, and tansy.

Blends: PanAway

- Helichrysum with clove
- Melaleuca with rosemary
- Mix birch, spruce, and black pepper

Recipe 1:
- 3 parts melaleuca
- 5 parts rosemary

Anemia

(See BLOOD DISORDERS)

Aneurysm

(See CARDIOVASCULAR CONDITIONS)

Aneurysms are weak spots on the blood vessel wall which balloon out and may eventually rupture. In cases of brain aneurysms, a bursting blood vessel can cause a hemorrhagic stroke, which can result in death or paralysis (with a fatality rate of over 50 percent).

See your physician for treatment if you have, or suspect you have, and aneurysm

Some nutritional supplements and essential oils that can be used to strengthen blood vessel walls include:

Single Oils: Helichrysum, sandalwood, Idaho tansy, cypress.

Blends: Aroma Life and Brain Power.

Recipe:
- 5 drops of frankincense
- 1 drop helichrysum
- 1 drop cypress

Supplements: Ultra Young, Essential Manna, and Rehemogen.

Some essential oils support the cardiovascular system. Cypress strengthens capillary and vascular walls. Helichrysum helps absorb blood back into tissue

Anorexia

(See ADDICTIONS)

Anorexia nervosa is an eating disorder characterized by total avoidance of food and virtual self-starvation. It may or may not be accompanied by bulimia (binge-purge behavior).

While psychotherapy remains indispensable, the inhalation of essential oils may alter emotions enough to effect a change in the underlying psychology or disturbed-thinking patterns which supports this self-destructive behavior. This is accomplished by the ability of fragrance to directly impact the emotional hub inside the brain.

Many anorexics suffer life-threatening nutrient and mineral deficiencies. The lack of magnesium and potassium can actually trigger heart rhythm abnormalities and cardiac arrest. So replacement of calcium, magnesium, potassium, and other minerals is absolutely essential.

Single Oils: Tarragon.

Blends: Christmas Spirit, Valor, Citrus Fresh, Motivation, and Brain Power.

Supplements: AuraLight, Ultra Young, Super Cal, Mineral Essence.

Anthrax

Caused by the bacteria *Bacillus anthracis,* anthrax is one of the oldest and deadliest diseases known. There are three predominant types: the **external** form acquired from contact with infected animal carcasses, the **internal** form is obtained from breathing airborne anthrax spores, and **battlefield anthrax**, which is a far more lethal variety of internal anthrax that was developed for biological warfare. When this anthrax invades the stomach and lungs, it causes fatal hemorrhaging. Symptoms include:

- Fever
- Prostration
- Skin pustules

Internal varieties of anthrax may be initiated by consumption of infected meat or milk, or exposure to animal hides and wool. While vaccination and antibiotics have stemmed anthrax infection in recent years, new strains have developed that are resistant to all countermeasures.

According to Jean Valnet, M.D., thyme oil is extremely effective for killing the anthrax bacillus. Two highly antimicrobial phenols in thyme, carvacrol and thymol, are responsible for this action.

Single Oils: Thyme, oregano, clove, cinnamon, and rosewood.

Blends: Thieves and Exodus II.

Supplements: Exodus, Radex, and Super C.

Antibiotics

Many essential oils have broad-spectrum antifungal, antibacterial and antiviral effects. For example, thyme oil was shown to exert powerful antimicrobial effects against 25 different types of bacteria (Deans and Richie, 1987).

Unlike synthetic antibiotics, which are composed of a single type of chemical, essential oils are composites of hundreds of chemicals.

Single Oils: Oregano, thyme, cinnamon, mountain savory, lemon, rosewood, melaleuca, clove, ravensara, and eucalyptus radiata.

Blends: Thieves, Exodus II, ImmuPower, Melrose, Inspiration, and Sacred Mountain.

Supplements: Royaldophilus, ImmuGel, Exodus, Super C, Radex, and ImmuneTune.

Antibiotic Reactions

Synthetic antibiotic drugs indiscriminately kill both beneficial and harmful bacteria. This can result in yeast infections, diarrhea, poor nutrient assimilation, fatigue, degenerative diseases, and many other conditions and symptoms.

The average adult has 3-4 pounds of beneficial bacteria permanently residing in the intestines. These beneficial flora:

• Constitute the first line of defense against bacterial and viral infection

• Produce B vitamins

• Maintain pH balance

• Combat yeast and fungus overgrowth

Supplements: Royaldophilus and Stevia Select.

During antibiotic treatment, take 5 grams of Stevia Select and 2-3 servings of acidophilus daily on an empty stomach before meals. After completing antibiotic treatment, continue for using acidophilus and Stevia Select for 10-15 days.

Antiseptic

Single Oils: Rosemary cineol, rosemary verbenon, thyme thymol, thyme linalol, eucalyptus (all types), mountain savory, melaleuca, lavandin, lemon, lemongrass, clove, cinnamon, clove, oregano.

• Birch with lavender, mountain savory, lavandin, peppermint, spearmint, ravensara, sage, clove, cinnamon, juniper, or nutmeg.

• Frankincense with lavender, cedarwood, rosemary, melaleuca, lemon, oregano, thyme, myrrh, geranium, cumin, Eucalyptus globulus and Eucalyptus radiata, or sandalwood.

• Lemongrass with melaleuca, lavandin, cedarwood, lemon, rosemary, citronella, basil, cypress, fennel, fir, pine, mandarin, tarragon, patchouly, rosewood, laurus nobilis, or vetiver.

Blends: Birch, frankincense, or lemongrass with Purification, Melrose, Christmas Spirit, Citrus Fresh, Thieves, ImmuPower, R.C., or Raven.

Skin Care: Rose Ointment and A D & E.

Melrose or other essential oils added to Rose Ointment makes an ideal disinfectant and healing agent.

Apnea

Apnea is a temporary cessation of breathing during sleep. It can degrade the quality of sleep resulting in chronic fatigue, lowered immune function, and lack of energy.

Blends: Clarity, Surrender, and Valor.

Supplements: Royal Essence, VitaGreen, Super B, AuraLight, and Thyromin.

- Diffuse Clarity in bedroom.
- Rub Valor on bottom of feet.
- Take 3 droppers of Royal Essence, 4 times daily.
- Take VitaGreen, 2 times daily.
- Take Super B, 3 times daily with meals.
- Take Thyromin at bedtime.

Appetite, Loss of

Single Oils: Bergamot, ginger, spearmint, orange, and nutmeg.

Ginger stimulates digestion and improves appetite.

Blends: Inner Child, Citrus Fresh, and Christmas Spirit.

Supplements: Megazyme, Mint Condition, and ComforTone.

Arteriosclerosis

Single Oils: Helichrysum, cypress, and frankincense.

Blends: Aroma Life.

Supplements: A.D.&E., Chelex, JuvaTone, and Rehemogen.

Arthritis (Osteoarthritis)

(See RHEUMATOID ARTHRITIS)

Osteoarthritis involves the breakdown of the cartilage that forms a cushion between two joints. As this cartilage is eaten away, the two bones of the joint start rubbing together and wearing down. (In contrast, rheumatoid arthritis is caused from a swelling and inflammation of the synovial membrane, the lining of the joint. (see RHEUMATOID ARTHRITIS)

Researchers have linked the increasing risk of many degenerative diseases to nutrient deficiencies, including a lack of sufficient minerals and trace minerals.

Single Oils: Birch with helichrysum, spruce, fir, pine, cypress, peppermint, vetiver, marjoram, rosemary cineol, *Eucalyptus citriodora*, basil, oregano, lemongrass, Idaho tansy, black pepper, elemi, or peppermint.

- Idaho tansy with birch, basil, rosemary, peppermint, marjoram, mountain savory, cypress, ginger, black pepper, or tarragon.
- Elemi with spruce, fir, pine, cedarwood, juniper, rosemary, peppermint, helichrysum, birch, basil, wild Idaho tansy, lemon, nutmeg, or oregano.
- Juniper with rosemary, Roman chamomile, lemon, or melaleuca alternifolia.

Blends: Aroma Siez, PanAway, Relieve It, Ortho Ease, Ortho Sport.

- Birch with Aroma Siez, PanAway, Relieve It, or Peace & Calming.
- Lavender with PanAway, Relieve It, or Aroma Siez.
- 1-2 drops cypress with Aroma Life, PanAway, Purification, Aroma Siez, or Sacred Mountain.

Dilute 1-3 drops in 1 tsp. massage oil and apply on location. Oils can also be applied undiluted and followed with massage oil.

Supplements: Super Cal, Super C, Mineral Essence, Goji Berry Tea, ArthroTune, Immune-Tune, Exodus, Sulfurzyme.

- Super Cal: 2-3 capsules, 2 times daily.
- Super C: 3-4 tablets, 3 time daily.
- Mineral Essence: 2 droppers, 3 times daily.
- Goji Berry Tea: 4-10 cups daily.
- ArthroTune: 2-6 capsules, 3 times daily.
- ImmuneTune: 2-3 capsules, 3 times daily.
- Exodus: 2-3 capsules, 2-3 times daily as needed.

Detoxification of the body and strengthening the joints is important. Cleanse the colon and liver. Rehemogen cleans and purifies the blood which may have toxins blocking nutrient and oxygen absorption into cells (see CIRCULATION).

Apply oils on location followed by massage oil or AromaSilk Satin Body Lotion. PanAway and Relieve It have cortisone-like action, which give relief of arthritic pain without the cortisone side effects.

Asthma

During an asthma attack, the bronchials (air tubes) in the lungs become swollen and clogged with a thick, sticky mucus. The muscles of the air tubes will also begin to constrict or tighten. This results in very difficult or labored breathing. If an attack is severe, it can actually be life-threatening.

Many asthma attacks are triggered by an allergic reaction to pollen, skin particles, dandruff, cat or dog dander, dust mites, and foods such as eggs, milk, flavorings, dyes, and preservatives. Asthma can also be triggered by respiratory infection, exercise, stress, and psychological factors. (see ALLERGIES)

Essential oils should not be inhaled for asthma-related problems, The oils should be applied to the soles of the feet or ingested (If they are GRAS list – Generally Regarded As Safe).

Single Oils:

- Lavender with Roman chamomile, Eucalyptus polybractea, myrtle, peppermint, frankincense, marjoram, or rose.

- Frankincense with ravensara, cypress, abies alba, spruce, pine, lemon, thyme, rosemary, eucalyptus, helichrysum, birch, or myrtle.

- Rosemary cineol with ravensara, eucalyptus radiata, mountain savory, lemon, or juniper.

- Sage with lavender, myrrh, hyssop, or eucalyptus.

Blends:

- Lavender or Roman chamomile with Melrose, Di-Tone, Purification, or Thieves.

- Frankincense (single oil) with R.C., Raven, Inspiration Blend, or Sacred Mountain.

- Rosemary (single oil) with R.C. or Raven.

Supplements: ImmuGel, Radex, Super C, Exodus, Royal Essence, VitaGreen, ImmuneTune, Ultra Young, Megazyme, and Royaldophilus.

Athlete's Foot

(See FUNGAL INFECTIONS)

Attention Deficit Disorder (ADD)

Attention deficit disorder may be caused by mineral deficiencies in the diet. Improper intake of magnesium and potassium, as well as other trace minerals, is linked to many kinds of similar cognitive disturbances.

The use of fragrance and essential oils can also have a significant effect in mitigating the problems of ADD through their effect on the limbic system of the brain.

Single Oils: Lavender, sandalwood, cardamom, basil, frankincense, and vetiver..

Blends: Brain Power and Joy. Diffuse Peace & Calming, Clarity, lavender, German chamomile, Joy, and Brain Power.

Supplements: Mineral Essence, Essential Manna, Ultra Young, and Power Meal.

The Power of Smell

Unlike other senses (such as sight, hearing, touch, and taste) the sense of smell can exert a direct effect on the limbic system of the brain, the hormonal and emotional center of the brain. This enables essential oils (through their aroma) to affect many types of neurological, emotional, or behavioral problems, including autism, ADD, cerebral palsy.

Autism

Autism is a childhood developmental disorder of the brain that is four times more common in boys than girls. It is characterized by:

- Social ineptness (loner)
- Nonverbal and verbal communication difficulties
- Repetitive behavior (rocking, hair twirling)
- Self injurious behavior (head-banging)
- Very limited or peculiar interests
- Reduced or abnormal responses to pain, noises, or other outside stimuli

Some researchers believe that gastrointestinal disorders may be linked to the brain dysfunctions that cause autism in children (Horvath et al., 1998). In fact, there have been several cases of successful treatment of autism using pancreatic enzymes.

Stimulation of the limbic region of the brain may also help treat autism. Aromas from essential oils have a powerful ability to stimulate this part of the brain since the sense of smell (olfaction) is tied directly into the mind's emotional and hormonal centers. As a result the aroma of an essential has the potential to exert a powerful influence on disorders such as ADD and autism.

Single Oils: Frankincense, sandalwood, melissa, and basil.

Blends: Brain Power, Clarity, and Peace & Calming

Supplements: Megazyme, Ultra Young, Mineral Essence, Master Formula Vitamins, and Power Meal

Back Injuries and Pain

(See Spine Injuries and Pain)

Bed Wetting

Blends: Valor and Harmony.

Supplements: K&B.

Use K&B tincture once in the afternoon and once before bedtime (2 droppers maximum).

Bell's Palsy

(See NEURITIS)

Benign Prostate Hyperplasia (BPH)

Almost all males over age 50 have some degree of prostate hyperplasia, a condition which worsens with age. BPH can severely restrict urine flow and result in frequent, small urinations.

Two herbs which are extremely effective for treating this condition are saw palmetto and *Pygeum africanum*. The mineral zinc is also important for normal prostate function and prostate health.

Supplements: ProGen.

Bites

(See SKIN DISORDERS, INSECT BITES)

Bladder Infection

(See URINARY/BLADDER INFECTION)

Bleeding

(See HEMORRHAGING)

Single Oils: Cypress, helichrysum, Idaho tansy, lavender, and geranium.

Blends: Aroma Life and PanAway.

Supplements: Rehemogen

Bleeding Gums

(See PERIODONTAL DISEASE)

Blisters

Single Oils: Melaleuca, lavender, melissa, and cistus.

Blends: Purification, Inspiration, and Melrose.

Supplements: AD&E, Power Meal, and Essential Manna.

Bloating

Bloating is usually a result of hormonal imbalances that trigger excess fluid retention in the body. Correcting hormone imbalances or using natural diuretics can both help.

Single Oils: Tarragon, peppermint, juniper, and fennel.

Blends: Di-Tone.

Supplements: Estro Tincture, Femalin, Megazyme, Mint Condition, and Royaldophilus.

Blood Disorders

(See CIRCULATION or CARDIOVASCULAR CONDITIONS)

Anemia

Anemia is a condition caused from the lack of red blood cells (or a lack of properly functioning ones). Nutritional deficiencies such as the lack of adequate iron or vitamin B12 can contribute to this disorder.

Anemia also may be caused by improper liver function. A liver cleanse and support may be effective in this case for rebuilding red blood cell counts.

There may be many different causes of anemia. Please see your physician for propper diagnosis.

Here are some rocommended oils and supports:

Single Oils: Lemon, lemongrass, and helichrysum.

Blends: Aroma Life, JuvaFlex.

Supplements: Super B, Master Formula Vitamins, Rehemogen, Mineral Essence, Royal Essence, JuvaTone, VitaGreen, and Chelex.

Blood Platelets (Low):

Supplements: Rehemogen

To enhance effects of Rehemogen use JuvaTone.

Blood Clots

Blood clots (also known as embolisms) can form anywhere in the body. If they block a blood vessel in the brain, they can cause a stroke; if they obstruct a coronary artery, they can cause an ischemic heart attack.

Those who have thicker blood or suffer from narrowed blood vessels due to diabetes, arteriosclerosis, atherosclerosis, or hypertension, are far more likely to suffer serious or fatal consequences from a blood clot.

Helichrysum is especially effective for preventing blood clot formation and promoting the dissolution of the clot. Natural blood thinners, such as clove oil, can also be effective. Clove oil occurs in high concentrations in the essential blend Thieves, which is the active ingredient in Dentarome Toothpaste.

Single Oils: Helichrysum, clove, lemon, orange, grapefruit, tangerine.

- Lavender and lemon.
- Thieves.

Take 1-3 drops diluted in 2 oz. of rice milk, or soy milk, three times daily. Oils can also be applied on location. Essential oils, such as clove, should be diluted in massage oil when used topically.

Massage lemon and lavender with helichrysum on location with or without hot packs.

Mix 1-3 drops helichrysum in water and take 2-3 times daily.

Supplements: A.D.&E., Super Cal, Ultra

Dr. J. Hofman, author of *The Missing Link*, asserted that the best way to maximize good health is to promote a free-flowing alkaline blood stream (see BODY pH, ACID/ALKALINE BALANCE).

Young, and Essential Manna.

Personal Care: Dentarome Toothpaste.

Blood Detoxification

Detoxified blood results in better nutrient and oxygen flow and is the key to begin combating many diseases.

Single Oils: Helichrysum, German chamomile, Roman chamomile, rosemary verbenon, geranium, orange, lemon.

- Helichrysum with German chamomile, Roman chamomile, rosemary, geranium, lemon, orange, or cardamom.

Blends:

- Helichrysum (single oil) with Di-Tone, JuvaFlex, Exodus, or EndoFlex.

Supplements: VitaGreen, Rehemogen, Chelex, Exodus, AlkaLime, and Sulfurzyme.

Rehemogen helps with any type of blood disorder including toxemia and blood toxicity.

Chelex helps remove heavy metals from blood/system. Use with cardamom and JuvaTone.

MSM (found in Sulfurzyme) purifies the body and blood.

Blood Oxygenation

Single Oils: Helichrysum, lemongrass, pepper, spruce, and anise.

Blends: Valor, R.C., En-R-Gee, and PanAway.

Supplements: Royal Essence, Super B.

Many essential oils are oxygenators. R.C. and Valor increase oxygen at the cellular level. Spruce enhances oxygen exchange in the lungs.

Hydrogen peroxide (H_2O_2) taken orally increases blood oxygen by 9.2 percent. Essential oils can increase circulation between 22 and 32 percent.

Royal Essence increases energy and blood oxygen very quickly. Put under tongue for fastest results.

Blood Pressure, High (Hypertension)

(See CARDIOVASCULAR CONDITIONS)

Single Oils: Marjoram.

- Lavender with ylang ylang, marjoram, cypress, mountain savory, or helichrysum.

- Rosemary with ylang ylang, marjoram, helichrysum, or lavender.

Blends:

- Lavender with Aroma Life, Aroma Siez, Peace & Calming, or Citrus Fresh.

- Ylang Ylang with Aroma Life, or Joy.

Supplements: Essential Manna, ImmuneTune, Super B, Mineral Essence, Super Cal, Stevia, AuraLight.

Regimens:

1. Increase intake of magnesium which acts as a smooth-muscle relaxant and acts as a natural calcium channel blocker for the heart, lowering blood pressure and dilating the heart blood vessels. Mineral Essence, Essential Manna, AuraLight, and Super Cal are good sources of magnesium.

2. Take 20 mg. daily of vitamin B3 (niacin). Niacin is also an excellent vasodilator and Super B is an excellent source of niacin.

4. AuraLight nutrient spray helps reduce stress due to its standardized content of St. John's wort.

5. Use therapeutic-grade Hawthorne berry extracts. Hawthorne berry (contained in HRT tincture provides powerful cardiovascular support.

6. Do a colon and liver cleanse.

7. For 3 minutes, massage 1-2 drops each of Aroma Life and ylang ylang on heart Vita Flex point and over the heart and carotid arteries. Blood pressure will drop for up to 20 minutes. Monitor the pressure and reapply as required. Lemon and helichrysum can also be used.

8. Inhalation of jasmine reduces anxiety and therefore, lowers blood pressure.

How to Use the Heart Vita Flex Point of the Hands and Feet

The heart Vita Flex point of the foot is behind the knuckle of the second smallest toe of the left foot. Vita Flex massaging this point is as effective as the hand and arm together (see VITA FLEX CHAPTER).

The hand point is in the palm of the left hand, one inch below the ring finger joint (at the life line), and the secondary point is on bottom of the left arm in line with the inside of the upturned arm (approximately two inches up the arm from the funny bone), not on the muscle, but up under the muscle. Have another person use thumbs and firmly press these two points alternately for three minutes, in a kind of pumping action. Work all three points when possible; start with the foot first, then go to the hand and arm.

Blood Pressure, Low (Hypotension)

Single Oils: Sage, pine and rosemary.

Blends: Rosemary with Aroma Life, EndoFlex, or Joy.

Use 1 drop each of Aroma Life and rosemary on heart Vita Flex points; for massage, dilute with vegetable oil. Place 2 drops of Aroma Life and rosemary in capsules to take internally.

Boils

Single Oils: Frankincense, lavender, Roman chamomile, patchouly, and myrrh.

Blends: 3 Wise Men, Exodus II, and Thieves.

Supplements: Rehemogen, JuvaTone, A.D.&E., and Essential Manna (Potassium).

Bone (Bruised, Broken, Spurs)

Single Oils:

- Birch with spruce, fir, pine, cypress, peppermint, Idaho tansy, rosemary, basil, or elemi.

- Cypress with spruce, fir, pine, cedarwood, rosemary, peppermint, helichrysum, birch, basil, lemongrass, clove, or ginger.

Blends:

- Birch with Aroma Siez, PanAway, or Peace & Calming.

- Cypress with Aroma Life, PanAway, Relieve It, Aroma Siez, Purification, Melrose, Release, or Sacred Mountain.

Recipe 1:
- 5 drops oregano
- 6-8 drops mountain savory
- 1 drop lemon.

Supplements: Ortho Ease, Relaxation massage oil, Super Cal, Arthro Plus, Mineral Essence, ArthroTune, and Ortho Sport.

NOTE: Be gentle on location of new breaks.

How to Speed Healing

With any damaged tissue, circulation should be increased to promote healing. The essential oil of cypress can increase circulation.

Anytime there is tissue damage, there is always inflammation which should be addressed first.

Bone ache

Single Oils: Birch, spruce, pine, and helichrysum.

Growing: Birch, spruce, Super Cal, ArthroTune, PanAway, and Sulfurzyme.

Joints: PanAway.

Muscle: Aroma Siez, Ortho Sport, Ortho Ease, marjoram, lavender, and elemi.

Ligaments: Lemongrass, lavender, Ortho Ease, Essential Manna, and Sulfurzyme.

Poor bone and muscle development can indicate hGH and potassium deficiency. To correct, use: Ultra Young, Essential Manna, Power Meal, Super Cal, and Sulfurzyme.

Acid pH: Too much acid in the body can create pain (See regimen for Acidosis).

Broken Bones

- 10 drops birch
- 3 drops helichrysum
- 2 drops lemongrass
- 3 drops pine
- 4 drops ginger

Prior to casting, mix in teaspoon and apply a few drops to local area neat. If there is any signs of skin sensitivity or irritation, be prepared to apply V-6 Mixing Oil or Massage Oil Base.

Bone Regeneration

Recipe 1 *(Mix in teaspoon)*:
- 8 drops helichrysum
- 4 drops clove
- 2 drops lemongrass
- 12 drops birch
- 6 drops pine

Recipe 2:
- 10 drops birch
- 8 drops marjoram
- 4 drops cypress
- 2 drops peppermint
- 1 drop basil

Mix in 1/2 ounce of massage oil or V-6 Mixing Oil or Massage Oil Base.

Supplements: ArthroTune and Super Cal

Seeing the Big Picture Can Produce Big Results

When selecting oils, particularly for injuries, think through the cause and type of injury and select oils for each segment. For instance, a broken bone could encompass muscle damage, nerve damage, ligament strain or tear, inflammation, infection, bone injury, and possibly an emotion. So select an oil or oils for each perceived problem and apply in rotation or prepare a blend to cover all of them. The emotion may be shock, anger, guilt, or the person may have had pain for a long time and need to release or relieve it or need some joy in their lives, etc. Try to work through all factors.

Bone Spurs

Bone spurs are a calcium deposit or growth that generally forms from the cartilage.

Single Oils:

- Cypress with birch, marjoram, or rosemary.
- Cypress with birch and marjoram.
- Cypress with marjoram and rosemary.

Blends: R.C.

Birch helps dissolve calcium deposits.

Apply oils neat on location, then massage using Vita Flex Technique.

Brain Disorders

(See NEUROLOGICAL DISEASES)

The fragrance of many essential oils exerts a powerful stimulus on the limbic system—a part of the brain located on the margin of the cerebral cortex, including the amygdala, hippocampus, and other components, which interact directly with the thalamus and hypothalamus. Acting together, these glands and brain components are the seat of memory, emotions, and sexual arousal, and govern aggressive behavior.

The ability of essential oils to pass the blood-brain barrier gives them enormous therapeutic potential against such neurological diseases like Parkinson's, Alzheimer's, Lou Gehrig's, and MS.

Right Brain vs. Left Brain

The left brain is logical, rational, and judgmental and not as responsive as the right. The right brain is the subconscious and superconscious part of the limbic system.

Using essential oils heightens right brain activity, according to D. Gary Young.

Dr. Richard Restick, a leading neurologist in Washington, D.C., stated that maintaining normal synaptic firing would forestall many types of deterioration in the body.

Other researchers believe that if a substance could pass the blood-brain barrier then a therapeutic solution could be devised to help neurological diseases like Parkinson's, Lou Gehrig's, MS, and Alzheimer's.

Essential oils high in sesquiterpenes, such as frankincense, cypress, myrrh, and sandalwood, have been documented to cross the blood-brain barrier.

Moreover, essential oils also increase oxygen levels in the brain. According to Dr. Asawa of Japan and Dr. Richardson of England, the inhalation of essential oils increases brain activity by increasing blood flow by 15 percent and oxygen by 25 percent.

Single Oils: Frankincense, myrrh, cypress, sandalwood, helichrysum.

- Helichrysum with frankincense, peppermint, melissa, or nutmeg.

Blends:

- Brain Power, Valor, Helichrysum or Frankincense with Aroma Life.

Action of Selected Essential oils:

- Helichrysum increases neurotransmitter activity.

- Nutmeg is a general cerebral stimulant and also has adrenal cortex-like activity

Put the oils directly onto the nerve centers as is practical. The brain reflex points include the forehead, temples, and mastoids (the bones just behind the ears). Use direct pressure application to the brainstem located on the center of the backbone, on the neck, and work down the spine.

You can also apply essential oils to a natural bristle brush (oils may dissolve plastic bristles). Rub and brush vigorously along the brain stem and spine.

Supplements: JuvaTone, VitaGreen, Chelex, A.D.&E., and Sulfurzyme.

Concentration (Poor)

Single Oils: Basil, lemon, and bergamot.

Blends: Brain Power, Clarity, Harmony, and Valor.

Inhale Clarity, rub Harmony on the crown and on throat, and rub Valor on the forehead.

Memory Problems

Single Oils: Peppermint, rosemary cineol, basil, rose.

- Lemongrass with basil, rosemary cineol, peppermint or rose.

- Rosemary cineol with basil, lemon, peppermint, clove, cardamom, or helichrysum.

Blends: Brain Power, Clarity.

- Lemongrass with Clarity.

- Rosemary with M-Grain.

- Clarity with En-R-Gee (indirectly helps because of boost in one's energy level).

Supplements: Essential Manna, Royal Essence, AuraLight, and VitaGreen.

These oils improve memory by stimulating an opening of emotional blocks.

Peppermint improves mental concentration and memory. Dr. Dember conducted a study at the University of Cincinnati in 1994 showing that inhaling peppermint increased mental accuracy by 28 percent.

The fragrance of diffused oils, such as lemon, have also been reported to increase memory retention and recall.

How to Tap the Full Therapeutic Potential of Essential Oils

An outstanding way to tap the full therapeutic potential of essential oils is to combine them with bath salts and use them in the shower. The RainSpa aromatherapy shower head has a specially designed chamber that can be filled with essential oils and bath salts. As the water passes through the mixture, it disperses the essential oils into the spray, creating a fragrant, antiseptic spa.

Recipe 1:
- 5 drops basil
- 10 drops rosemary
- 2 drops peppermint
- 4 drops helichrysum

Recipe 2:
- 4 drops lavender
- 3 drops geranium
- 3 drops rosewood
- 3 drops rosemary
- 2 drops tangerine
- 1 drop spearmint
- 2 drops Idaho tansy

Blend in 1/2 to 1 ounce V-6 Mixing Oil or Massage Oil Base. Rub on temples, forehead, mastoids (bone behind ears), brainstem (back of neck).

Supplements: Rehemogen.

Vascular cleansing will allow better and unimpeded blood flow, giving improved distribution of oxygen and nutrients (see VASCULAR CLEANSING).

Mental Fatigue

Single Oils: Cardamom, rosemary cineol, peppermint, and frankincense.

Blends: Brain Power, Acceptance, and Clarity.

Supplements: Stevia Select

Diffuse and wear as a cologne or perfume. Dilute 1-3 drops in 1 tsp. V6 Mixing Oil or massage oil and rub on temples, neck, and shoulders.

Stimulate Pineal/Pituitary Gland

Single Oils: Sandalwood, lavender, and frankincense.

Blends: Dream Catcher, Forgiveness, Gathering, Harmony, Humility, 3 Wise Men, and ImmuPower.

These blends contain frankincense and sandalwood, which oxygenate the pineal/pituitary gland, thus improving attitude and frequency balance.

Supplements: Ultra Young, AuraLight.

Stroke

There are two different kinds of strokes: thrombotic strokes and hemorrhagic strokes. Thrombotic strokes are caused from a blood clot lodging in a cerebral blood vessel and cutting blood supply to a part of the brain. A hemorrhagic stroke is caused by an aneurysm, or a weakness in the blood vessel wall that balloons out and ruptures, spilling blood into the surrounding brain tissue.

For Thrombotic Strokes:

(See BLOOD CLOTS)

Single Oils: Helichrysum, cypress, juniper, peppermint, clove, lemon, grapefruit, orange, tangerine.

Blends: Thieves, ImmuPower.

- Helichrysum with cypress, juniper, peppermint, Aroma Life, Brain Power, or Clarity.
- Lemon with ImmuPower.

Take 1-3 drops as a dietary supplement or massage on back of neck, brainstem, and Vita Flex points of the feet and hands. Apply ImmuPower over the thymus.

Supplements: Sulfurzyme, Essential Manna, Super Cal.

These supplements are rich in the essential minerals, fatty acids, and nutrients necessary for helping to regenerate and rebuild damaged nerve tissues.

For Hemorrhagic Strokes:

(See HEMORRHAGING or BRUISING)

The essential oil of cypress may help strengthen vascular walls.

Single Oils: Cypress, helichrysum.

Supplements: Sulfurzyme, Essential Manna, Super Cal.

These supplements are rich in the essential minerals, fatty acids, and nutrients necessary for helping to regenerate and rebuild damaged nerve tissues.

Bronchitis

Bronchitis is characterized by inflammation of the bronchial tube tube lining accompanied by a heavy mucus discharge. Bronchitis can be caused by an infection or exposure to dust, chemicals, air pollution, or cigarette smoke.

When bronchitis occurs regularly over a long periods (i.e. 3 months out of the year for several years) it is known as chronic bronchitis. It can eventually lead to emphysema.

Symptoms:
• Persistent, hacking cough
• Mucus discharge from the lungs
• Difficulty breathing

Avoiding air pollution is an easy way to reduce bronchitis symptoms. In cases where bronchitis is caused by a bacteria or virus, the inhalation of high antimicrobial essential oils may help combat the infection.

How Essential Oils Benefit the Respiratory Tract

• Myrrh is very effective for throat problems and hoarseness.

• Pine dilates and opens bronchial tubes.

• Raven strengthens the respiratory system, dilates and opens the pulmonary tract, fights respiratory infections.

• Rose, sage, and sandalwood help chronic bronchitis.

• Fresh Essence oral rinse is effective for killing a broad spectrum of viruses and bacteria.

Single Oils: Cypress, rosemary, lemon, cinnamon, eucalyptus radiata, frankincense, marjoram, sandalwood, ravensara, thyme, birch, myrrh, dill, fir, spruce, pine, oregano, helichrysum, rose, melaleuca, clove, lavender, spearmint, clary sage, hyssop, and myrtle.

• Cypress with rosemary, lemon, cinnamon, eucalyptus radiata, frankincense, marjoram, or sandalwood.

• Frankincense with ravensara, cypress, lemon, thyme, rosemary, eucalyptus radiata, birch, myrtle, or hyssop.

• Lavender with lemon, lemongrass, ginger, tarragon, peppermint, frankincense, oregano, thyme, spearmint, clary sage, dill, myrrh, or rose.

• Melaleuca or rosemary verbenon with fir, spruce, pine, oregano, helichrysum, thyme, or cinnamon.

• Thyme with ravensara, oregano, melaleuca, frankincense, clove, cinnamon, or lavender.

Blends: Exodus II, ImmuPower, R.C., Raven, Melrose, Thieves, and Purification.

• Lavender with Melrose or Thieves.

• Cypress or frankincense with Raven, or R.C.

• Melaleuca or rosemary verbenon with Melrose, Purification, R.C., or Brain Power.

• Sage with R.C., Thieves, or Raven.

• Thyme with Melrose, Purification, Thieves, or Brain Power.

Add 1-2 drops of essential oil to 2-4 oz. of water or Fresh Essence mouthwash and gargle every hour.

Dilute 1-2 drops of essential oil in 1 Tbsp. massage oil and apply on the neck and chest or apply neat to the Vita Flex points of the feet and hands. The blends Exodus II, ImmuPower, R.C., Raven, Melrose, Thieves, and Purification work especially in these applications.

Supplements: ImmuGel, Radex, Super C, ImmuneTune, Exodus, Cleansing Trio, and Fresh Essence.

Regimen:

• ImmuGel: 1/2 tsp. every 3-4 hours. Hold in mouth for 30 seconds for better absorption.

• Fresh Essence: Gargle whenever needed.

• Diffuse: Raven, Thieves, R.C., ImmuPower, Exodus II, and Purification. Alternate the oils every hour, but diffuse for about 15 minutes or as needed. Alternate Raven and R.C.

- For respiratory conditions combine 1 drop each of myrtle, mountain savory, and eucalyptus radiata with 4 drops Raven in 1 Tbsp. V-6 Mixing Oil or Massage Oil Base and insert as a rectal implant. An easy way to do a rectal implant is to buy a small enema syringe, empty out the contents, fill with oil mixture, and insert before going to sleep. Retain throughout the night.

Bruising

(See BLOOD CLOTS under BLOOD)

Some people bruise easily because the capillary walls are weak and break easily, particularly in the skin. Those who bruise easily may be deficient in vitamin C.

Essential oils can help speed the healing of bruises and reduce the risk of blood clot formation. Oils like cypress help to strengthen capillary walls, while oils like helichrysum help speed the reabsorption of the blood. that has collected in the tissue.

Single Oils: Cypress, helichrysum

- Helichrysum or lavender with cypress, Idaho tansy, lemongrass, geranium, peppermint, rosemary, or Roman chamomile.

- Clove with black pepper, peppermint, cypress, marjoram, or geranium.

Mix 3-4 drops of essential oil in 1/2 oz. V-6 Mixing Oil or Massage Oil Base and spread over the area.

Supplements: Master Formula vitamins, Vita-Green, JuvaTone, and Super C.

Regimen:

- Apply 2-3 drops of helichrysum on location neat or put in 2 oz. water and take as a dietary supplement.

- Super C: 2-6 tablets, 3 times daily.

- Master Formula Vitamin: 2-6 tablets, 3 times daily.

- VitaGreen: 2-6 capsules 3 times daily.

Recipe 1:
- 1 drop helichrysum
- 3 drops lavender
- 2 drops lemongrass
- 2 drops geranium
- 1 drop peppermint

Recipe 2 (deep tissue bruising and pain):
- 8 drops clove
- 8 drops black pepper oil
- 4 drops peppermint
- 5 drops cypress
- 8 drops marjoram
- 5 drops geranium

Recipe 3:
- 2 drops lavender
- 3 drops rosemary
- 1 drop geranium

Apply 1-4 drops on location neat or mix in 1-2 Tbsp. V-6 Mixing Oil or Massage Oil Base.

Essential oils can also be mixed in water to saturate wash cloth or towel and applied as compress

Burns

(See SKIN DISORDERS or SHOCK)

There are three types of burns:

- First-degree burns only damage the outer layer of the skin.

- Second-degree burns damage both the outer layer and the underlying layer known as the dermis.

- Third-degree burns not only destroy or damage skin but can even affect underlying tissues.

Burns can be caused by sunlight, chemicals, electricity, radiation, or heat. Thermal burns are the most common type.

Aloe vera gel (contained in LavaDerm) has been extensively used in the treatment of burns and has been studied for its anti-inflammatory and tissue-regenerating properties. Helichrysum is a tissue regenerator and reduces scarring and discoloration.

NOTE: All burns can be serious, so seek medical attention if necessary. If the burn is large or severe, the individual may go into shock. Inhaling oils may help reduce the shock. (See SHOCK)

The Deadly Dehydration of Burns

The reason that burns tend to swell and blister is due to fluid loss from the damaged blood vessels. This is why it is important to keep the burn well hydrated and to drink plenty of water.

In cases of serious burns, fluid loss can become so drastic as to send the victim into shock and requiring intravenous transfusions of saline solution to bring up blood pressure.

Single Oils: Lavender

• Lavender with peppermint, Idaho tansy, helichrysum, and rose. Use peppermint sparingly: 1 drop to 5 to 10 drops lavender.

Blends:

• Lavender with Gentle Baby or Sunsation with LavaDerm Cooling Mist.

Skin Care: LavaDerm Cooling Mist and Rose Ointment.

Apply LavaDerm every 15 minutes the first day (Keep LavaDerm refrigerated). Apply 3 to 5 drops of lavender as needed immediately after misting.

On days 2 through 5, mist every 1/2 to 1 hour and follow with lavender.

Continue using cooling mist 3 to 6 times daily until healed. Apply Rose Ointment to keep tissue soft.

After a burn has started to heal and is drying and cracking, use Rose Ointment or body lotion with a few drops of lavender to keep skin soft and to promote faster healing.

Using Peppermint Oil on Burns

Peppermint is highly effective for reducing inflammation in damaged tissue. Unfortunately, it stings when applied to a fresh burn.

So to avoid any stinging or discomfort, you might want to first dilute the peppermint oil with lavender oil (equal parts) and mix well in water. Moisten a cloth with the mixture and apply as a cold compress on location.

You can also wait 1-2 days after receiving the burn before applying peppermint. Once the burn has started to heal, peppermint can be applied with minimal discomfort.

Peppermint can also be applied to the sealed over burn to reduce inflammation and speed healing.

Sunburn

The best prevention for sunburn is to avoid prolonged exposure to the sun. When you do go outdoors, it is smart to always wear sunblock or lotion with an SPF greater than 15—especially during the summer and when you expect to be outdoors a good deal.

In the event you do suffer a sunburn, essential oils like lavender can offer excellent pain-relieving and healing benefits.

Single Oils: Lavender, peppermint.

• Lavender, helichrysum, peppermint with LavaDerm Cooling Mist.

To cool tissue and reduce inflammation, apply 1 drop of peppermint oil mixed with V-6 Mixing Oil, or Massage Oil Base on location.

Blends:

• Lavender with Gentle Baby or Melrose.

Spray burn immediately with LavaDerm Cooling Mist and continue misting when necessary to cool the area. Spray 4-5 times every hour and follow with 2-3 drops of lavender.

Third-Degree Burns

For third-degree burns, seek medical attention. Spray LavaDerm on burn every 10 minutes for the first 24 hours until the tissue appears to be well rehydrated. Apply a few drops of lavender oil after misting.

As burn heals, continue to apply Lavaderm with or without other undiluted oils, 2 or more times daily for 3-4 days.

Bursitis

Bursitis is in an inflammation of the bursa, which are small, fluid-filled sacs located near the joints. Bursa act as shock absorbers when muscles or tendons come into contact with bone. As the bursa become swollen, they result in pain, particularly when the affected joint is used.

Bursitis can be caused by injury, infection, or arthritis, and usually involves the joints of the knees, elbows, shoulders, and Achilles tendon. Occasionally bursitis can occur in the base of the big toe. Bursitis may signal the beginning of arthritis.

Single Oils: Marjoram, basil, lavender, pepper, spruce, fir, pine, birch, Idaho tansy, and elemi.

Blends: Relieve It and PanAway.

• Birch with oregano.

Supplements: Arthro Plus, ArthroTune, AlkaLime, Super Cal, Essential Manna, and Sulfurzyme.

Cancer

Researchers have linked most degenerative diseases to lack of nutrients in the body. Minerals and trace minerals play a large part in nutritional deficiencies.

Oils rich in d-limonene have been shown in animal studies to have potent anticarcinogeic effects. According to a study at the University of Indiana, "monoterpenes would appear to act through multiple mechanisms in the chemoprevention and chemotherapy of cancer."

Cancer requires strong cleansing and nutritional building programs. The programs suggested here can be tailored to fit your particular needs.

1. Intensive cleanse with Cleansing Trio with JuvaTone.

2. The Burrough's Cleanse using cayenne pepper, lemon juice, and grade C maple syrup. (See Health Programs, Chapter 20)

3. The Megazyme program (See box).

Megazyme Program

This program should be monitored by a health care professional:

Phase 1: Start with 3 tablets, 3 times daily. Increase amount by 1 tablet every day until vomiting starts. At this point, stop Megazyme for 24-36 hours.

Phase 2: Start again with 4 tablets, 3 times daily. Increase daily amount until vomiting starts again. Stop and rest for 24-36 hours.

Phase 3: Start with 5 tablets, 3 times daily. Increase amount by one tablet every day until vomiting starts. Rest for 24-36 hours.

Phase 4: Go back to the amount taken before vomiting occurred the third time. Continue this amount for 6 weeks.

Phase 5: Start enzyme saturation again.

NOTE: Anyone with cancer should skip phase 3 and rest at least 1 day per week.

Single Oils: Helichrysm, lemon, orange, lavender, clove.

• Frankincense with helichrysum, clove, lavender, inula, Idaho tansy, or clary sage.

Blends: ImmuPower.

• ImmuPower and Grounding (for emotions related to the disease).

Recipe 1:
• 12 drops frankincense
• 5 drops lavender
• 6 drops bergamot
• 6 drops helichrysum

Use neat for serious conditions or in 1 oz. V-6 Mixing Oil or Massage Oil Base for maintenance and long-term use.

Apply oils neat direct on skin cancers, cancerous nodes, or on Vita Flex points for internal cancers. Apply on the spine up to 3 times daily.

When people have terminal illness, their minds are fractured, and they have difficulty focusing and collecting their thoughts. Gathering promotes greater focus and the ability to gather feelings.

Supplements: Master Formula vitamins, VitaGreen, Super C, Radex, ImmuneTune, Ultra Young, AuraLight, Essential Manna, Power Meal, Thyromin, Exodus, Sulfurzyme, Mineral Essence, and Royaldophilus.

Blood Types

O blood types may require larger amounts of supplements. They can also tolerate more supplements without overdoing.

Gary Young Daily Maintenance Program

- Master Formula: 6-8 tablets daily.
- VitaGreen: 8-18 capsules daily.
- Super C: 8-18 tablets daily.
- Radex: 8-12 tablets daily.
- ImmuneTune : 6-12 capsules daily.
- Ultra Young: 3 squirts, 3 times daily.
- Power Meal: 2-3 scoops, 3 times daily.
- Megazyme: 2-6 tablets, 3 times daily according to blood type.
- Thyromin: Start 1 before bedtime and increase as needed.
- Exodus: 6-8 capsules daily.
- Sulfurzyme: Begin with 1 tsp., 3 times daily and work up to 1-3 Tbsp. daily.
- Rehemogen: 3 droppers, 3 times daily. Rehemogen cleans blood, restoring nutrients and oxygen to the cells. Cleansed blood helps overcome disease.

- Mineral Essence: 3-4 droppers, 3 times daily.
- Royaldophilus: 2-3 capsules, 3 times daily for good digestion and assimilation.
- Super B is a good source of all B vitamins including pantothenic acid (vitamin B5). Many cancer patients evidence a deficiency in vitamin B5.

Friedmann Program

Terry S. Friedmann, M.D., conducted an experimental cancer program on ten patients. All those who followed the program are now healthy. One little girl had a massive tumor on her forehead, spinal problems, and was on morphine. Three days into the program she went off morphine, and 2 weeks later went off Tylenol. One month later her tumor was gone, and she had gained 7 pounds with her spine 75 percent regenerated. Dr. Friedmann's program is as follows:

- ImmuneTune: 1 capsule
- Super C: 6 tablets
- Radex: 3 tablets
- Master Formula vitamin: 1 tablet
- VitaGreen: 2 capsules

Take 6 to 7 times daily.

Apply frankincense on tumorous growths and ImmuPower on spine and bottom of feet 2 times daily. Massage a blend of 6-10 drops each of frankincense and clove on tumor location.

Brain Tumors

Single Oils: Frankincense, lemon, orange, clove.

Supplements: Take as suggested under Cancer.

Inhale frankincense until nauseated and massage frankincense on brainstem and carotid arteries. Apply frankincense on the roof of the mouth and the buccal cavity (inside of cheeks) with your finger.

Megazyme program:

- Take 20 Radex, 15 to 20 ImmuneTune, 15 Exodus, and 20 Super C daily.

- Maintain a concentrated carrot juice diet. Potassium is critical. Drink plenty of dandelion tea (diuretic) and yellow dock tea (iron).

Increase blood flow to the brain:

- Mix 4 drops frankincense and 5 drops ImmuPower and massage on the neck.

- Mix 15 drops frankincense and 6 drops clove in 1/2 oz. V-6 Mixing Oil or Massage Oil Base and rub several times daily on the brain stem (spine at base of skull), temples, mastoids (behind the ears), forehead, and crown (top of head).

- Put 10 drops frankincense and 1 drop clove in diffuser. Sit in front of the diffuser and breathe vapors for 1/2 hour, 3 times a day. If you get a headache or feel nauseous, reduce to what is tolerable, but do not quit.

- AlkaLime: 1 Tbsp. in water 1 hour before or after meals to help restore pH balance.

Bone Cancer

Single Oils: Frankincense, lemon, orange, and clove.

When taking essential oils internally, always dilute – 1 drop oil in 1 tsp. vegetable oil.

Recipe 1:
- 15 drops frankincense
- 6 drops clove

Mix in 1/2 oz. V-6 Mixing Oil or Massage Oil Base and massage on location daily.

Blends: ImmuPower

Apply 2-3 drops each of frankincense and ImmuPower on the spine, 3 times daily.

Supplements: Cleansing Trio.

Cleanse: Cleansing Trio.

Breast Cancer

Single Oils: Frankincense, lavender, clove.

Blends: Present Time and Brain Power.

Supplements: Cleansing Trio, JuvaTone, Femi-Gen, Femalin, Power Meal, Body Balance, Mineral Essence, and Super Cal.

Program:

1. Start with a colon and liver cleanse.

2. Massage frankincense on breast Vita Flex point on feet, which is on top of the foot at the base of the three middle toes. Continue massaging the Vita Flex areas after applying the oils. (See VITA FLEX)

3. Massage oils for 4 days and rest for 4 days. Layer on 15 drops frankincense, 10 drops lavender, and 3 drops clove. Apply 3 drops Present Time on the sternum. Put 3-6 drops of frankincense in a capsule and swallow daily. Diffuse frankincense and Brain Power.

Prevention and Remission:

1. Keep lymphatics open with deep breathing exercise and aerobics.

2. Have a body massage with Cel-lite Magic once per month to work the lymph nodes in the abdomen and the thoracic region.

3. The soy in the Body Balance helps balance estrogen hormones. Take 2-3 Tbsp. Body Balance with water or juice 1-2 times daily. *Do not use for estrogen-based cancers.*

4. Discontinue use of antiperspirants and monitor calcium levels.

Colon Cancer

Single Oils: Clove, frankincense, lemon, orange, and lavender.

When taking essential oils internally, always dilute – 1 drop oil in 1 tsp. vegetable oil.

Essential Oil Program:

Day 1: Put 6 drops of frankincense in a capsule and swallow 3 to 4 times daily

Day 2: Mix 6 drops frankincense and 3 drops clove, diluted in vegetable oil, and put in capsule. Take orally 3 to 4 times daily.

Day 3: Put equal parts frankincense and lavender in a capsule and take 3 to 4 times a day

Day 4: Take frankincense capsules 3 to 4 times daily.

Day 5: Rest for 4 days and restart program.

Supplement Program:

1. Begin with Megazyme to digest toxic waste.

2. Take 2 capsules ComforTone, 3 times daily. Increase by one daily until the bowels move. Then begin reducing. If diarrhea occurs, reduce amount and increase I.C.P. Drink plenty of purified or distilled water.

3. I.C.P. fiber cleanse: Begin with 1 Tbsp. in water, 3 times daily. Increase to 2 Tbsp., 3 times daily or as needed until bowels are moving regularly.

Leukemia

Single Oils: Frankincense.

Apply in a full body massage.

Blends: Thieves.

Use: Apply on bottom of the feet.

Supplements: Rehemogen, Radex, Super C, ImmuneTune, VitaGreen, and Royal Essence.

Take the following throughout the day, for 39 days:

- Radex: 10 tablets daily.
- Rehemogen: 3 droppers, 3 times daily.
- Super C: 12 tablets daily.
- ImmuneTune: 15 capsules daily.
- VitaGreen: 9 capsules daily.
- Royal Essence: 9 droppers daily in water.
- Fresh carrot juice: 1/2 gallon.

Do not eat white flour, sugar, salt, or red meat.

Liver Cancer

Single Oils: Frankincense, lavender, clove.

- 30 drops frankincense

- 20 drops lavender

- 10 drops clove

Combine with castor oil and use in a compress over liver 5 nights per week.

Blends: JuvaFlex

- *Rub JuvaFlex over the liver, with or without compresses or hot packs. Massage JuvaFlex on liver Vita Flex points on the feet.*

Supplements: JuvaTone and Ultra Young in addition to supplement program as stated.

Cleansing is extremely important since an optimally functioning liver is necessary to rid the body of toxins. Anger and hate are stored in the liver and cause extreme toxicity and eventually trigger disease.

Lung Cancer

Single Oils:

- Frankincense with sage, myrrh, clove, ravensara, or hyssop.

Blends: Raven

- Frankincense with ImmuPower.

Essential Oil Program:

Day 1: Begin diffusing frankincense and R.C. Use 20 drops frankincense and R.C. in rectal implant.

Day 2: Use equal parts frankincense and Raven in rectal implant.

Day 3: Use equal parts frankincense and lavender in rectal implant.

Day 4: rectal implant: frankincense.

Day 5: Use equal parts frankincense and R.C. in rectal implant.

Rest 2 days before continuing. If an improvement is not detected, do not rest.

Alternate in rectal implant:

- Eucalyptus globulus: 10 drops
- Frankincense: 10 drops
- Peppermint and frankincense: 10 drops
- Tangerine: 40 drops
- Cypress: 10 drops
- Peppermint: 5 drops

Diffuse oil combinations used in rectal implants consistently.

Recipe 1:
- 4 drops clove
- 2 drops frankincense

Dilute in vegetable oil. Put in a capsule and take as dietary supplement or dilute in 1 tsp. V-6 Mixing Oil or Massage Oil Base and use in a full body massage. Alternate with clove and lavender every day for a minimum of 7 days in massage therapy.

Recipe 2:
- 2 drops sage
- 4 drops myrrh
- 5 drops clove
- 6 drops Raven
- 5 drops frankincense

Mix in 1/2 oz. (1 Tbsp.) V-6 Mixing Oil or Massage Oil Base. Use enema syringe to implant and retain through the night.

Rub ImmuPower up the spine, daily. Apply compress on back and chest twice daily.

Supplements: Super C, K & B, Goji Berry Tea, Super Cal, and Essential Manna.

Take daily Super C, 30 to 40 capsules, dandelion tea, raw lemon juice, red clover tea, K & B, and Goji Berry Tea.

Edema: Super Cal, Essential Manna, pomegranate juice, or organic bananas.

Lymphoma (Cancer of Lymph Nodes)

Both Hodgkin's disease and non-Hodgkin's disease are characterized by swollen lymph gland nodes, generally first appearing on the neck, armpit or groin.

Lymphoma may be caused from petrochemical pollution in the air and water. After prolonged exposure, toxins such as benzene, styrene, and toluene begin to accumulate in the lymphatic system, eventually triggering cellular mutations and cancer.

Symptoms for non-Hodgkin's lymphoma

- Generally ill, loss of appetite, loss of weight, fever, and night sweats.

Symptoms of Hodgkin's lymphoma

- Fever, fatigue, weakness, itching.

Single Oils:

- Frankincense with myrrh and sage.

Recipe 1:
- 10 drops frankincense
- 5 drops myrrh
- 3 drops sage
- 1/2 to 1 oz. V-6 Mixing Oil or Massage Oil Base.

Apply on swollen nodes daily. Every second day apply 1-2 drops of frankincense. For faster results apply in a rectal implant.

Rub along spine twice daily. Every other day rub frankincense, neat, along spine. Rub Immu-Power 3 times daily on spine.

A program for lymphoma stage 4 (very fatty bone marrow):

Recipe 2 (body massage):
- 15 drops frankincense
- 6 drops clove
- 1 oz. V-6 Mixing Oil or Massage Oil Base.

Supplements: ImmuneTune, Super C, Vita-Green, Cleansing Trio, and Radex.

Regimen:

- Take 4 ImmuneTune, 3 times daily
- Take 6 Super C, 3 times daily
- Take 6 VitaGreen, 3 times daily
- Take 3 Radex, 4 times daily.

Follow this program for one month, then gradually reduce. If lymphoma goes into remission, continue program for another month, then gradually reduce. It is best eat a total vegetarian diet. O-blood types, who need more protein, should eat fresh stream trout or Arctic salmon.

Melanoma (Skin Cancer)

Melanoma is the most lethal form of skin cancer. It tends to aggressively spread and metastasize, quickly colonizing the lymph nodes and internal organs. It has a high rate of fatality.

A sudden change in the appearance of an old mole or the appearance of red lesions, may indicate melanoma. If you suspect that you have melanoma or any skin cancer, you should immediately contact your physician.

Single Oils:

• Frankincense with inula, lavender, Idaho tansy, melaleuca, lemongrass, or tarragon.

Blends:

• Frankincense with Release, JuvaFlex, Endo-Flex, Purification, or Gentle Baby.

Apply 1-2 drops frankincense neat on location, 2-3 times daily.

Recipe 1:
• 3 drops lavender
• 4 drops frankincense

Mix in 3/4 oz. V-6 Mixing Oil or Massage Oil Base. Apply 3 times daily.

Ovarian Cancer

Single Oils:

• Frankincense with myrrh and geranium.

Blends:

• Frankincense with ImmuPower.

Supplements: FemiGen, Femalin, Body Balance, Protec, and ArthroTune

Daily Regimen:

• Drink 3-4 cups Goji Berry Tea.

• Use essential oils in rectal or vaginal implants. Use a vaginal retention implants one night and a rectal retention implant the second night. Alternate as needed.

　—15 drops frankincense
　—5 drops myrrh
　—6 drops geranium
　—1/2 oz. V-6 Mixing Oil

• Rub 3-4 drops ImmuPower up the spine, on the feet, and on the throat, daily.

• Rub Protec topically over the abdomen, over the ovaries, and also over the reproductive Vita Flex areas on hands and feet.

• Use Protec as a nighly retention douche. Start with 1/2 tsp. and build up to 1 Tbsp. If irritation occurs, discontinue for 3 days and start again with a smaller amount.

To increase Protec's strength, add extra oils and use for alternating applications:

• *NIGHT 1: Add 3 to 4 drops of frankincense.*
• *NIGHT 2: Add 3 to 4 drops of clove.*
• *NIGHT 3: Add 3 to 4 drops of myrrh.*

Prostate Cancer

Many prostate cancers may be testosterone-dependent, so it may be necessary to avoid taking anything that can raise testosterone levels, such as DHEA or androstenedione.

Single Oils:

• Frankincense with myrrh, sage, or anise seed.

Blends: Mister, Protec.

Use Protec as a nighly retention enema. Start with 1/2 tsp. and build up to 1 Tbsp. If irritation occurs, discontinue for 3 days and start again with a smaller amount.

To increase Protec's strength, add extra oils and use for alternating applications:

• *NIGHT 1: Add 3 to 4 drops of frankincense.*
• *NIGHT 2: Add 3 to 4 drops of clove.*
• *NIGHT 3: Add 3 to 4 drops of myrrh.*

Supplements: Super B, ProGen, Cleansing Trio, and JuvaTone.

- -

Regimen:

This regimen reduced PSA (prostate specific antigen) counts over 70 percent in 2 months:

• 10 drops frankincense
• 5 drops myrrh
• 3 drops sage

Mix in 1 Tbsp. V-6 Mixing Oil or Massage Oil Base for rectal implant. Rub topically between the rectum and scrotum and on the reproductive Vita Flex areas on hands and feet.

- -

Uterine Cancer

Environmental pollutants become lodged in tissues, such as the breasts, thyroid, ovaries, and uterus. Many chemicals mimic or imitate our natural hormones and can fit the hormone receptors, thus tricking and over-stimulating these organs. This can become a major source of cancer of the breast, uterus, and lymph nodes.

(Same program as OVARIAN CANCER)

Candida

(See FUNGAL INFECTIONS)

Canker Sores

These tend to occur because of stress, illness, weakened immune system, injury caused by such things as hot food, rough brushing of teeth, or dentures.

Single Oils:

• Melissa, Sage with clove or lavender.

Blends:

• Sage with Thieves.

Carbon Monoxide Poisoning

Almost everyone who lives in a large metropolitan area will suffer varying degrees of subtle carbon monoxide poisoning. The more polluted or stagnant the air, the more likely that carbon monoxide levels in the blood may be elevated.

NOTE: Someone who has suffered serious carbon monoxide poisoning should be immediately exposed to fresh air while a doctor, paramedic, or other professional is contacted.

Blends:

• Myrtle with R.C., Inspiration, Sacred Mountain, Purification, Valor, or Harmony.

Supplements: Master Formula vitamins, Royal Essence, VitaGreen, Super B, Super C, and Radex.

Regimen:

(Perform every 3-4 hours)

Massage Valor on the bottom of feet.

• Apply Purification through Raindrop Technique on the spine and back.

• Diffuse Purification, rub on the feet.

• Inhale R.C., Purification, Inspiration, and Sacred Mountain, and rub on the lung Vita Flex areas on bottom of the feet and on top of the feet at the base of the toes.

Cardiovascular Conditions

High Cholesterol

Single Oils: Rosemary, Roman chamomile, and helichrysum italicum.

• Rosemary with helichrysum.

• Helichrysum with German chamomile, Roman chamomile, clary sage, geranium, or fennel.

Blends:

• Rosemary with Clarity, Aroma Life, or JuvaFlex.

• Helichrysum with Di-Tone, JuvaFlex, or EndoFlex.

Apply neat on arteries at pulse points where the arteries are close to the surface, or mix with V-6 Mixing Oil or Massage Oil Base for body massage.

Recipe 1:
• 2 to 5 drops rosemary cineol
• 5 drops Roman chamomile
• 3 drops helichrysum

Dilute with vegetable oil and place in capsule and take 3 times daily

Rub along spine twice daily. Every other day rub frankincense, neat, along spine. Rub Immu-Power 3 times daily on spine.

Aroma Life regulates and lowers blood pressure and breaks down plaque on the blood vessel walls.

Helichrysum is a chelator that lowers and regulates cholesterol and reduce blood clotting. *(For tips on application, see Heart Vita Flex under Blood Pressure.)*

Supplements: JuvaTone, Cleansing Trio, Vita-Green, Radex, Super C, Super Cal, ImmuGel, Royal Essence, Mineral Essence, Chelex, Goji Berry Tea, and I.C.P. (work up to 2 Tbsp. twice daily).

Do a colon and liver cleanse using the Cleansing Trio, JuvaTone, and JuvaFlex. JuvaTone is particularly useful for high cholesterol. I.C.P. helps break down plaque.

Mix 25 drops of HRT in 6 ounces of distilled water, 3 times daily. Supports blood system and circulation deficiency.

Magnesium acts as a smooth muscle relaxant and supports the cardiovascular system. It acts as a natural calcium channel blocker for the heart, lowering blood pressure and dilating the heart blood vessels *(Dr. Terry Friedmann)*. Mineral Essence and Super Cal are good sources of magnesium.

Hardening of the Arteries

Singles: Helichrysum and cypress.

Blends: Aroma Life.

Phlebitis (Inflammation of Veins)

Single Oils:

- Helichrysum with lavender, German chamomile, Roman chamomile, or geranium.

Blends:

- Helichrysum or lavender with Aroma Life.

Helichrysum with lavender is excellent. Helichrysum prevents phlebitis. Use the oil on location with cold packs.

Carpal Tunnel Syndrome

(See NERVOUS SYSTEM)

Cataracts/Glaucoma

(See EYE DISORDERS)

Cellulite

Cellulite is one of the harder types of fats to dissolve in the body. Cellulite is an accumulation of old fat cell clusters that solidify and harden as the surrounding tissue loses its elasticity.

Excess fat is undesirable for two reasons:

1. The extra weight puts an extra load on all body systems, particularly the heart and cardiovascular system, as well as the joints (knees, hips, spine).

2. Toxins and petrochemicals (pesticides, herbicides, metallics) tend to accumulate in fatty tissue. This can contribute to hormone imbalance, neurological problems, and a higher risk of cancer.

Essential oils such as tangerine and grapefruit may help digest fat cells. Cypress enhances circulation to enhance the elimination of fatty deposits. The essential oils of lemongrass and spearmint and Goji Tea also may help burn fat and Cel-Lite Magic Massage Oil may help dissolve cellulite deposits.

Single Oils:

- Rosemary with grapefruit*, lemon*, cypress, fennel, juniper, spearmint, tangerine, lemongrass, or cedarwood.

  Grapefruit and Lemon are photo-sensitizing. Do not expose the skin to UV rays after using these oils.

Blends:

- Rosemary with Citrus Fresh or EndoFlex.

241

Supplements: Thyromin, Power Meal, Cel-Lite Magic Massage Oil, and Goji Berry Tea.

Recipe 1:
- 5 drops rosemary
- 10 drops grapefruit
- 2 drops cypress

Massage oils into the skin at least once daily and before exercising. Cellulite is slow to dissolve, so target areas should be worked for a month or more in conjunction with weight training and a weight loss program.

Recipe 2:
- 9 drops lemon
- 9 drops cypress
- 2 ounces of jojoba oil

Recipe 3:
- 10 drops grapefruit
- 5 drops lavender
- 3 drops helichrysum
- 3 drops patchouly
- 4 drops cypress
- *1/2 to 1 oz. V-6 Mixing Oil or Massage Oil Base.*

Add 3-5 drops of grapefruit to increase fat-dissolving action in areas of fat rolls, puckers, and dimples.

Apply 1-3 times daily, depending on extent of problem and the person's age. Old fat and cellulite take longer to dissolve, so be patient. You should begin to see results in 6 to 8 weeks when used in combination with a muscle-building and weigh-loss regime.

Recipe 4 (Bath):
- 5 drops juniper
- 3 drops orange
- 3 drops cypress
- 3 drops lemon
- 2 tbsp. honey

Dissolve in warm bath water. Massage with Cel-Lite Magic afterwards.

Thyromin helps to balance or increase metabolism.

Chemical Sensitivity Reaction

Environmental poisoning and chemical sensitivity are fast becoming a major cause of discomfort and disease. Strong chemical compounds, such as insecticides, herbicides, and formaldehyde found in paints, glues, cosmetics, and finger nail polish, easily enter the body. Symptoms include indigestion, upper and lower gas, poor assimilation, poor electrolyte balance, rashes, hypoglycemia, allergic reaction to foods and other substances, along with emotional mood swings, fatigue, irritability, lack of motivation, lack of discipline and creativity.

Single Oils: Frankincense and sandalwood.

Blends: Purification, Clarity, Brain Power, and JuvaFlex.

Supplements: Radex, ImmuneTune, Exodus, Rehemogen, Chelex, JuvaTone, and Cleansing Trio.

For headache relief:
- 6 Radex
- 4 ImmuneTune or ArthroTune

Drink 2-3 large glasses of water.

(See VASCULAR CLEANSING)

Absorption of Chemicals

Handling refuse or any type of contaminant without protective gloves may cause discoloration of hands.

Single Oils: Lavender and lemon.

Blends: Purification

Use good rubber gloves and change them often or at least wash them out with strong soap, rinse well, and dry well. If hands become discolored through chemical absorption, soak them in a solution of hydrogen peroxide 3 percent, available at drug stores. This helps remove chemicals from the skin. Rub lavender, lemon, or Purification neat on hands and cover with clean cotton gloves or wrap lightly with cotton bandages all night.

Chicken Pox

Single Oils: Lavender

Add lavender to calamine lotion and dab on spots.

Cholecystitis

(See GALLBLADDER)

Inflammation of the gallbladder due to excessive pooling of concentrated bile.

Cholera

Single Oils: Clove, ravensara, rosemary, and sage

Cholesterol

(See CARDIOVASCULAR CONDITIONS)

Chronic Fatigue Syndrome

Single Oils: Rosemary, melaleuca, thyme, nutmeg, and blue tansy.

Blends: EndoFlex, Exodus II, Thieves, Di-Tone, and ImmuPower.

Supplements: Cleansing Trio, Thyromin, Exodus, ImmuGel, Master Formula, VitaGreen, Ultra Young, Power Meal, and Mineral Essence.

Circulation Problems

(See BLOOD AND CARDIOVASCULAR)

While good circulation is undoubtedly the foundation of good health, sluggish or inadequate circulation can result in tissue toxicity, starvation, and eventually, cellular death. The damage that poor or inadequate circulation can cause is best illustrated in the gangrene that often develops in the legs and arms of many advanced diabetic patients. Because the blood cannot efficiently circulate in these areas, parts of the tissues literally rot away.

Niacin (nicotinic acid) is a B vitamin that is extremely powerful for dilating blood vessels and increasing circulation. The amino acid L-arginine has similar properties.

Essential oils may be extremely useful for promoting circulation. For example, myrtle, lemon, and cypress have been used to strengthen and dilate capillaries and increase circulation. Helichrysum and clove are natural blood thinners, balancing the viscosity or thickness of the blood, and it amplifies the effects of cypress. Marjoram relaxes muscles and dilates blood vessels, while nutmeg acts as a circulatory stimulant.

Essential oils like clove and citrus rind oils can enhance circulation through their ability to reduce the thickness or viscosity of blood.

Single Oils: Helichrysum, marjoram, cypress, myrtle, lemon, orange, grapefruit, clove.

- Cypress with basil, rosemary, thyme, lavender, peppermint, helichrysum, ginger, lemon, geranium, clary sage, sandalwood, black pepper, Idaho tansy, birch, or orange.

Blends:

- Cypress with Aroma Life, Citrus Fresh, Harmony, Di-Tone, En-R-Gee, Harmony, and PanAway.

Rub Harmony over areas of poor circulation. Add Aroma Life and cypress to the Cel-Lite Magic and perform body massage starting at feet, working up towards heart.

Supplements: Super B, Cel-Lite Magic, HRT, Cardia Care, VitaGreen, Royal Essence, Rehemogen, and JuvaTone.

Regimen:

1. Put 25 drops HRT in 1 oz. distilled water and take 3 times a day.

2. Rub Aroma Life on the carotid arteries and pulse points, wherever an artery comes close to the skin.

3. Rub Harmony over areas of poor circulation.

4. Take cayenne pepper with a glass of water but avoid using at bedtime.

Cold Sores (Herpes Simplex Type 1)

Single Oils:

- Melissa
- Lavender with peppermint, melaleuca, Idaho tansy, melissa, ravensara, bergamot, lemon, helichrysum, oregano, thyme, or mountain savory.

Apply mesissa three times a day neat on location

Dilute with V-6 Mixing Oil or Massage Oil Base.

Blends: Melissa, Hope, and Purification.

- Lavender with Melrose.

As soon as a cold sore appears, apply neat 1 drop each of lavender and melaleuca or melrose.

To reduce discomfort or drying of the skin when applying essential oils to an open sore, dilute in V-6 Mixing Oil or Massage Oil Base.

Supplements: Super C, ImmuGel, Radex, Royal Essence, VitaGreen, ImmuneTune, Stevia, Cleansing Trio, and JuvaTone.

Apply Stevia directly on lip sores to help heal without scarring.

Colds and Flu

(See INFECTION)

The best treatment for a cold or flu is prevention. Because many essential oils have strong antimicrobial properties, they can be diffused to prevent the spread of airborne germs. Essential oils and blends such as Thieves, Purification, Raven, R.C, and Sacred Mountain are extremely effective for killing germs.

The First Step Is to Cleanse the Blood

Clean, healthy, and detoxified blood assists in the recovery from any disease. Rehemogen cleanses the blood, which carries nutrients and oxygen to the cells to help the healing process. Toxins block nutrient and oxygen flow into cells.

Single Oils:

- Lavender with lemon, lemongrass, Roman and German chamomile, marjoram, ginger, tarragon, peppermint, oregano, frankincense, thyme, fennel, or *Laurus nobilis*.
- Frankincense with cypress, oregano, thyme, lemon, rosewood, eucalyptus, myrrh, hyssop, or mountain savory.
- Melaleuca with thyme, Idaho tansy, myrrh, eucalyptus, ravensara, or rosemary.
- Rosemary with ravensara, eucalyptus, lemon, or juniper.
- Sage with mountain savory, fir, spruce, oregano, clary sage, helichrysum, thyme, cinnamon, cedarwood, or spearmint.

Blends:

- Lavender with Melrose, Di-Tone, Immu-Power or Thieves.
- Frankincense with Peace & Calming, R.C., Raven, Sacred Mountain, Inspiration, or Exodus II.
- Melaleuca with Raven, R.C., Thieves, or ImmuPower.
- Rosemary with R.C. or Raven.
- Sage with Melrose, Purification, R.C., Christmas Spirit, Di-Tone, or Sacred Mountain.

Massage oils on the Vita Flex points on the feet and hands. Apply 4 drops oregano and 4 drops thyme using Raindrop Technique. Other oils and blends may be substituted for oregano and thyme.

For congestion:

Single Oils: Cedarwood, R.C., frankincense, and lemon.

These oils can be mixed together or used separately. Inhale, diffuse, or put 1 drop in honey and take as a dietary supplement.

To reduce mucus and fight infection:

Single Oils: Peppermint, myrrh.

Inhale, diffuse, or put 1 drop in honey and take as a dietary supplement.

(See MUCUS)

For coughs:

Single Oils: Myrtle, cedarwood.

Inhale, diffuse, or put 1 drop in honey and take as a dietary supplement.

For laryngitis:

Put 1 drop Melrose and lemon in 1 tsp. honey, swirl in mouth for 1-2 minutes and swallow.

For relief of general cold symptoms:

Recipe 1:
- 2 drops rosemary
- 2 drops melaleuca
- 1 drop eucalyptus radiata
- 3 drops lemon.

Recipe 2:
- 1 drop lemon
- 2 drops eucalyptus radiata
- 3 drops rosemary
- 2 drops peppermint

Inhale as needed or use in a steam vaporizer. Oils can also be added to bath gel base or Epsom salts for use in a bath or shower. The RainSpa shower head enables essential oils and bath salts to be used in the shower.

Mix 1 tsp. V-6 Mixing Oil or Massage Oil Base, massage around sinuses, forehead, nose, cheek bones, chest, and upper back.

Rub 6 drops R.C. and 2 drops Raven on chest, neck, and throat. Works well with cypress, birch, lemon, peppermint, and eucalyptus.

Recipe 3:
- 10 drops rosemary verbenon
- 8 drops Raven
- 8 drops frankincense
- 2 drops oregano
- 2 drops peppermint

Gargle 2-4 times daily,

Recipe 4:
- 2 drops Raven
- 1 drop thyme
- 3 drops frankincense
- 3 drops lemon
- 3 drops rosemary verbenon

Mix in 3/4 tsp. honey. The first week gargle 4 times daily, 2nd week 2 times daily, 3rd week 3 times daily, and 4th week 1 time daily. Stop for 1 month and repeat if necessary.

(See INFECTION or MUCUS).

Supplements: ImmuGel, Radex, Super C, Royal Essence, VitaGreen, ImmuneTune, Royaldophilus, Rehemogen, Stevia, and Exodus.

How to Shake Off the Cold or Flu Faster

The following program is designed to support all systems of the body to accelerate recovery from a cold or flu:

- Take 2 tsp. ImmuGel to support the immune system (do not mix with citrus juices).

- Take 2 capsules Royaldophilus 3 times daily to help fortify the healthy bacteria in intestinal tract and bowels.

- Do a colon and liver cleanse.

- Take 3 droppers of Rehemogen, 3 times daily to cleanse the blood.

- Take 2 to 6 Exodus capsules, 3 times daily to stimulate the immune system. The companion oil blend Exodus II can be inhaled or applied topically.

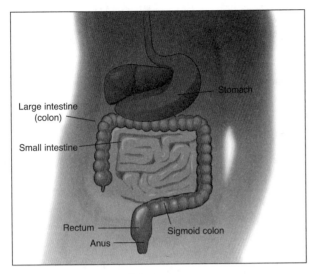

Colitis (ulcerative)

Also known as ileitis or proctitis, ulcerative colitis is marked by the inflammation of the top layers of the lining of the large intestine (colon) It is a different from both irritable bowel syndrome (which has no inflammation) and Crohn's disease (which occurs deeper in the colon wall).

The inflammation and ulcerous sores that are characteristic of ulcerative colitis occur most frequently in the lower colon and rectum and occasionally throughout the entire colon.

Symptoms include:
Fatigue
Nausea
Weight loss
Loss of appetite
Bloody diarrhea
Loss of body fluids and nutrients
Frequent fever
Abdominal cramps
Arthritis
Liver disease
Skin rashes

Single Oils: Peppermint, spearmint, tarragon, anise seed oil, and fennel.

Blends: Di-Tone, 20 drops in a capsule, 2 times daily.

Supplements: Royaldophilus, Kefir, AlkaLime, Mint Condition, and ImmuGel.

Take oils orally diluted in honey or vegetable oil or use topically.

Colitis, Viral

In cases where colitis is caused by a virus rather than a bacteria, the following treatments are recommended:

Single Oils:

- Oregano with thyme, Roman chamomile, clove, cinnamon, or peppermint.

- Thyme with melaleuca, lemon, basil, lemongrass, rosemary, lavender, eucalyptus, geranium, bergamot, patchouly, clove, or cinnamon.

- Helichrysum with myrrh, German chamomile, Roman chamomile, lavender, or tarragon.

Blends:

- Thyme with Di-Tone, Melrose, Purification, Thieves, or 3 Wise Men.

- Helichrysum with Di-Tone.

- Oregano with Purification or Di-Tone

Take 1-3 drops as a dietary supplement. Massage Di-Tone on abdomen as needed. Massage on Vita Flex points on feet, or apply oils using Raindrop Technique on the spine: Use helichrysum with tarragon or Di-Tone in a hot compress.

Recipe 1:
- 2 drops oregano
- 2 drops thyme
- 3 drops Purification
- 2 drops Roman chamomile
- 2 drops clove or cinnamon
- 2 drops Di-Tone

Mix with 1 oz. V-6 Mixing Oil or Massage Oil Base and use in a rectal implant.

Supplements: Mint Condition, ImmuGel, VitaGreen, Master HERS and Master HIS.

Colon and Liver Cleanse: Cleansing Trio, JuvaTone, and JuvaFlex. Take Mint Condition, along with ComforTone. Wait about 2 weeks or more before adding I.C.P. Start with a small amount of the I.C.P. and increase slowly. If any discomfort is experienced, reduce to a level of comfort and take it slower. Listen to your body.

Coma

Single Oils: Frankincense, sandalwood, cypress, pepper, and peppermint.

Blends: Trauma Life, Hope, and Surrender.

Supplements: Mineral Essence and Ultra Young.

Confusion

Single Oils: Peppermint, rosemary, basil, and cardamom.

Blends: Clarity, Brain Power, M-Grain, and Gathering.

Supplements: Mineral Essence, Super B, and Ultra Young.

Congestion (Sinus)

(See COLDS)

Single Oils: Sandalwood, coriander, cypress, eucalyptus radiata, fennel, and rosemary.

Blends: Di-Tone, R.C., Raven, and Exodus II.

Supplements: Cleansing Trio and Cel-Lite Magic Massage Oil.

Congestive Heart Failure

Coenzyme Q10 is one of the most effective supplements for supporting the heart muscle.

Single Oils: Helichrysum, cypress.

Blends: Aroma Life.

Supplements: HRT, CardiaCare, Super Cal, Mineral Essence.

Connective Tissue - Sprains, Tendonitis

Connective tissue is an essential part of every structure in the body.

Tendonitis, often called Tennis Elbow and Golfer's Elbow, is a torn or inflamed tendon. Tenosynovitis, sometimes called "Trigger Finger," is a tendon being restricted by its sheath (particularly thumbs and fingers) by being swollen and inflamed. Repetitive use or infection may be the cause.

ArthroTune and Super Cal help the repair process. Sulfurzyme, formulated with MSM (methylsulfonylmethane), equalizes water pressure inside the cells so that the cell protein envelope will allow water transfer in and out freely. When water pressure is higher inside the cells than outside, it creates pain.

PanAway and lemongrass make a potent combination. PanAway keeps the pain down and lemongrass promotes the repair of connective tissue.

Helichrysum and lemongrass also make a powerful combination for repairing torn ligaments. Lavender and lemongrass, and marjoram and lemongrass work well together for inflamed tendons. Ortho Sport and Ortho Ease Massage Oils also help with the healing.

Single Oils:

- Basil with lemongrass, lavender, marjoram, helichrysum, birch, or Idaho tansy.
- Lemongrass with helichrysum, cypress, lavender, or ginger.
- Helichrysum with lemongrass, cypress, or rose.
- Rosemary with eucalyptus or peppermint.

Bone: Birch, spruce, fir, PanAway, Relieve It on location, multiple times daily.

Muscle: Basil, marjoram, lavender, Relieve It, PanAway.

Ligament: Lemongrass, lavender (equal parts), PanAway, Relieve It, elemi, Idaho tansy.

Spasms: Aroma Siez with Ortho Ease or Ortho Sport Massage Oils.

Blends:

- Basil with PanAway.
- Lemongrass with Aroma Life, PanAway, R.C., or Citrus Fresh.
- Helichrysum with Relieve It or Release.

Supplements: Master Formula, ArthroTune, Super Cal, Super B, Super C, VitaGreen, Royal Essence, Mineral Essence, Sulfurzyme, Cel-Lite Magic, Ortho Ease, and Ortho Sport Massage Oils.

Rub 4 to 5 drops of oils over the area and then cover with massage oil.

Tendonitis

Recipe:
- 10 drops basil
- 8 drops birch
- 6 drops cypress
- 3 drops peppermint

Rub neat on location. Mix with V-6 Mixing Oil or Massage Oil Base to massage larger areas. For general pain, use Raindrop Technique.

Recipe (Pain Relief):
- 10 drops rosemary
- 10 drops eucalyptus
- 10 drops peppermint

Mix with 2 Tbsp. V-6 Mixing Oil or Massage Oil Base and use with ice packs.

Sprain - Torn Ligament Blend

Pain Relief:
- 1 drop lemongrass,
- 2 to 3 drops Aroma Siez.

Mix with V-6 Mixing Oil or Massage Oil Base and apply.

NOTE: For sprains, use cold packs. For any serious sprain or constant pain, always consult a health care professional.

When selecting oils, particularly for injuries, think through the cause and type of injury and select oils for each segment. For instance, tendonitis could encompass muscle damage, nerve damage, ligament strain or tear, inflammation, infection, fever on location, and possibly an emotion. Therefore, select an oil or oils for each perceived problem and apply in rotation or prepare a blend to cover all problems. The emotional distress may be anger or guilt, or the person may have had pain for a long time and needs to release.

Any time there is tissue damage, there is always inflammation, which needs to be reduced first.

Constipation

The principle causes of constipation are inadequate fluid intake and low fiber consumption. Constipation can eventually lead to diverticulosis and diverticulitis, conditions common among older people.

(see DIVERTICULOSIS and DIVERTICULITIS)

Why Constipation Can Produce Problems Later in Life

The reason constipation creates diverticulosis is due to the fact that the muscles of the colon must strain to move an overly-hard stool, which puts excess pressure on the colon. Eventually weak spots in the colon walls form, resulting in the creation of abnormal pouches called diverticula.

Single Oils: Ginger, peppermint, fennel, and anise seed oil.

Blends: Di-Tone.

Supplements: Cleansing Trio, AlkaLime, Royaldophilus, Goji Berry Tea, Body Balance, Royal Essence, and Power Meal.

- Megazyme: 3 to 6 capsules, 3 times daily.
- AlkaLime: 1 Tbsp. in water, 2 times daily before or after meals.
- ComforTone: Start with 1 capsule and increase next day to 1 more capsule. Continue to increase 1 capsule each day until bowels start moving.
- I.C.P.: One week after beginning Comfor-Tone, start with 1 Tbsp., 2 times daily and then increase to 3 times daily, up to 2 Tbsp., 3 times daily.
- Drink aloe vera juice, water, prune juice, and other raw fruit and vegetable juices.

Convulsions

(See BRAIN DISORDERS)

Monitor diet. Discontinue sugar and dairy products.

Blends: Brain Power and Valor.

Apply these oils at base of skull, across the neck, C1 to C6 receptors, and bottom of feet (for relief only).

Supplements: Master Formula CHILDREN'S and Ultra Young.

Corns

(See FOOT PROBLEMS)

Coughs

(See COLDS)

Cramps (Abdominal)

(See DIGESTIVE PROBLEMS)

Cramps (Muscle)

(See MUSCLES)

Crohn's Disease

Crohn's disease creates inflammation, sores, and ulcers on the intestinal wall. These sore occur deeper than ulcerative colitis. Moreover, unlike other forms of colitis, Crohn's disease can also occur in other areas of the body including large intestine, appendix, stomach, and mouth.

Symptoms include:
- Abdominal cramping
- Lower right abdominal pain
- Diarrhea
- A general sense of feeling ill

Attacks may occur once or twice a day for life. If the disease continues for years, it can cause deterioration of bowel function, leaking bowel, poor absorption of nutrients, loss of appetite and weight, intestinal obstruction, severe bleeding, and increased susceptibility to intestinal cancer.

Some researchers believe that Crohn's disease is caused by an overreacting immune system and is actually an autoimmune disease (where the immune system mistakenly attacks the body's own tissues). MSM has been extensively researched for its ability to treat many autoimmune disease, and is the subject of research by University of Oregon researcher Stanley Jacobs. (MSM is included in Sulfurzyme).

Single Oils: Peppermint.

Blends: Di-Tone.

Supplements: Sulfurzyme, Mint Condition, Royaldophilus, ImmuGel, AlkaLime, Body Balance, VitaGreen, Goji Berry Tea, Cleansing Trio, Power Meal, and Mineral Essence.

- Mint Condition: 2-4 capsules, 3 times daily.
- Royaldophilus: 2-4 capsules, 3 times daily. Empty capsules and add to water or yogurt if needed twice daily.
- ImmuGel: 1/2 tsp., 5 times daily.

Each phase lasts 1 week and should be added to the previous phases.

Phase I: Take Mint Condition in yogurt or kefir, liquid acidophilus, and charcoal tablets. Do not use ICP, ComforTone, or Megazyme.

Phase II: Add AlkaLime if no diarrhea. Body Balance for 2 to 3 weeks.

Raw juices (5 oz. celery and 2 oz carrot).

Phase III: VitaGreen, Goji Berry Tea.

Phase IV: (One week after blood spots stop).

- ComforTone (1 capsule morning and night) until stools loosen.
- I.C.P.: Start with 1 level tsp., 2 times daily and gradually increase.
- Megazyme: Start 1 tablet, 3 times daily.

If irritation occurs, rest from Cleansing Trio for a few days and start again. Switch from Body Balance to Power Meal.

- Mineral Essence: Start the second week: 1 dropper, 2 times daily.

Raindrop Technique on the spine with ImmuPower.

Chronic Fatigue Syndrome

(See HYPOGLYCEMIA)

Symptoms can include indigestion, upper and lower gas, poor assimilation, poor electrolyte balance, allergic reaction to food and other substances, mood swings, fatigue, irritability, and a lack of motivation, discipline, and creativity. Hypoglycemia is a precursor and even causes chronic fatigue syndrome. Overcome hypoglycemia, and the symptoms of chronic fatigue syndrome will probably disappear.

Cushing's Disease

(See ADRENAL GLAND IMBALANCE)

Cuts

(See WOUNDS)

Cyst (Ganglion)

2 drops Oregano, 2 drops thyme. Rotate every other day on location.

Cystitis

(See URINARY/BLADDER INFECTION)

Dandruff

Dandruff may be caused from allergies, parasites, and chemicals.

Single Oils: Melaleuca, cedarwood, lavender, rosemary, and sage.

Blends: Citrus Fresh, Melrose.

Supplements: Lavender Shampoo and Lemon Sage Shampoo.

Decongestants

(See MUCUS)

Dental

Prior to visiting the dentist, rub helichrysum with PanAway on gums and jaw.

Tooth Extraction (Pain and infection control)

Single Oils: Birch, helichrysum, melaleuca, eucalyptus, clove, thyme, and oregano. May be diluted if necessary.

Blends:

• Helichrysum with Thieves and R.C.

Before having teeth pulled, rub helichrysum with Thieves and R.C. around gums.

Rub R.C. on gums to bring back feeling from numbness of Novocaine.

Deodorant

Excessive body odor indicates putrefaction in the system and possibly poor digestion from the lack of enzymes in the digestive tract. A colon and liver cleanse may be needed.

The essential oils of lavender, lavendin, citronella, geranium, and melaleuca inhibit proliferation of odor-causing bacteria on the skin.

Single Oils: Lavender, geranium, bergamot, cypress, eucalyptus, and myrtle.

Blends: Aroma Siez, Acceptance, Dragon Time, EndoFlex, Harmony, Joy, Mister, R.C., Release, White Angelica, and Peace & Calming.

Skin Care: Dragon Time and Relaxation Massage Oils, AromaSilk Satin Body Lotion, Sandalwood Moisture Cream, Dragon Time Bath and Shower Gel, and Evening Peace.

You can also use oils under your arms or on the skin, neat or in the V-6 Mixing Oil or Massage Oil Base. You can also put a couple of drops on a face cloth when washing.

Deodorant Recipe 1:

• 4 ounces of unscented talcum powder

• 2 ounces of baking soda

• 3 drops lavender

Mix well. Use under arms, on the feet (or in shoes), or any other place on the body.

Dermatitis - Eczema

Eczema and dermatitis are both inflammations of the skin and are most often due to allergies, but also can be a sign of liver disease (See LIVER).

Dermatitis usually results from external factors, such as sunburn or contact with poison ivy, metals (wristwatch, earrings, jewelry, etc.). Eczema usually results from internal factors, such as irritant chemicals, soaps and shampoos, allergy to wheat (gluten), etc. In both dermatitis and eczema, skin becomes red, flaky and itchy, small blisters may form and if broken by scratching, can become infected.

Single Oils: Lavender and cistus.

- Lavender with Roman or German chamomile, helichrysum, geranium, rosewood, patchouly, sage, or thyme.

Blends: JuvaFlex.

- Lavender with Purification, Melrose, Sensation, or Gentle Baby.

Oils for treating dermatitis and eczema are probably best if applied when diluted in V-6 Mixing Oil or Massage Oil Base.

Supplements: Cleansing Trio, JuvaTone, Rehemogen, and Rose Ointment.

Most skin problems are a result of a toxic liver. It is therefore, extremely important to cleanse the liver and blood and make certain that the elimination system is working properly.

Diabetes - Blood Sugar Imbalance

The pancreas produces insulin, which enables the body to use glucose. If there is no insulin, or not enough insulin is produced, the body cannot regulate the sugar levels in the body. This disorder is called diabetes mellitus, which causes low energy and abnormally high blood glucose (sugar).

Single Oils:

- Coriander with cinnamon, fennel, dill, cypress, rosemary, pine or ylang ylang.

Blends:

- Cypress with Thieves or EndoFlex.

- Lavender with Thieves, JuvaFlex, or Di-Tone.

- Helichrysum with Thieves.

Supplements: VitaGreen, Stevia, Master HIS/HERS, Megazyme, Super B, Body Balance, Power Meal, Royal Essence, Mineral Essence, Sulfurzyme, Goji Berry Tea, and Wolfberry Power Bars.

- Body Balance and Power Meal.

- VitaGreen: 8 to 16 capsules daily.

- Sulfurzyme: 1 to 4 Tbsp. daily.

- Massage on pancreas Vita Flex points on bottom of feet: Thieves, coriander, fennel, and dill to lower glucose levels. Apply as compress over pancreas area.

- Cleansing Trio, JuvaTone, and JuvaFlex.

NOTE: Do not use fennel longer than 10 days at a time, since it excessively increases flow through the urinary tract.

VitaGreen is high in plant protein, which helps balance blood glucose. The MSM/sulfur found in the Sulfurzyme promotes insulin production.

Megazyme supports enzyme production, which helps keep the pancreas from premature wasting and enlargement, a condition linked to diabetes and premature aging.

Super B is a good source of B vitamins to support pancreas function.

The Stevia leaf extract is one of the most health-restoring plants known. It is a natural sweetener, has no calories, and does not have the harmful side effects of processed sugar or sugar substitutes. Stevia increases glucose tolerance and helps normalize blood sugar fluctuations.

Goji Berry Tea helps prevent diabetes. Wolfberry balances the pancreas and is a detoxifier and cleanser. Diabetes is not common in China, where wolfberry is consumed regularly.

Digestion Problems - Diarrhea, Constipation, Intestinal Infections

Any of the following indicate that the digestive system is not digesting properly:

- Belching, flatulence, and bloating.
- Rumbling or gurgling sounds in the abdomen.
- Heartburn (may be a possible indication of candida).
- Constipation and diarrhea.
- Constant hunger or fatigue after eating.
- Food intolerance or food allergies.
- Intestinal parasites.

Poor bowel function is linked to enzyme deficiency, low fiber, insufficient liquid, bad diet, and stress.

General Gastrointestinal Complaints:

Single Oils:

- Basil with tarragon, peppermint, fennel, juniper, ginger, geranium, cumin, or pepper.
- Lavender with patchouly, peppermint, Idaho tansy, tarragon, sandalwood, lemon, bergamot, eucalyptus, myrrh, oregano, thyme, spearmint, mandarin, melaleuca, nutmeg, orange, tangerine, *Laurus nobilis*, or rose.
- Lemongrass with tarragon, ginger, peppermint, patchouly, cinnamon, spearmint, grapefruit, mandarin, or spikenard.
- Rosemary with clary sage, sage, marjoram, lavender, Roman chamomile, German chamomile, caraway seed, or neroli.

Blends:

- Basil with Di-Tone.
- Lavender with Di-Tone or JuvaFlex.
- Lemongrass with Di-Tone or JuvaFlex.
- Sage with Di-Tone.

Supplements: Megazyme, Royaldophilus, Royal Essence, Mineral Essence, Master Formula vitamins, Mint Condition, Body Balance, Vita-Green, AlkaLime, Stevia, and Sulfurzyme.

Bloating, Gas, Flatulence:

Single Oils: Peppermint, tarragon, nutmeg, anise seed, fennel, carrot seed oil.

Blends: Di-Tone.

Take 1-2 drops as dietary supplement or place up to 15 drops Di-Tone or 4-6 drops peppermint in the palm and rub over stomach and around navel. In severe cases apply hot compress over stomach. Massage 3 drops on stomach Vita Flex points on bottom of each foot.

Supplements: Megazyme, Mint Condition, AlkaLime, and Royaldophilus.

Cramps (stomach)

Single Oils: Rosemary cineol, ginger

Detoxification of Intestines

Single Oils:

- Helichrysum with tangerine, ginger, peppermint, or tarragon.

Blends:

- Di-Tone with EndoFlex, JuvaFlex, or helichrysum.

Supplements: I.C.P., ComforTone, Megazyme, Mint Condition.

Diarrhea

Single Oils: Peppermint, cinnamon, clove, nutmeg, orange.

Blends: Thieves, Di-Tone.

Take 2-4 drops Thieves in capsule.

If you can't tolerate cinnamon or clove, substitute.

For oral and topical use always dilute. One drop essential oil per tsp. vegetable oil.

Recipe 1 (diarrhea):
- 4 drops lemon
- 3 drops mountain savory
- 2 drops oregano.

Dilute in vegetable oil, put 2 drops in capsule. Rub Di-Tone or peppermint over the stomach around the navel.

Supplements: I.C.P., ComforTone, Megazyme, Mint Condition

Flatulence

(See BLOATING, GAS, FLATULENCE)

Gas

(See BLOATING, GAS, FLATULENCE)

Heartburn

Lemon juice is one of the best remedies for heartburn. Place several drops in water and sip slowly.

Recipe 1:
- 2 drops basil
- 2 drops Idaho tansy
- 8 drops sage
- 3 drops sandalwood

Blend in 1/2 to 1 oz. V-6 Mixing Oil or Massage Oil Base. Rub over your navel and on the colon Vita Flex area on bottom of feet.

Hiccups

Single Oils: Tarragon.

Indigestion

(See UPSET STOMACH)

Poor Digestion

Single Oils: Peppermint, tarragon, sage, marjoram, nutmeg, and tangerine.

Blends: Di-Tone.

Take 1-2 drops as dietary supplement or place up to 15 drops Di-Tone or 4-6 drops peppermint in the palm and rub over stomach and around navel. In severe cases apply hot compress over

stomach. Massage 3 drops on stomach Vita Flex points on bottom of each foot.

Supplements: Megazyme, Mint Condition, Stevia.

Upset Stomach (Indigestion)

Singles: Peppermint, nutmeg, orange, grapefruit seed oil (vegetable oil).

Blends: Di-Tone.

Supplements: Stevia, I.C.P., ComforTone, Megazyme, Mint Condition.

Mint Condition taken before eating helps with digestion and upset stomach. When heaviness is felt in the stomach, Mint Condition is a beneficial synergistic companion to Di-Tone.

- Lemongrass helps eliminate lactic acid (from fermentation of lactose in milk).

Traveler's Diarrhea

Single Oils: Peppermint, ginger, lemon, mountain savory, and oregano.

Blends: Di-Tone.

Supplements: Royaldophilus, ComforTone, I.C.P., Megazyme, and JuvaTone.

A maintenance dosage of ComforTone has protected travelers going to other countries from diarrhea, and other digestive discomforts.

Travel Sickness

Single Oils:

- Peppermint with ginger.

Mix 4 drops peppermint and 4 drops ginger in 1 ounce V-6 Mixing Oil or Massage Oil Base. Rub on chest and stomach before traveling.

Disinfectant

(See ANTISEPTIC)

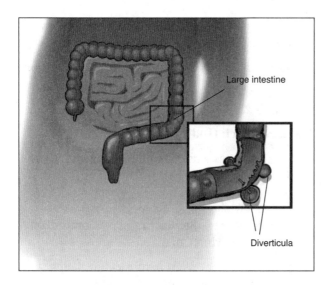

Large intestine

Diverticula

Diverticulitis

While diverticulosis involves the condition of merely having colon abnormalities, diverticulitis occurs when these abnormalities or diverticula become infected or inflamed. Diverticulitis is present in 10 to 25 percent of people with diverticulosis.

Symptoms:
- Tenderness on lower left of abdomen
- Fever and chills
- Constipation
- Cramping

Many of these symptoms are similar to those of irritable bowel syndrome.

(See IRRITABLE BOWEL SYNDROME)

Single Oils: Patchouly, anise seed oil, tarragon, rosemary, fennel, peppermint, mountain savory, oregano, thyme linalol.

Blends: Di-Tone.

Supplements: I.C.P., Essential Manna, Cleansing Trio, Mineral Essence, ImmuneTune, Exodus.

Diverticulosis

Diverticulosis is one of the most common conditions in the U.S. Caused by a lack of fiber in the diet, diverticulosis is characterized by small, abnormal pouches (diverticula) that bulge out through weak spots in the wall of the intestine. It is estimated that half of all Americans from age 60 to 80 have diverticulosis.

Symptoms:
- Cramping
- Bloating
- Constipation

Upping fiber intake to 20-30 grams daily is one of the easiest ways to resolve this condition. Because peppermint oil stimulates contractions in the colon, it also can be of value.

Single Oils: Peppermint.

Best taken in an enteric-coated capsule. Start with 2-4 drops.

Blends:

- Frankincense with Di-Tone or Melrose.

Supplements: I.C.P., Essential Manna, ComforTone, Mint Condition, ImmuGel, and Royaldophilus.

Recipe 1:
- 15 drops Di-Tone
- 5 drops Melrose

Mix in 1 Tbsp. of V-6 Mixing Oil or Massage Oil Base.

Recipe 2:
- 10 drops Di-Tone
- 15 drops frankincense

Mix in 1 Tbsp. of V-6 Mixing Oil or Massage Oil Base.

Rub on feet, use as a hot compress on stomach, as a rectal implant, or as a dietary supplement (mix 1 drop peppermint in 1 tsp. of honey).

Dizziness

Single Oils: Cypress, tangerine, peppermint, basil, and cardamom.

Blends: Aroma Life, Clarity, Brain Power, and Thieves.

Apply Thieves to pancreas point on bottom of foot.

Supplements: Cel-Lite Magic Massage Oil, VitaGreen, and Essential Manna.

Blood circulation can be a factor (see CIRCULATION).

Dysentery

Single Oils: Lemon, mountain savory, oregano, and peppermint.

Blends: Thieves and Di-Tone.

Mix Thieves with 5 drops of peppermint and take orally.

Supplements: Mint Condition, Royaldophilus, Megazyme, I.C.P., and Mineral Essence.

Dyspepsia

(See DIGESTIVE PROBLEMS)

Ear Infection (Otitis Media)

Single Oils:

- Lavender with melaleuca, rosemary, helichrysum, Roman chamomile, hyssop, peppermint, or eucalyptus radiata.

- Helichrysum with ravensara.

Blends: Lavender with Melrose, Purification, PanAway, Thieves (diluted), or ImmuPower.

Mix 1-2 drops of essential oil in 1 tsp. of warm olive oil. Apply in the opening of the ear with cotton swab and externally around the ear and the corresponding Vita Flex points on the feet.

Additional therapy: Put 2-3 drops of the diluted essential oil on a cotton ball and insert carefully into the opening of the ear as a plug. Then lay a hot pack over the ear.

NOTE: Do not drop oil directly on the eardrum. First place oil on a cotton swab or put on finger and then place into ear.

Ear pain can be very serious. Always seek medical attention if pain persists.

Supplements: Super C, ImmuGel, Radex, Royal Essence, VitaGreen, ImmuneTune, Rehemogen, Cleansing Trio, and JuvaTone.

Perforated Eardrum

Single Oils: Lavender, Melrose

Use cotton swab soaked in lavender on canal opening. Repeat, alternating lavender with Melrose

Ear Mites

Blends: Purification.

Put one drop Purification oil on a piece of cotton and put in ear.

Ebola Virus

(See INFECTION)

Single Oils:

- Rosemary with Geranium and Lemon.

Recipe 1:
- 10 drops rosemary
- 10 drops geranium
- 10 drops lemon
- 1/2 raw lemon
- 1 tablespoon honey

Mix in 8 oz. warm water. Drink every 2 hours. Every hour take 2 JuvaTone. Do a rectal implant of 2 tablespoons of Protec. Drink a mixture of 1/2 cup sauerkraut juice, 1/2 cup tomato juice, and 2 Tbsp. olive oil.

Eczema

(See SKIN DISORDERS)

Edema

(See KIDNEY DISORDERS)

Emotional Trauma

Single Oils:

- Frankincense with lavender, orange, tangerine, lemon, German chamomile, patchouly, sandalwood, myrrh, juniper, or geranium.

Blends:

- Frankincense with Present Time, Valor, Peace & Calming, Citrus Fresh, Christmas Spirit, White Angelica, 3 Wise Men, Sacred Mountain, or Trauma Life.

Supplements: Royaldophilus.

Apply oils by anointing the crown of the head and the forehead and also by diffusing (see EMOTIONAL CLEARING). It is best if done in a quiet and dark room or at least in a low-lit room.

Place 1-3 drops of Present Time over the thymus and rub clockwise 3 times, up to 3 times daily as needed. This is important to help people move out of the past and out of their negative thinking.

The synergistic combination of frankincense with Valor applied at night for a couple of days helps one to wake up in the morning ready to face the world and get on with life.

The effect of heavy emotional trauma can disrupt the stomach and digestive system. You may need 2 capsules of Royaldophilus, 2 or 3 times daily during the period of trauma and for 10 to 15 days thereafter (see DIGESTION).

Emphysema

A condition of the lung marked by abnormal dilation of its air spaces, frequently with impaired heart action.

Endocrine Balancing

Essential oils both increase and enable the transport of oxygen to the brain. This enables the pituitary and other glands to secrete neural transmitters and endorphins that support the endocrine and immune systems.

The thyroid is one of the most important glands for regulating the body systems. The hypothalamus plays an even more important role, since it not only regulates the thyroid, but the adrenals and the pituitary gland as well.

To balance the endocrine system:

Place EndoFlex on the tongue, roof of the mouth, thyroid, kidneys, liver, all of the glands, and the Vita Flex points for these glands on the feet and hands.

Use helichrysum on the Vita Flex points on the bottom of the feet and hands to stimulate the pineal and pituitary glands, which are considered the most important of the endocrine system.

Endocrine System

The endocrine system encompasses the hormone-producing glands of the body. These glands cluster around blood vessels and release their hormones directly into the bloodstream. The pituitary gland exerts wide range of control over the hormonal (endocrine) system and is often called the master gland. Other glands include the pancreas, adrenals, thyroid and parathyroid, ovaries, and testes. The limbic system lies along the margin of the cerebral cortex (brain) and is the hormone-producing system of the brain. It includes the amygdala, hippocampus, pineal, pituitary, thalamus, and hypothalamus.

Single Oils:

- Helichrysum with nutmeg, clove, rosemary, bergamot, spearmint, blue tansy, melissa, spruce, or pepper.

Blends:

- Helichrysum with EndoFlex, En-R-Gee, or Humility.

Supplements: Thyromin.

Energy, Lack of

(See THYROID IMBALANCES or ADRENAL GLAND IMBALANCES)

A lack of energy can be due to a host of factors, including low thyroid hormone activity or adrenal hormone imbalance. Other factors may also play a part, including diabetes, cancer, and other conditions.

Single Oils:

- Lemongrass or juniper with basil, lemon, peppermint, rosemary, nutmeg, pepper, geranium, rosemary, Roman chamomile, melissa, ylang ylang, cypress, patchouly, or thyme.

Blends:

- Lemongrass or juniper with En-R-Gee, Clarity, Hope, or Citrus Fresh.

- Ylang Ylang with Joy, Motivation, or Awaken.

Supplements: Royal Essence, VitaGreen, Master Formula vitamins, Thyromin, Super B.

Place Royal Essence under the tongue for quick energy boost by increasing blood oxygen.

Epilepsy

Single Oils: Clary Sage

Blends: Brain Power.

Apply on brainstem (back of the neck at base of skull) and on brain Vita Flex points on the bottom of the feet.

Supplements: Cleansing Trio

Note: If epileptic, you may choose to avoid basil, birch, fennel, hyssop, Idaho tansy, and sage.

Epstein-Barr Syndrome or Virus

(See HYPOGLYCEMIA)

Symptoms include indigestion, upper and lower gas, poor assimilation, poor electrolyte balance, allergic reaction to foods and other substances, emotional mood swings, fatigue, irritability, and a lack of motivation, discipline and creativity.

Hypoglycemia is a precursor and can render the body susceptible to the Epstein-Barr virus. Treat the hypoglycemia, and the symptoms of the Epstein-Barr virus will probably disappear.

Blends: ImmuPower.

Supplements: Radex, ImmuGel, Super C, ImmuneTune, Cleansing Trio, and JuvaTone.

Use Raindrop Technique on the spine with a mixture of ImmuneTune.

Exhaustion (Physical) - Fatigue

Single Oils:

- Lemongrass with lavender, peppermint, mountain savory, sage, thyme, rosemary, or clove.

Mountain savory is a tonic and stimulant for the body.

Blends:

- Lemongrass with En-R-Gee

En-R-Gee helps with alertness.

Supplements: VitaGreen, Power Meal, Master Formula, Mineral Essence, Royal Essence, Super B, Thyromin.

VitaGreen is a plant-derived high-protein energy formula that athletes use to boost endurance. Royal Essence increases energy and endurance.

Digestion and colon problems may cause fatigue. A colon and liver cleanse unburdens the gut and increases energy

Expectorant

(See MUCUS)

Eye Disorders

Supplements: Mineral Essence, Royal Essence, A.D.&E., Chelex, and VitaGreen.

Selenium supports the eyes. Mineral Essence and Royal Essence are good sources of all minerals, including selenium. A.D.&E. is beneficial for all eye problems.

Dr. Terry Friedmann no longer needs his glasses after using sandalwood and juniper around the opening of his eyes in a wide circle (above the eyebrow and around cheeks). He also used the supplements of Chelex, VitaGreen, the Cleansing Trio, and JuvaTone for a complete colon and liver cleanse.

Note: Never place oils in eyes or on eyelids.

Blocked Tear Ducts

Single Oils: Lavender.

1 drop lavender oil rubbed over the bridge of the nose has been reported to work in seconds.

Cataracts and Glaucoma

Single Oils:

- Lemongrass or lemon with cypress and eucalyptus.

Recipe 1:
- 10 drops lemongrass
- 5 drops cypress
- 3 drops eucalyptus radiata

Mix in 1 oz. V-6 Mixing Oil or Massage Oil Base and apply in a wide circle around the eye. Never apply directly to eyelid or eye. Also apply on temples and Vita Flex points on the hands and feet (the undersides of your two largest toes, index and middle fingers). This will also help with puffiness.

Recipe 2:
- 10 drops lemon
- 5 drops cypress
- 3 drops eucalyptus

Mix in 1 oz. V-6 Mixing Oil or Massage Oil Base. Apply daily as above.

Recipe 3 (Eyewash formula):
- 2 parts pure honey
- 1 part pure apple cider vinegar
- 5 parts distilled water

Use as an eye wash, 3 or 4 times a day, while using the above oils. Apply as needed for maintenance.

NOTE: *Do not get into eyes. If this happens, dilute with V-6, milk, butter, or any other oil based substance. NEVER rinse with water.*

Drooping Eyelids

Single Oils: Lavender and helichrysum.

Blends:

- Lavender or helichrysum with Aroma Life.

Recipe 1:
- 5 drops lavender
- 1 drop helichrysum
- 2 drops Aroma Life

Mix in 1/2 oz. V-6 Mixing Oil or Massage Oil Base.

Supplements: VitaGreen.

Inflamed Eyes

Single Oils: Idaho tansy, lavender, and lemon (dilute in V-6 Mixing Oil or Massage Oil Base).

Apply in a wide circle around eyes and massage.

Note: Never apply directly to eyelid or eye

Recipe:
- 10 drops lemongrass
- 5 drops cypress
- 3 drops eucalyptus radiata
- 1/2-oz. V-6 Mixing Oil or Massage Oil Base

Massage neat into fingertips and end of toes.

Supplements: A.D.&E., Ultra Young, and Sulfurzyme.

Bleeding

Single Oils: Idaho tansy, helichrysum, lavender, and peppermint.

Blends: Aroma Life or PanAway.

Supplements: Master Formula vitamins, VitaGreen, and Sulfurzyme.

Blurred Vision

Single Oils: Idaho Tansy, helichrysum, lavender, and peppermint.

Blends: Aroma Life or PanAway.

Supplements: Master Formula Vitamins, VitaGreen, Sulfurzyme, Super B, Super Cal, and Power Meal.

Fainting

(See SHOCK)

Single Oils: Peppermint, spearmint.

Blends: Clarity, Brain Power, and Trauma Life.

Fatigue (Mental)

Single Oils: Pepper, peppermint, and nutmeg.

Blends: En-R-Gee and Motivation.

Supplements: Thyromin, Power Meal, Vita-Green, Master Formula, Mineral Essence, and Royal Essence.

Fertility

Single Oils:

• Clary sage with sage, fennel, yarrow, geranium, or bergamot.

Blends: Dragon Time, Mister, and Sensation.

Application: Rub on the reproductive Vita Flex areas on the hands and feet. These areas are inside of wrists, around the front of the ankles in line with the anklebone, particularly inside and outside of the foot on either side of the anklebone, and along the Achilles tendon.

In addition, women may rub on the lower back and area of lower bowels near the pubic bone or use as a vaginal retention implant.

Women: FemiGen 3-6 capsules daily to nourish reproductive system.

Use VitaGreen 3-8 capsules, 2-3 times a day and Essential Manna.

Men: Progen 2-4 capsules daily to nourish reproductive system.

Use VitaGreen and Essential Manna.

In addition for men, rub on the lower bowel near the pubic bone and in the area between the scrotum and rectum or use as a rectal implant.

Fever

Fevers are one of the most powerful healing responses orchestrated by the human body, and are especially valuable in fighting infectious diseases. However, if fever raises body temperature excessively (over 104°F) then neurological damage can occur.

Some essential oils are very cooling when applied to the skin and can help reduce fevers. Because of its menthol content, peppermint is one the most-used oils in fever control.

Single Oils:

• Lavender with peppermint, eucalyptus radiata, sandalwood, and rosemary CT cineol.

Blends:

• Lavender with Melrose.

Supplements: AlkaLime, Super C, ImmuGel, Radex, Royal Essence, and Cinnamint Lip Balm.

Sip 1-2 drops of lemon or peppermint diluted in soy milk.

Drink 1-2 drops of lemon or peppermint in an 8 oz. glass of water and sip slowly.

Fibroids

Fibroids are fairly common benign tumors of the female pelvis that are composed of smooth muscle cells and fibrous connective tissue. Fibroids are not cancerous and neither develop into cancer nor increase a women's cancer risk in the uterus.

Fibroids can have a diameter as small as 1 mm or as large as 8 inches. They can develop in clusters or alone as a single knot or nodule.

Fibroids frequently occur in premenopausal women and are seldom seen in young women who have not begun menstruation. Fibroids usually stabilize or even regress in women who have passed menopause.

Single Oils: Frankincense, inula, cistus, lavender, Idaho tansy, oregano, pine, and helichrysum.

Blends: Valor, EndoFlex, Cel-Lite Magic, and Protec.

Supplements: Ultra Young, Thyromin, Vita-Green, AlkaLime, Power Meal, and Megazyme.

Fibromyalgia

Fibromyalgia is a autoimmmune disorder of soft tissues. (In contrast arthritis occurs in the joints.) Symptoms include general body pain, in some parts worse than others, brought on by only short periods of exercise. The pain is ubiquitous and continuous. It interrupts sleep patterns so that the fourth stage of sleep is never attained, and thus the body cannot rejuvenate and heal. Fibromyalgia is an acid condition in which the liver is toxic (see LIVER DISORDERS).

Fibromyalgia may be linked to a deficiency of minerals and trace minerals, including organic sulfur, which naturally occurs in MSM. According to UCLA researcher, Ronald Lawrence, M.D. Ph.D., supplementation with MSM offers a breakthrough in the treatment of fibromyalgia.

Blends: PanAway, Relieve It, ImmuPower, Ortho Ease, and Ortho Sport.

- Birch or spruce with PanAway, Relieve It, or ImmuPower.

Mix 20 drops PanAway in 1 oz V-6 Mixing Oil or Massage Oil Base. Massage wherever there is pain. Follow with Ortho Ease or Ortho Sport Massage Oils. Add 3-4 drops of birch or spruce to make it stronger if needed. Massage small areas with PanAway, neat (undiluted).

Recipe 1:
- 10 drops PanAway
- 8 drops birch
- 8 drops marjoram
- 6 drops spruce

Dilute in 1/2 oz. of V-6 Massage Oil or Massage Oil Base and massage the entire body.

Supplements: Sulfurzyme, Ultra Young, Essential Manna, Power Meal, Super B, Super C, VitaGreen, Megazyme, ImmuneTune, Super Cal, Royal Essence, Mineral Essence, Royaldophilus, Stevia Select.

Regimen:

1. Start cleansing using Cleansing Trio

2. Use 2 Tbsp. a day Sulfurzyme

3. Eat less acidic-ash foods and more alkaline-ash foods such as wheat sprouts or barley sprouts. The following are a list of alkalinizing supplements:

   - VitaGreen: up to 4 times daily.

   - Super C: 4-6 tablets daily.

   - ImmuneTune: 2-6 times daily.

   - Mineral Essence: 2-3 droppers 2 times daily in water or cold apple juice will supply the trace minerals needed without increasing the acid condition.

- Super Cal: 2-4 daily or as needed.

- ImmuPower: Apply 4-6 drops along the spine and back with using Raindrop Technique (See RAINDROP TECHNIQUE).

Flatulence (See Digestive Problems)

Flu

Single Oils: Idaho tansy, lemon, mountain savory, oregano, eucalyptus radiata and peppermint.

Blends: Di-Tone, Thieves, ParaFree, Megazyme, and Mint Condition.

Tansy should be applied topically on stomach and bottom of feet.

Food Poisoning

Single Oils: Tarragon, patchouly, and rosemary cineol.

Blends: Di-Tone, Exodus II, and Thieves.

Supplements: Megazyme and Exodus.

Foot Problems

Athlete's Foot

Athlete's foot is a fungal infection of the skin similar to ringworm (See FUNGAL INFECTIONS). It thrives in the warm moist environment to which many feet are subjected.

The best remedy is to keep feet cool and dry and avoid wearing tight-fitting shoes or heavy socks. Instead wear sandals, and socks woven from a light, breathable fabric.

It is especially important to control this fungus infection during showering or bathing, since the moist, warm environment favors the growth of the *Tinea* culture responsible for athlete's foot. Antifungal essential oils such as melaleuca and Melrose can be added to bath salts or Epsom salts and used in a the RainSpa shower head to create a mild, antifungal shower.

Single Oils: Melaleuca, lavender.

- Melaleuca with peppermint

- Melaleuca with lemon, lemongrass, thyme, basil, rosemary, lavender, eucalyptus, geranium, or bergamot.

- Lavender with melaleuca, frankincense, rosemary, thyme, geranium, bergamot, patchouly, tarragon, myrrh, Melrose, Purification, Mister, Di-Tone, or Thieves

- Melaleuca with Thieves.

Blends: Melrose.

Recipe 1:
- 4 drops melaleuca
- 1 drop lavender.

Recipe 2:
- 11 drops geranium
- 6 drops myrrh
- 13 drops melaleuca
- 6 drops patchouly

Use undiluted or mix in 1 tsp. V-6 Mixing Oil or Massage Oil Base. Apply to infected areas between toes and around toenails. Oils can also be added to bath salts and used in the shower with the RainSpa shower head.

Supplements: ImmuGel, Exodus, and Rose Ointment.

Blisters on Feet

Mix 1 drop lavender with 1 drop Roman chamomile. Mix 1 drop lavender with 1 drop melaleuca. Gently pat on thoroughly, but carefully.

Bunions

Bunions are caused from bursitis at the base of a toe. (See BURSITIS)

Recipe 1:
- 6 drops eucalyptus
- 3 drops lemon
- 4 drops raven
- 1 drop birch

Apply over area. Dilute if needed with 1 oz. V-6 Mixing Oil or Massage Oil Base if concerned about skin sensitivity.

Corns

Single Oils: Lemon, tangerine, grapefruit, and myrrh.

Blends: Citrus Fresh.

Apply 1 drop of oil directly on the corn.

Sore Feet

Single Oils: Peppermint, lavender, patchouly, myrrh, frankincense, sandalwood, and vetiver.

Blends: Melrose, PanAway, and Relieve It.

Supplements: A.D.&E., Essential Manna (high in potassium, which is extremely important), Super Cal, Master Formula, and Mineral Essence.

Mix peppermint in footbath; keep water agitated while soaking feet.

Frigidity

(See SEXUAL PROBLEMS)

Fungal Infections (Candida)

Fungi and yeast feed on decomposing or dead tissues. They exist everywhere: inside our stomachs, on our skin, and out on the lawn. When kept under control, the yeast and fungi populating our bodies are harmless and digest what our bodies cannot or do not use.

When we feed the naturally-occurring fungi in our bodies too many acid-ash foods, such as sugar, animal proteins, and dairy products, the fungi population grows out of control. This condition is known as systemic candidiasis and is marked by fungi invading the blood, gastrointestinal tract, and tissues.

Fungal cultures like candida excrete large amounts of poisons called mycotoxins as part of their life cycles. These poisons must be detoxified by the liver and immune system.

Eventually they can wreak enormous damage on the tissues and organs and are believed to be an aggravating factor in many degenerative diseases, such as cancer, arteriosclerosis, and diabetes.

Insufficient intake minerals and trace minerals like magnesium, potassium, and zinc may also stimulate candida and fungal overgrowth in the body.

Symptoms of Systemic Fungal Infection:

- Fatigue/low energy
- Overweight
- Low resistance to illness
- Allergies
- Unbalanced blood sugar
- Headaches
- Irritability
- Mood swings
- Indigestion
- Colitis and ulcers
- Diarrhea/constipation
- Urinary tract infections
- Rectal or vaginal itch

Two Powerful Fungus Fighters

Two of the most powerful weapons for fighting fundus infections such as candida are FOS (fructoligosaccharides) and *L. acidophilus* cultures.

FOS has been clinically documented in dozens of peer-reviewed studies for its ability to build up the healthy intestinal flora in the colon and combat the overgrowth of negative bacteria and fungi (See APPENDIX G).

Acidophilus cultures have also been shown to combat fungus overgrowth in the gastrointestinal tract. Royaldophilus is an excellent source of *L. acidophilus* cultures, and Stevia Select is a superior source of plant-derived FOS.

Seven Tips For Combating Systemic Fungal Infections

1. Use both probiotics and prebiotics. Probiotics like Royaldophilus are supplements containing live cultures of beneficial bacteria such as acidophilus and bifidus. Prebiotics include supplements like Stevia Select that help feed them, but do not include any live bacteria.

2. Avoid yeast-promoting (acidic) foods such as meats, sugars, dairy products, mushrooms, and pickled and malted products.

3. Eat an alkaline diet. The optimum ratio should be 4 parts alkaline-ash food to 1 part acid-ash food. Garlic is excellent for controlling fungi and yeast. Other high-alkaline, fungus-inhibiting foods include green and yellow vegetables, beans, and whole, uncracked nuts. VitaGreen is a high-energy, mineral rich alkaline supplement, and AlkaLime is an extremely alkaline complex of mineral salts.

4. Avoid excessive use of antibiotics. Antibiotics wipe out the beneficial bacteria in our bodies while leaving the mycotoxin-generating yeast and fungi intact (see ANTIBIOTICS).

5. Avoid stress. Emotional turmoil stresses the immune system and opens the door for fungal overgrowth. This is why Type A personalities are especially vulnerable to candida. Reduce stress by diffusing or inhaling essential oils such as lavender, lemon, or Peace & Calming.

6. Healthy thyroid function can counteract Candida overgrowth (see THYROID).

7. Use digestive enzyme supplements, such as Megazyme, to maximize protein assimilation. Inadequate digestion of protein can worsen candida overgrowth and amplify symptoms. (see DIGESTION PROBLEMS).

Single Oils: Melaleuca, lavender, lemongrass, rosemary verbenon, geranium, rosewood.

- Lavender with melaleuca, frankincense, Roman chamomile, rosemary verbenon, thyme, geranium, bergamot, cumin, patchouly, mountain savory, ravensara, tarragon, rosewood, peppermint, spearmint, lemongrass, or *Laurus nobilis*.

- Melaleuca with rosemary verbenon, tarragon, lavender, spruce, thyme, eucalyptus (all varieties), clove, lemon, lemongrass, basil, geranium, bergamot, cinnamon, or spikenard.

- Thyme with rosemary cineol, tarragon, lavender, myrrh, spruce, eucalyptus, clove, or cinnamon.

- Rosemary with clary sage, sage, mountain savory, fennel, bergamot, sandalwood, rosewood, geranium, myrrh, peppermint, spearmint, or cistus.

Dilute 1-2 drops in 1 tsp. V-6 Mixing Oil or Massage Oil Base. Take daily as a dietary supplement or apply topically on location. These oils can also be added to bath or Epsom salts and used during showering with the RainSpa shower head.

Blends: Melrose, R.C., Raven, ImmuPower.

- Lavender with Melrose, Purification, Mister, ImmuPower, Inspiration, Di-Tone, Thieves, Abundance, Acceptance, or Exodus II.

- Melaleuca with Melrose, Purification, Thieves, R.C., Di-Tone, or Raven.

- Rosemary with Melrose, Purification, R.C., Di-Tone, Raven, Christmas Spirit, or Clarity.

- Thyme with Melrose, Purification, Thieves, Sensation, or 3 Wise Men.

Use as above. Take 3 drops ImmuPower in 4 oz. of water, 3 times daily after meals. Massage 5-10 drops Di-Tone over stomach and 3 drops on the feet.

Dilute 1-2 drops Thieves in 1 Tbsp. V-6 Mixing Oil or Massage Oil Base and massage on the thymus to stimulate the immune system.

ImmuPower: Apply 1-3 drops diluted in massage oil to the bottom of the feet, on the throat, and chest.

Supplements: Master Formula, FemiGen, Royaldophilus, Stevia Select, Megazyme, ImmuGel, ImmuneTune, VitaGreen, Thyromin, Super C, Radex, Mineral Essence, AlkaLime, Exodus.

Combating Ringworm

Using antifungal essential oils while bathing or showering is especially important because fungal infections thrive in moist, warm environments. Essential oils like melaleuca or Melrose can easily be added to bath salts or Epsom salts to combat fungal infections.

The RainSpa aromatherapy shower head has a specially-designed chamber that can be filled with bath salts and essential oils. As the water passes over the mixture, it disperses the essential oils and salts into the shower spray, creating an antiseptic spa.

Ringworm and Skin Candida

The ringworm fungus infects the skin causing scaly round itchy patches. It is infectious and can be spread from an animal or human host alike. Skin candida is a fungal infection that can erupt almost anywhere on the skin. It shows up in various places, such as behind the knees, inside the elbows, behind the ears, on temple area, and between the breasts.

Single Oils: Melaleuca, lavender, rosemary verbenon, geranium, rosewood, myrrh.

Blends: Melrose, R.C., Raven, Ortho Ease.

Recipe 1:
- 3 drops melaleuca
- 3 drops spearmint
- 1 drop peppermint

Recipe 2:
- 2 drops tansy
- 10 drops melaleuca
- 1 drop oregano
- 2 drops patchouly

Apply undiluted on location or mix 2-3 drops in 1 tsp. V-6 Mixing Oil or Massage Oil Base. and layer on Rose Ointment. Apply to spinal Vita Flex points on the feet and hands.

In severe cases, use 35 percent food-grade hydrogen peroxide to clean infected areas before applying Melrose and Rose Ointment. Saturate gauze with oils and wrap infected area.

Thrush (*Candida albicans*)

Thrush is a fungal infection of the mouth and throat marked by creamy, curd-like patches in the oral cavity. Even though it appears in the mouth, thrush is usually a sign of systemic fungal overgrowth throughout the body. Thrush can usually be treated locally through the use of antifungal essential oils like clove, cinnamon, rosemary cineol, peppermint, and rosewood.

Single Oils: Cinnamon, clove, peppermint, rosemary cineol, geranium, rosewood, orange, and lavender.

Blends and Personal Care: Thieves, Melrose, Purification, ImmuPower, Fresh Essence Mouthwash.

Add 1-3 drops to 2 oz. of Fresh Essence mouthwash and gargle for two minutes. Add 4-6 drops to a bottle of Fresh Essence and rinse five times a day.

Vaginal Yeast Infection

Essential oils like melaleuca have been documented to have highly antifungal activity. Outstanding results have been obtained against vaginal yeast infections using them in douches. Equally excellent results have been achieved by inserting a capsule of Royaldophilus into the vagina after douching.

Single Oils: Lavender, melaleuca, rosemary verbenon, Roman chamomile, geranium, rosewood, peppermint, spearmint, or *Laurus nobilis.*

Blends: Melrose.

- Thyme with Melrose, Purification, R.C., or Di-Tone.

- Aroma Siez with Dragon Time or Mister.

Dilute 1-2 drops in 1 oz. V6 Mixing Oil or Massage Oil Base and use in a douche once daily for two weeks.

Recipe 1:
- 1 drop bergamot
- 1 drop lavender
- 2 drops melaleuca

Recipe 2:
- 7 drops Purification
- 2 drops frankincense

Recipe 3:
- 2 drops juniper
- 2 drops lavender
- 2 drops melaleuca

Recipe 4:
- 12 drops melaleuca
- 12 drops Purification
- 12 drops juniper

Mix in 1-2 Tbsp. V-6 Mixing Oil or Massage Oil Base and apply as a douche or vaginal retention implant every night.

Recipe 5:
- 10 drops cinnamon
- 10 drops clove
- 10 drops melaleuca

Dilute in 1-2 oz. V-6 Mixing Oil or Massage Oil Base and massage over entire body. Massage and rub on bottom of feet once a day.

Using Raindrop Technique to Purge Pathogenic Fungi

Pathogenic microorganisms have a tendency to hibernate along the spinal cord and in the lymphatic system. The body has the ability to hold them in a suspended state for long periods of time. When the immune system becomes compromised from stress, fatigue or other factors, they can be released and manifest illness and disease.

Oregano, thyme, or hyssop along the spine using Raindrop Technique may help to drive the dormant fungi out of the spinal fluid.

Lymphatic pump therapy will cleanse a sluggish lymphatic system and help remove dormant fungi.

Gallbladder

The gallbladder stores bile created by the liver and releases it through the biliary ducts into the duodenum to promote digestion. Bile is extremely important for fat digestion and the absorption of vitamins such as A, D, and E.

When bile flow is obstructed due to gallstones or inflamed due to infection, serious consequences can ensue, including poor digestion, jaundice, and severe abdominal pain.

Single Oils: Geranium, juniper, Roman chamomile, German chamomile.

- Lavender with geranium, juniper, Roman chamomile, German chamomile, rosemary, or eucalyptus.

Blends: JuvaFlex

- Lavender with JuvaFlex, PanAway, or Release.

Use as dietary supplement or apply on Vita Flex points on feet and hands, on location, and around navel.

JuvaFlex stimulates the gallbladder.

Supplements: Sulfurzyme, Megazyme, Mint Condition.

Gallstones

When bile contains excessive cholesterol, bilirubin, or bile salts, gallstones can form. Stones made from hardened cholesterol account for the vast majority of gallstones, while stones made from bilirubin, the brownish pigment in bile, constitute only about 20 percent of gallstones.

Gallstones can block both bile flow and the passage of pancreatic enzymes. This can result in inflammation in the gallbladder (cholecystitis) or pancreas (pancreatitis) and jaundice. In some cases, gallstones can be life-threatening, depending where they are lodged.

Single Oils:

- Lavender with rosemary, geranium, juniper or nutmeg.

Blends: JuvaFlex stimulates the gall bladder. Rosemary and/or nutmeg are supportive.

Rub oils over gallbladder or apply a hot compress over area, massage Vita Flex points on bottom of feet.

Recipe:
- 1 drop lavender
- 1 drop rosemary
- 1 drop geranium
- 1 drop juniper

Mix in juice or vegetable oil.

Risk Factors For Gallstones

- Being overweight. Obesity decreases gallbladder emptying and results in a dramatically higher risk for gallstones.

- Being over 60 years old or being female and middle-aged (age 20-60)

- Using excess estrogen from hormone replacement or birth control pills.

- Using cholesterol-lowering drugs. While these drugs can lower cholesterol in the bloodstream, they can raise cholesterol in the gallbladder.

- Being diabetic. Diabetics suffer higher levels of triglycerides, which can increase the likelihood of getting gallstones.

- Rapid weight loss. This forces the liver to pump out extra cholesterol, which can become concentrated in the bile.

Gangrene

Gangrene is the death or decay of living tissue caused by a lack of blood supply. A shortage of blood can result from a blood clot, arteriosclerosis, frostbite, diabetes, infection, or some other obstruction in the arterial blood supply, Gas gangrene (also known as acute or moist gangrene) occurs when tissues are infected with *Clostridium* bacteria. Unless the limb is amputated or treated with antibiotics, the gangrene can be fatal.

The part of the body affected with gangrene becomes evidences the following symptoms:

- Coldness
- Becomes darker in color
- Begins rotting or decomposing
- Emits putrid smell
- Fever
- Anemia

Dr. René Gattefossé suffered gas gangrene as a result of burns from a chemical explosion at the turn of the century. He successfully engineered his own recovery solely with the use of pure lavender oil.

Single Oils: Oregano, lavender, mountain savory, thyme, ravensara, and cistus.

Blends: Exodus II, Thieves, ImmuPower, and Melrose.

Supplements: Exodus, Radex, ImmuGel, ImmuneTune, and Super C.

Gastritis

(See DIGESTIVE PROBLEMS)

Gastritis occurs when the stomach's mucosal lining becomes inflamed and the cells become eroded. This can lead to bleeding ulcers and severe digestive disturbances. Gastritis may be caused by excess acid production in the stomach, alcohol consumption, stress, and fungal or bacterial infections.

Symptoms of gastritis:
- Weight loss
- Abdominal pain
- Cramping

Single Oils: Tarragon, peppermint, and fennel.

Blends: Di-Tone.

Supplements: AlkaLime, Megazyme, Royal-dophilus.

- Megazyme: 3-4 capsules, 3 times daily.

- Mint Condition: 3-4 capsules, 3 times daily.

- Royaldophilus: 2-4 capsules, 3 times daily.

- Mineral Essence: 2-3 droppers, 3 times daily.

- ComforTone and I.C.P.: Begin after 2 weeks.

Gingivitis, Pyorrhea

Essential oils make some of the best treatments against gum diseases such as gingivitis and pyorrhea. Clove oil, for example, is used as dental disinfectant, and the active principle in clove oil, eugenol, is one of the best-studied germ-killers available.

(See PERIODONTAL DISEASE)

Glaucoma

Common among people over 30 years of age, glaucoma is an eye disease in which escalating pressure within the fluid of the eye eventually damages the optic nerve and causes blindness. Many people are unaware of that they have the disease until their peripheral vision is permanently lost.

Glaucoma usually develops in middle age or later, although glaucoma in newborns, children, and teenagers can occur.

(See EYES)

Gout

Gout is a disease marked by abrupt, temporary bouts of joint pain and swelling that are most evident in the joint of the big toe. It can also affect the wrist, elbow, knee, ankle, hand, and foot. As the disease progresses, pain and swelling in the joints becomes more frequent and chronic, with deposits called tophi appearing over many joints, including the elbows and on ears

Gout is characterized by accumulation of uric acid crystals in the joints caused by excess uric acid in the blood. Uric acid is a byproduct of the breakdown of protein that is normally excreted by the kidneys into the urine. To reduce uric acid concentrations, it is necessary to support the kidneys, adrenal, and immune functions and detoxify by cleansing and drinking plenty of fluids.

Excess alcohol, allergy-producing foods, or strict diets can cause outbreaks of gout. Foods rich in purines, such as wine, anchovies and liver, can also cause gout.

Single Oils: Geranium, juniper, rosemary, Roman chamomile, lemon, melaleuca, nutmeg, and Idaho tansy.

Blends: PanAway and JuvaFlex.

Recipe 1:
* 10 drops geranium
* 8 drops juniper
* 5 drops rosemary
* 3 drops Roman chamomile
* 4 drops lemon
* 8 drops melaleuca

Dilute 6 drops in an oil-soluble liquid like honey or soy milk, and take 3 times daily.

Mix in 1 teaspoon of V-6 Mixing Oil or Massage Oil Base for massage on affected areas. May be applied neat 1-3 drops.

Recipe 2:
* 10 drops birch
* 6 drops fennel
* 2 drops tansy
* 3 drops patchouly
* 10 drops tangerine

Mix with 1/2 to 1 teaspoon. V-6 Mixing Oil or Massage Oil Base. This is helpful for liver, kidneys, and water retention.

Supplements: Thyromin, Essential Manna, Mineral Essence, Super C, Super Cal, Arthro-Tune, VitaGreen, Sulfurzyme, Cleansing Trio, JuvaTone, Ortho Ease Massage Oil, and Ortho Sport Massage Oil.

* Mineral Essence: 3 droppers, 3 times daily.

* ArthroTune: 3 capsules, 3 times daily.

* JuvaTone: up to 18 daily, reduce after 2 weeks.

* Super Cal: 2-4 capsules, 1-2 times daily.

* Super C: 2-4 tablets, 2-3 times daily.

* VitaGreen: 2-6 capsules, 2-3 times daily.

Graves Disease

(See THYROID IMBALANCES)

Gum Disease

(See PERIODONTAL DISEASE)

Hair and Scalp Problems

Sulfur is the single most important mineral for maintaining the strength and integrity of the hair and hair follicle.

Single Oils: Rosemary or lavender with clary sage, sage, fennel, cedarwood, juniper, ylang ylang, sandalwood, lemon, Roman chamomile, German chamomile, cypress, rose, rosewood, geranium, or patchouly.

Supplements: ParaFree, Thyromin, Super B, Master Formula, Royal Essence,

Skin and Hair Care: Morning Start Bath Gel, Lavender Shampoo.

Massage: 4-8 drops of the single oils listed above into the scalp or add to any AromaSilk Hair and Scalp Wash. Sandalwood helps restore hair color by helping the body utilize nutrients. Sage supports the hair follicle and helps deliver nutrients to the hair shaft.

Premature Graying

Thought to be from a deficiency of biotin. Super B is a good source of all B vitamins.

NOTE: Shampoos containing essential oils do not lather up because they do not contain harmful foaming chemicals.

Lemongrass has been reported to clear acne and balance oily skin and scalp conditions. Lavender shampoo helps to balance skin pH, decongest the lymphatics, and stimulate circulation.

Sandalwood oil rinse retards graying. Rosewood will lighten hair color.

A rinse to help restore the acid mantle of the hair:

* 1 drop rosemary, 1 tsp. pure apple cider vinegar, and 8 oz. water. Use as a final rinse on hair. Rosemary adds body and conditions the hair. Rub 1 or 2 drops on as hairdressing or on hairbrush to prevent static electricity.

Dandruff:

Single Oils: Melaleuca, rosemary cineol.

- 5 drops lemon
- 1 drop rosemary or sage
- 1 drop lavender
- 1 quart/liter of water

Dry Hair:
- 2 drops ylang ylang
- 8 drops rosewood
- 4 drops geranium

Oily Hair:
- 6 drops patchouly
- 2 to 5 oz. of lavender shampoo
- 6 drops lemon

Split Ends:
- 1 drop rosemary
- 3 drops sandalwood
- 1 drop ylang ylang

To darken hair:
- 1 drop geranium
- 5 drops sandalwood
- 1 quart/liter of water

To lighten hair:
- 2 drops Roman chamomile
- 1 drop lemon
- 2 drops rosemary
- 1 quart/liter of water

Hair Loss

(See ALOPECIA AREATA)

Hair loss by hormonal imbalances (such as increase in testosterone) or auto-immune conditions (as in the case of alopecia areata).

Essential oils are excellent for cleansing, nourishing, and strengthening the hair follicle and shaft. Rosemary (cineol chemotype) encourages hair growth.

Single Oils:

- Lavender or rosemary with any of the following: ylang ylang, sage, cedarwood, sandalwood, sage, or clary sage.

Prevent premature balding:
- 3 drops rosemary
- 5 drops lavender
- 4 drops cypress
- 2 drops clary sage
- 2 drops juniper

Add a drop of the above blend to 1 tsp. of water and massage into scalp where balding; then rub gently into rest of scalp. Best used at night.

To prevent hair loss:
- 10 drops cedarwood
- 8 drops rosemary
- 10 drops sandalwood
- 10 drops lavender

Combine and mix in shampoo base or massage individually into scalp, one oil daily.

Stimulate hair growth:
- 3-4 drops rosemary
- 4 drops ylang ylang
- 6 drops cedarwood
- 6 drops clary sage

Stimulate hair growth:
- 10 drops rosemary
- 3 drops cedarwood
- 3 drops birch
- 2 drops ylang ylang

Mix in V-6 Mixing Oil or Massage Oil Base. Rub into scalp at night.

Supplements: Super B, Thyromin, Sulfurzyme.

Halitosis (Bad Breath)

Persistent bad breath or gum disease, may be a sign of poor digestion or other health problems. One should consult a physician.

(See DIGESTION PROBLEMS and GUMS).

Single Oils: Nutmeg, peppermint, and tarragon.

- Peppermint or spearmint with lemon, mandarin, or cinnamon.

Blends: Thieves, Fresh Essence Mouthwash

Disinfectant mouthwash or gargle:

- 3 drops peppermint
- 2 drops lemon
- 1 drop mandarin

Thoroughly stir essential oil blend into one bottle of Fresh Essence Mouthwash or dilute blend in 2 Tbsp. honey and 4 oz. of hot water.

Oral Hygiene: Dentarome Toothpaste, Fresh Essence Mouthwash.

Hashimoto's Thyroiditis

(See THYROID CONDITIONS)

Head Lice

Single Oils: Eucalyptus with lavender, peppermint, thyme, or geranium.

Recipe 1:
• 2 drops eucalyptus
• 1 drop lavender
• 1 drop geranium

Mix into 1 tsp. of V-6 Mixing Oil or Massage Oil Base. Massage into scalp. Leave for 1/2 hour. Shampoo and rinse well.

Antiseptic rinse:
• 2 drops eucalyptus
• 2 drops lavender
• 2 drops geranium
• 1/2 ounce vinegar
• 8 oz. water

Pour over hair making sure every hair is rinsed. Dry naturally. Repeat daily until lice and eggs are gone.

How to Tap the Full Therapeutic Potential of Essential Oils

An outstanding way to tap the full therapeutic potential of essential oils is to combine them with bath salts and use them in the shower. The RainSpa aromatherapy shower head has a specially designed chamber that can be filled with essential oils and bath salts. As the water passes through the mixture, it disperses the essential oils into the spray, creating a fragrant, antiseptic spa.

Headaches

Headaches can be due to hormone imbalances, shortage of oxygen, stress, and sugar imbalance (hypoglycemia).

Essential oils boost the oxygen-carrying capacity of the blood and oxygen infusion into the cell.

Single Oils: Idaho tansy, Roman chamomile, peppermint, lavender, basil, spearmint, bergamot, lemon, and rosemary.

Blends: M-Grain, Brain Power, Clarity, and Thieves.

Diffuse, rub on back of neck, temples, or put under nose.

Recipe 1:
• 4 drops Idaho tansy
• 5 drops Roman chamomile
• 2 drops peppermint
• 2 drops lavender
• 1 drop basil
• 3 drops rosemary

Mix the above in 1 tsp. of V-6 Mixing Oil or Massage Oil Base.

Recipe 2:
• 2 drops Idaho tansy
• 1 drop Roman chamomile
• 3 drops spearmint
• 7 drops lavender
• 9 drops basil

*Mix the above in 1 tsp. of V-6 Mixing Oil or Massage Oil Base.*Recipe 3:

• 12 drops bergamot
• 2 drops lavender
• 3 drops geranium
• 2 drops rosemary
• 5 drops lemon

Mix the above in 1 tsp. of V-6 Mixing Oil or Massage Oil Base.

• Thieves: 1 drop on tongue and push against roof of mouth.

• Clarity: 1-2 drops on back of neck, under nose, and on temples. Put 1-2 drops in palm of hands, rub hands together, cup over nose, and breathe deeply.

Supplements: VitaGreen, Power Meal, Body Balance, and Brain Power.

Stress

Single Oils:

- Lavender with patchouly, birch, spruce, lemongrass, rosemary, or basil.

Blends:

- Lavender with Valor or Aroma Siez.
- Lemongrass with Valor or Aroma Siez.

Children's Migraine

Single Oils: German chamomile, grapefruit, peppermint, and rosemary.

Recipe 1:
- 1 drop German chamomile
- 10 drops grapefruit
- 5 drops peppermint
- 3 drops rosemary

Mix in 1 teaspoon of V-6 Mixing Oil or Massage Oil Base. Rub on temples, forehead, and brainstem. Also massage on thumbs and big toes.

Headache from Diffusing - (Clarity, Brain Power)

People who get an instant headache from diffusing usually have a blockage related to metallics or synthetic chemicals in the brain.

Single Oils: Helichrysum with rosemary.

Blends: Aroma Life, M-Grain, and Clarity.

Apply helichrysum, rosemary, Aroma Life and M-Grain to the arteries in the neck on the pulse points where arteries are closest to the surface.

Continue to diffuse Clarity or the offending oil, but in small amounts until the body clears itself and the diffused oil does not cause the headache any more. Clarity will also help the chelation process.

Hormonal Imbalance

Single Oils:

- Lavender with clary sage, sage, fennel, bergamot, or geranium.

Blends:

- Lavender or basil with Mister, Dragon Time, EndoFlex, or M-Grain.

Supplements: Femalin, Thyromin, Super B, VitaGreen, Royal Essence, Dragon Time Massage Oil, and Dragon Time Bath and Shower Gel.

Oils may be rubbed on the reproductive Vita Flex areas on hands and feet. These areas are inside of wrists and around the front of the ankles in line with the anklebone and particularly inside and outside of the foot just above the anklebone and up along the Achilles tendon. They may also be rubbed on the lower back and groin (see MENOPAUSE and HORMONAL IMBALANCE).

Hypoglycemic Migraine

Single Oils: Peppermint, lavender, lemongrass, clove, caraway, thyme, or geranium.

Blends: Clarity.

- Lavender or peppermint with Thieves, M-Grain, JuvaFlex, or Di-Tone.

Supplements: Power Meal, Body Balance, VitaGreen, Royal Essence, and Estro Tincture.

Migraine

Single Oils:

- Rosemary with basil, peppermint, melissa, lavender, ylang ylang, German chamomile, eucalyptus, or marjoram.
- Helichrysum with sandalwood.

Blends:

- Rosemary or peppermint with M-Grain or Clarity.

Supplements: A.D.&E. and Megazyme.

The vast majority of migraine headaches may be due to colon congestion or poor digestion. The Cleansing Trio is most important for cleansing the colon.

M-Grain is specially formulated for migraine headaches. Put a couple of drops in your palm (can also add a drop of peppermint). Rub hands together clockwise; then cup hands over your nose and breathe deeply. Put on temples, forehead, and brain stem (back of neck at skull). Massage on thumbs and big toes. Lavender and basil, layered on temples and forehead, have relieved migraine headaches.

Apply 1 drop helichrysum and 1 drop sandal-wood to the inside of nasal passages, also on temples and brainstem.

A.D.&E. vitamin supplement is important for vision. Eye strain and decreased vision can accompany migraine headaches.

Muscle-Related Headache

Single Oils:

- Lavender with marjoram, rosemary, peppermint, lemongrass, basil, valerian, marjoram, or cardamom.

Blends:

- Lavender or lemongrass with M-Grain or Aroma Siez.

Supplements: Relaxation, Ortho Ease and Ortho Sport Massage Oils.

Use peppermint around the hairline, on the back of the neck, and across the forehead.

Sinus-Related Headache

Single Oils:

- Rosemary with bergamot, Melaleuca ericifolia with eucalyptus, lavender, lemon, or geranium.

Recipe 1:
- 5 drops Melaleuca ericifolia
- 9 drops rosemary
- 2 drops bergamot
- 7 drops lavender
- 3 drops lemon
- 4 drops geranium

Mix in 1 oz. V-6 Mixing Oil or Massage Oil Base

Structural - Bone-Related Headache

Single Oils:

- Lavender with birch, basil, marjoram, lemongrass, or rosemary.

Blends:

- Lavender or lemongrass with M-Grain and Aroma Siez or PanAway.

Supplements: Ortho Ease, Relaxation and, Sensation Massage Oils, Evening Peace Bath and Shower Gel.

Hearing Impairment

Single Oils:

- Helichrysum with juniper, peppermint, or geranium.

- Lavender with basil.

Blends:

- Helichrysum with Purification, ImmuPower, and Melrose.

Drop ImmuPower on a cotton ball and place in the ear.

Lavender and basil, layered on temples and forehead, has helped ringing (tinnitus).

NOTE: Never place any essential oil, including helichrysum, directly into the ear canal. Only rub on the opening of the ear.

Hearing Vita Flex Regimen

- Make sure that your fingernails are short. Place 1-2 drops of helichrysum, on each index finger.

- Standing behind the person, gently insert index fingers into the person's ears. Have the person hold head firmly against your chest.

- Rotate your hands (with the index fingers still inserted in ears) until the palms face upward. Lift fingers alternately (in a rocking motion) 10 times in each ear to a count of 20.

- Rotate hands 90 degrees until the palms face backwards. Pull back alternately 5 times in each ear to a count of 10.

- Rotate hands 90 degrees until the palms face downward. Press down alternately 5 times in each ear to a count of 10.

- Rotate hands 90 degrees until the palms face backward. Put thumbs behind the fingers. Push forward alternately 5 times in each ear to a count of 10.

- Rotate hands 90 degrees back to starting position (palms facing upward). Lift both fingers up once and let down slowly.

- Rotate fingers 90 degrees back and remove slowly.

- Grasp ear lobes, pull down and release.

For the average hearing loss problem, massage Purification on ear lobe, behind the ears, and down the jaw line (along the Eustachian tube).

For ringing in the ears (Tinnitus)

Massage helichrysum or juniper. Additionally, apply juniper with peppermint and geranium on tips of toes and fingers, and on the brainstem, so that the oils get into the nerve pathways. It generally takes 12 to 15 minutes to notice a change in hearing. Apply 1 drop of helichrysum on the opening of each ear.

Heart

Heart Vita Flex

The foot Vita Flex point related to the heart is on the sole of the left foot, on the ring toe (second toe) and behind the knuckle. Massaging this point is as effective as massaging the hand and arm together. The hand Vita Flex point related to the heart is in the palm of the left hand, one inch below the ring finger joint (at the lifeline). The secondary point is on the bottom of the left arm in line with the inside of the up-turned arm (approximately 2 inches up the arm from the funny bone), not on the muscle but up under the muscle. Have another person use thumbs and firmly press these two points alternately for 3 minutes, in a kind of pumping action. Work all 3 points when possible. Start with the foot first; then go to the hand and arm.

Heart Attack - Myocardial Infarction

Interruption of blood supply to an area.

Single Oils:

- Lavender with Roman chamomile, helichrysum, Idaho tansy, or rose.

Blends:

- Lavender or marjoram with Aroma Life, Valor, Peace & Calming, Harmony, PanAway, or Relieve It.

Supplements: Cardia Care, HRT Tincture, CardiaCare, Mineral Essence, Super Cal, Power Meal, and, Sulfurzyme.

Apply to heart Vita Flex points on feet, hand, and arm as described above. If there is not enough time to remove shoes to get at the feet, apply pumping action to left hand and arm points. Using 1 drop of Aroma Life on each point will increase effectiveness and may even revive an individual having a heat attack while waiting for medical attention.

Applying Valor on bottom of feet improves effectiveness of other oils. Apply Harmony to the energy or chakra points (crown of head, forehead, throat (thyroid), thymus, navel, stomach, groin) to balance body frequencies. Inhale Peace & Calming to relax the individual.

Magnesium, the most important mineral for the heart, acts as a smooth muscle relaxant and supports the cardiovascular system. Magnesium will act as a natural calcium channel blocker for the heart, lowering blood pressure and dilating the heart blood vessels (Dr. Terry Friedmann). Mineral Essence along with Super Cal are good sources of magnesium.

MSM (methylsulfonylmethane), found in Sulfurzyme, normalizes heart function.

Angina

Single Oils: Ginger

False Angina

Single Oils: Orange

Arrhythmia (Heart Rhythm Disorders)

Marjoram and Aroma Life stimulate regeneration of smooth muscle tissue, particularly in the heart which can counteract both tachycardia (rapid heartbeat) or bradycardia (slow heartbeat).

Single Oils: Ylang ylang, marjoram, rosemary verbenon, and Idaho tansy

- Ylang ylang with marjoram or Idaho tansy.

Blends:

- Ylang ylang or marjoram with Aroma Life or Joy.

Massage 1 drop of each oil on heart Vita Flex points. Rub Joy over the heart or diffuse.

Supplements: CardiaCare, Mineral Essence, Super Cal, Sulfurzyme, and HRT Tincture.

Atrial Fibrillation

This is when the upper heart chambers contract at a rate of over 300 pulsations per minute. The lower chambers cannot keep this pace, so efficiency is reduced, and not enough blood is pumped. Palpitations, a feeling that the heart is beating irregularly, more strongly, or more rapidly than normal, is the most common symptom.

Single Oils:

- Ylang Ylang with marjoram, helichrysum, or orange.

Blends: Aroma Life.

Supplements: HRT, CardiaCare, Mineral Essence, Super Cal, and Sulfurzyme.

Place 1 drop of each oil on heart Vita Flex points and do Vita Flex (see HEART).

Cardiac Spasm and Tension

Single Oils: Marjoram, basil, and valerian.

- Lavender with marjoram, ylang ylang, vetiver, Roman chamomile, valerian or basil.

Blends:

- Lavender with Aroma Life, Peace & Calming, Valor, Joy, or Harmony.

Supplements: HRT tincture.

Rub Joy over heart every day as needed (see BLOOD PRESSURE, CARDIOVASCULAR CONDITIONS).

Shortness of Breath

(Due to enlarged heart valve)

Blends: Aroma Siez and R.C.

Supplements: HRT Tincture, CardiaCare.

Tachycardia

Heart rate that suddenly increases to 160 beats per minute or faster for no reason.

Single Oils: Lavender, ylang ylang, and Idaho tansy.

Blends:

- Ylang ylang with Aroma Life or Joy.

Supplements: CardiaCare, HRT Tincture, and Sulfurzyme.

Place 1 drop of each oil on heart Vita Flex points and do heart Vita Flex.

Rub Joy over the heart and diffuse in the room.

Tonic - Stimulant

Single Oils: Anise, mandarin, rosemary, peppermint, and thyme.

Anise is a tonic and stimulant to the heart.

Blends:

- Marjoram with Aroma Life.

Supplements: HRT Tincture, CardiaCare

Heart Attack – Myocardial Infarction

Magnesium acts as a smooth-muscle relaxant and supports the cardiovascular system. It acts as a natural calcium channel blocker for the heart, lowering blood pressure and dilating the heart blood vessels. Mineral Essence, Essential Manna, and Super Cal are good sources of magnesium.

Single Oils: Helichrysum, lavender, peppermint, lemon, and cypress.

Blends: Aroma Life.

- Lavender with Roman Chamomile, rose, or Aroma Life.

Supplements: CardiaCare, Mineral Essence, Super Cal, and Sulfurzyme.

Apply on the Vita Flex point for the heart. If there is not enough time to remove shoes to work on feet, apply pumping action to left hand and arm points. A drop of Aroma Life on each point will increase effectiveness.

Heartburn

Single Oils: Peppermint, spearmint

Blends: Di-Tone.

Supplements: AlkaLime and Mint Condition.

Heat Stroke

Single Oils: Helichrysum, cypress, sandalwood, and peppermint.

- Rub 1 drop lavender with 1 drop peppermint on back of neck and on forehead.

Supplements: CardiaCare and HRT Tincture.

Heavy Metals

(See CHEMICAL POISONING)

Hematoma

A hematoma is a tumor-like mass of coagulated blood, caused by a break in the blood vessel or capillary wall. Essential oils such as helichrysum are excellent for balancing blood viscosity and dissolving clots. Clove oil and citrus rind oils, like lemon and grapefruit, exert a mild blood-thinning effect that can help speed the dissolution of the clot.

Those who bruise easily are usually low in vitamin C, which may be caused by insufficient intake or poor absorption.

Single Oils: Cypress, helichrysum, lemon, grapefruit, clove.

- Helichrysum with German chamomile, rose, cypress, Roman chamomile, or geranium.

Blends:

- Helichrysum with Aroma Life.

Supplements: Super C, A.D.&E., and Mineral Essence.

Dilute 2-4 drops in a tsp. of vegetable oil, take three times daily as a dietary supplement. Apply diluted on location, with or without hot compresses.

Hemorrhaging (Bleeding)

Essential oils that are topically applied or used on pressure bandages are excellent for slowing bleeding and initiating healing.

Single Oils: Helichrysum, geranium, and cypress.

Hemorrhoids

Single Oils:

- Cypress with helichrysum, birch, patchouly, myrrh, myrtle, or clary sage.

- Basil with cypress or peppermint.

Blends:

- Basil with Aroma Siez, Citrus Fresh, Aroma Life, or PanAway.

- Cypress with PanAway.

Supplements: Cel-Lite Magic, Royaldophilus, Megazyme, Mint Condition, VitaGreen, Super B, and Royal Essence.

Mix with V-6 Mixing Oil or Massage Oil Base.

Cleanse using the Cleansing Trio

Recipe 1:
- 3 or 4 drops of basil
- 1 drop of birch
- 1 drop of cypress
- 1 drop of helichrysum

Mix with V-6 Mixing Oil or Massage Oil Base and place on location. This may sting, but one application works on hemorrhoids.

Recipe 2:
- 3 drops cypress
- 2 drops helichrysum
- 10 drops myrtle

Mix in V-6 Mixing Oil or Massage Oil Base.

Hepatitis

(See HEPATITIS under LIVER)

Hernia (Hiatal)

Single Oils:

- Peppermint with lavender, lemongrass, or helichrysum.

Supplements: Megazyme, Mint Condition, and Cleansing Trio.

Herpes

(See SEXUAL DISEASES)

Hiccups

This is usually caused by irritated nerves of the diaphragm, possibly caused from a full stomach or indigestion. (See DIGESTIVE PROBLEMS)

Single Oils: Tarragon, peppermint.

Tarragon (2-4 drops either topically applied or taken as a dietary supplement) may relax intestinal spasms, nervous digestion, and hiccups.

Hives

Hives refer to a generalized itching or dermatitis that can be due allergies, damaged liver, chemicals, or other factors.

Single Oils: Peppermint, patchouly

Supplements: Super Cal

(See ITCHING under SKIN)

Hodgkin's Disease

Single Oils: Clove, lavender, frankincense, and cistus.

Homocysteine

Elevated levels of homocysteine have been strongly linked to cardiovascular disease and arteriosclerosis. Certain B vitamins, including B12, B6, and folic acid, have been shown to reduce homocysteine levels and reduce the risk of heart disease.

Supplements: Super B, Master Formula vitamins.

(See HEART)

Hormone Imbalance (Women)

(See MENOPAUSE)

Hot Flashes

(See MENOPAUSE)

Huntington's Chorea

(See NEUROLOGICAL DISEASES)

Hyperactivity

Single Oils: Lavender, Roman chamomile, peppermint, and valerian.

Hypoglycemia

Hypoglycemia may also be caused by low thyroid function (See THYROID).

Excessive consumption of sugar or honey will also cause reactive hypoglycemia, in which a rapid rise in blood sugar is followed by abnormally low levels.

In some cases, hypoglycemia may be a precursor to candida, allergies, chronic fatigue syndrome, depression, and chemical sensitivities.

Signs of hypoglycemia (low blood sugar) include:

- Fatigue, drowsiness, and sleepiness after meals.
- Headache or dizziness if periods between meals are too long.
- Craving for sweets.
- Allergic reaction to foods.
- Palpitations, tremors, sweats, rapid heart beat.
- Inattentiveness, mood swings, irritability, anxiety, nervousness, inability to cope with stress, and feelings of emotional depression,
- Lack of motivation, discipline, and creativity.
- Hunger that cannot be satisfied.

Often people with some of these symptoms are misdiagnosed as suffering either chronic fatigue or neurosis. Instead, they may be hypoglycemic.

To treat chronic hypoglycemia, it may be necessary to first treat the underlying candida or yeast over growth (See FUNGUS INFECTION).

Single Oils:

- Lavender with cinnamon, cumin, clove, caraway, thyme, lemongrass, geranium, coriander or dill.

Blends:

- Lavender with Thieves, JuvaFlex, or Di-Tone.
- Ylang Ylang with Thieves, JuvaFlex, Di-Tone, or Exodus II.

Apply neat on pancreas Vita Flex points on feet. Thieves will boost blood sugar levels.

Supplements: Power Meal, Body Balance, VitaGreen, Stevia, Exodus, Mineral Essence, and Essential Manna.

Hysterectomy

(See MENOPAUSE)

How to Stimulate the Immune System

Apply Thieves or Exodus II to bottom of feet.

Apply ImmuPower on the throat and chest.

Apply 1-2 drops of Thieves in V-6 Mixing Oil or Massage Oil Base massaged on the thymus gland (located in upper chest area).

Recipe:
- 10 drops lemon
- 8 drops oregano
- 5 drops mountain savory

Apply 1-2 drops of blend in V-6 Mixing Oil or Massage Oil Base and use topically or as dietary supplement.

Immune Deficiency Syndrome

(See AIDS)

Single Oils: Cistus

Blends: Brain Power, Exodus, Valor, Thieves, and ImmuPower.

Exodus II: 6-8 drops on spine alternating days with Raindrop Technique.

Valor and Thieves: 4-6 drops on feet for 3 weeks.

ImmuPower: Take 6 drops daily in water.

Raindrop Technique: 3 times weekly for virus.

Supplements: Cleansing Trio, JuvaTone, ImmuGel, Thyromin, ImmuneTune, VitaGreen, Sulfurzyme, Exodus, Super B, Ultra Young, and Goji Berry Tea.

Cleansing Trio for 120 days with JuvaTone.

ImmuGel: 1/2 tsp., 3 times daily. Retain in mouth for better absorption.

Thyromin: Start by taking 2 at night and 1 in morning.

ImmuneTune: 6-8 capsules daily.

VitaGreen: 6-10 capsules daily.

Sulfurzyme: 1 tablespoon.

Exodus: Up to 18 capsules daily.

Super B: 1 capsule daily.

Ultra Young: 3 squirts on each inside of each cheek, 4-5 times daily.

Eat 5-6 mini-meals daily, primarily Power Meal (3 times daily) and fish for protein. Do not eat chicken for first 3-6 weeks to allow more energy for immune building.

Impotence

(See SEXUAL DYSFUNCTION)

Impotence (the inability to perform sexually) can be caused by physical limitations (an accident or injury) or psychological factors (inhibitions, trauma, stress, etc.) In males, impotence is often linked to problems with the prostate or prosate surgery (See BENIGN PROSTATE HYPERPLASIA).

If impotence is related to psychological trauma or unresolved emotional issues, it may be necessary to deal with these issues before any meaningful progress can be made. (See TRAUMA)

There is an extensive historical basis for the ability of fragrance to amplify desire and create a mood that can overcome frigidity or impotence. In fact, aromas like rose and jasmine have been used since antiquity to attract the opposite sex and create a romantic atmosphere.

Modern research has shown that the fragrance of some essential oils can stimulate the emotional center of the brain. This may explain why essential oils have the potential to help people overcome impotence based on emotional factors or inhibitions.

Single Oils: Ylang ylang, clary sage, sandalwood, clove, frankincense, myrrh, ginger, nutmeg, rose, jasmine, and pepper.

Supplements: ProGen.

Indigestion

(See DIGESTIVE DISORDERS)

Infection (Bacterial and Viral)

Diffusing essential oils is on of the best ways to prevent the spread of airborne bacteria and viruses. Many essential oils, like oregano, mountain savory, and rosemary cineol, exert highly antimicrobial effects and can effectively eliminate many kinds of pathogens.

Mountain savory, ravensara, and thyme applied by Raindrop Technique on the spine are beneficial for most infections, particularly chest-related.

(See COLDS)

Clean, healthy, and detoxified blood helps to overcome most diseases. Rehemogen cleans and purifies blood so that nutrients and oxygen may be delivered to the cells.

Single Oils:

- Cypress with rosemary cineol, rose, lavender, lemongrass, basil, thyme, oregano, nutmeg, rosewood, mountain savory, frankincense, myrrh, cistus, or marjoram.

- Melaleuca or sage or rosemary with lemongrass, lemon, Idaho tansy, German chamomile, thyme, basil, lavender, clary sage, eucalyptus (globulus and radiata), geranium, bergamot, pine, spruce, or tarragon. Thyme with ravensara, melissa, petitgrain, oregano, frankincense, clove, cinnamon, or lavender.

Blends:

- Cypress with Purification, Melrose, or R.C.

- Melaleuca or rosemary with Thieves, Melrose, Purification, ImmuPower, R.C., or Di-Tone.

- Thyme or sage with Melrose, Purification, Exodus, Raven, Thieves, or 3 Wise Men.

Supplements: Radex, Super C, Exodus, Immu-Gel, Royal Essence, VitaGreen, ImmuneTune, Rehemogen.

To Kill Airborne Viruses and Bacteria

Periodically alternate diffusing ImmuPower and Thieves.

Topically apply 1 drop melaleuca and 1 drop rosemary cineol to stem infection.

Single Oils: Melaleuca with cinnamon, clove, thyme, oregano, ravensara, or frankincense.

Blends: Melaleuca with Thieves.

Strep Throat

Single Oils:

- Cinnamon with lavender, chamomile, hyssop, myrrh, myrtle, or nutmeg.

Recipe 1:
- 1 drop cinnamon
- 6 drops lavender or chamomile
- 2 drops hyssop

Use up to 3 drops neat on the Vita Flex points of the feet or Mix into 1/2 oz. V-6 Mixing Oil or Massage Oil Base and apply topically on throat.

Blends:

- Cypress with Purification, Melrose, or R.C.

- Melaleuca or rosemary with Thieves, Melrose, Purification, ImmuPower, R.C., or Di-Tone.

- Thyme or sage with Melrose, Purification, Exodus, Raven, Thieves, or 3 Wise Men.

Supplements: Radex, Super C, Exodus, Immu-Gel, Royal Essence, VitaGreen, ImmuneTune, and Rehemogen.

Mountain savory, ravensara, and thyme applied by Raindrop Technique on the spine are beneficial for any and all infections, particularly chest-related infections.

Mix 1 drop melaleuca and 1 drop rosemary for antiseptic and healing benefits for infectious cuts, wounds, rashes, cleansing, and purifying.

Whooping Cough

A contagious disease affecting the respiratory system mainly in children. Lungs become infected, as the air passages become clogged with thick mucus. Over the course of several days, the condition worsens, resulting in long coughing bouts (up to 1 minute). The continual coughing makes breathing difficult and labored.

Single Oils:

- Cypress with rosemary, rose, lavender, lemongrass, basil, thyme, oregano, myrtle, or nutmeg.

- Melaleuca or sage or rosemary with lemongrass, lemon, Idaho tansy, Roman chamomile, thyme, basil, lavender, eucalyptus, geranium, or bergamot.

- Thyme with ravensara, melissa, petitgrain, oregano, frankincense, clove, cinnamon, lavender, myrrh, or ginger.

Blends:

- Cypress with R.C.

- *Melaleuca ericifolia* or rosemary with Thieves, Melrose, Purification, ImmuPower, R.C., or Di-Tone.

- Thyme or sage with Melrose, Purification, Thieves, or 3 Wise Men.

Supplements: Radex, Super C, ImmuGel, Royal Essence, VitaGreen, ImmuneTune, and Rehemogen.

NOTE: *Because whooping cough usually affects children, always dilute essential oils in massage oil or V-6 Mixing Oil before topically applying. Start with low concentrations until response is observed. Diffuse intermittently and observe reaction. Do not overdo.*

Viral Infection in the Spine (see SPINE).

Viruses and bacteria have a tendency to hibernate along the spine. The body may hold a virus in a suspended state for long periods of time. When the immune system is compromised, these viruses may be released and then manifest into illness. Raindrop Technique along the spine helps to bring out these microorganisms and rid them from the body.

Oregano and thyme are generally used first for the Raindrop application. However, other oils may also be used and may be more desirable for some people. ImmuPower, Raven, and Purification all work well in the Raindrop application method. Other oils and blends may be used depending on perceived requirements.

Infertility

Infertility could be caused be a mineral deficiency. It could also be caused by a hormone imbalance.

Supplements: Estro Tincture, Femalin, Vita-Green, Mineral Essence, Super Cal, Essential Manna, Ultra Young, and Thyromin.

Inflammation

Certain essential oils have been documented to be excellent for reducing inflammation. German chamomile contains azulene, a blue compound with highly anti-inflammatory properties. Peppermint is also highly anti-inflammatory. Other oils also have anti-inflammatory properties: Helichrysum, spruce, birch, and valerian.

There are different types of inflammation for which one oil might be better than another:

Myrrh: Tissue and capillary damage, bruising or loss of oxygen.

Roman chamomile and lavender: Inflammation due to infection.

Ravensara, hyssop, or oregano: Viral.

Single Oils:

- Birch with helichrysum, frankincense, hyssop, myrrh, marjoram, ravensara, lavender, oregano, Roman chamomile, cypress, peppermint, spearmint, or spruce.

- Mountain savory, clary sage, lemongrass, sandalwood, rose, spikenard, or fir.

- Melaleuca with German chamomile, tangerine, thyme, hyssop, eucalyptus radiata, jasmine, pepper, petitgrain, Idaho tansy, tarragon, yarrow, citronella, or coriander.

Blends:

- Birch with Purification, PanAway, Aroma Siez, Exodus II, Melrose, Abundance, Relieve It, or ImmuPower.

Supplements: Ortho Ease, Relaxation, and Ortho Sport Massage Oils.

Recipe 1:
- 10 drops fir
- 6 drops melaleuca
- 4 drops German chamomile
- 2 drops peppermint
- 2 drops lemongrass

Recipe 2:
- 6 drops frankincense
- 6 drops fir
- 6 drops *Eucalyptus citriodora*
- 4 drops ravensara
- 3 drops birch
- 1 drop peppermint

Mix in 1/2 to 1 oz.massage oil or V-6 Mixing Oil or Massage Oil Base.

Insect Bites

(See INSECT REPELLENT)

Because of their outstanding antiseptic and oil-soluble properties, essential oils are ideal for treating most kinds of insect bites. Essential oils like lavender and peppermint also help reduce insect-bite-induced itching.

Singles oils: Lavender, citronella, melaleuca, peppermint, and rosemary.

- Lavender with melaleuca, rosemary, Idaho tansy, clary sage, Roman chamomile, German chamomile, basil, patchouly, or bergamot.

Blends: Purification, Melrose, or PanAway

- Lavender with Purification, R.C., PanAway, or Melrose.

Recipe 1 (stings and bites):
- 1 drop thyme
- 10 drops lavender
- 4 drops eucalyptus
- 3 drops chamomile

Use neat or mix in 1 tsp. massage oil or V-6 Mixing Oil or Massage Oil Base and apply on location.

Bee Stings

Single Oils: Lavender, Idaho tansy.

Blends: Purification, Melrose, PanAway.

Recipe 1:
- 2 drops lavender
- 1 drop helichrysum
- 1 drop chamomile
- 1 drop birch

Regimen:

- Flick or scrape stinger out with credit card or knife, taking care not to squeeze the venom sack.

- Apply 1-2 drops Purification, Melrose, lavender, or Idaho tansy on location. Repeat until the venom spread has stopped.

- Apply lavender with or without one or more of the single oils listed, 2-3 times daily until redness abates. PanAway may be substituted for Purification.

Black Widow Spider Bite

Rub 1 drop lavender every 2-3 minutes over the bite until you reach the hospital.

Brown Recluse Spider Bite

The blend Purification neutralizes the venom of this spider's bite.

Recipe 1:
- 1 drop lavender
- 1 drop helichrysum
- 1 drop Melrose
- Cover with oatmeal poultice.

Chigger (Mite) Bites

Single Oils: Lavender.

Blends: R.C.

Massage undiluted on location.

Ticks

Single Oils: Thyme, oregan, peppermint.

Blends: R.C.

Regimen:

- Apply thyme oil to tick to loosen from skin.

- Apply Purification on site to detoxify wound.

- Apply 1 drop peppermint every 5 minutes for 50 minutes to reduce pain and infection

----

Insect Repellent

Single Oils: Peppermint, eucalyptus, lemon, lime, lavender, melaleuca, cedarwood, geranium, Idaho tansy, rosemary, patchouly, citronella, lemongrass, and thyme.

- Lemongrass with citronella

- Idaho tansy floral water

Blends: Purification, Thieves, Melrose.

Recipe 1:
- 6 drops peppermint
- 6 drops melaleuca
- 9 drops eucalyptus

Using Essential Oils As Insect Repellents

Mosquito-repellent: Lemon, peppermint, eucalyptus, lemongrass.

Moth-repellent: Patchouly.

Horse-fly-repellent: Idaho tansy floral water.

Aphids-repellent: Mix 20 drops essential oil in 2 quarts salt water, shake well, and spray on plants.

Cockroach-repellent: Mix 10 drops peppermint and 5 drops cypress in 1/2 cup salt water. Shake well and spray where roaches live.

Silverfish-repellent: Eucalyptus, citriadora

To repel insects, essential oils can be diffused or put on cotton balls or cedar chips (for use in closets or drawers).

Insomnia

Insomnia may be caused by bowel or liver toxicity, poor heart function, negative memories and trauma, depression, mineral deficiencies, hormone imbalance, or underactive thyroid.

The fragrance of many essential oils can exert a powerful calming effect on the mind through their influence on the limbic region of the brain.

Single Oils: Lavender, German chamomile, Roman chamomile, orange, and rosemary verbenon.

- Lavender and Roman chamomile

- Lavender with Roman chamomile, marjoram, myrtle, German chamomile, ravensara, basil, ylang ylang, tangerine, bergamot, mandarin, orange, or valerian.

- Cypress with marjoram, lavender, basil, geranium, rosemary verbenon, clary sage, German chamomile, rosewood, or angelica.

Blends: Peace & Calming, Harmony, Dream Catcher.

- Lavender with Peace & Calming, Valor, Aroma Siez, Present Time, Motivation, Harmony, Surrender, or White Angelica.

- Lavender with marjoram and Peace & Calming,

- Cypress with Peace & Calming, Valor, 3 Wise Men, Gentle Baby, or Citrus Fresh.

Recipe 1:
- 12 drops orange
- 8 drops lavender
- 4 drops bergamot
- 3 drops geranium
- 2 drops Roman chamomile

Recipe 2:
- 9 drops lavender
- 3 drops tansy
- 3 drops marjoram

Recipe 3 (calming):
- 15 drops lavender
- 15 drops Peace & Calming

Diffuse:
Essential oils can be diffused using a cold air diffuser. Place several drops of essential oil on a cotton towel and place under or on your pillow.

Topical application:
Mix in 1/2 to 1 oz. V-6 Mixing Oil or Massage Oil Base (more or less dilution may be needed depending on your sensitivity). Rub on shoulders, stomach, around the navel, or on the bottom of the feet.

Bath and shower:
Add 10 drops of lavender or geranium in 1/2 cup bath or Epsom salts. Use in RainSpa shower head or run bath water through the salts and soak.

Supplements: AuraLight, Evening Peace Bath and Shower Gel, Relaxation Massage Oil, Super Cal, Thyromin, HRT tincture, CardiaCare.

> Rub Peace & Calming or Dream Catcher across the shoulders along with a little lavender or Roman chamomile if needed.
>
> Put 1 drop of Harmony on energy meridians to help balance the energy flow in the body. (1 drop on stomach, navel, thymus, throat, forehead, and crown of head).

Thyroid Imbalance

Hyperthyroidism (having an overactive thyroid) can trigger insomnia.

(See THYROID)

Supplements: Thyromin.

Depression

Depression is a major cause of insomnia. St. John's wort has been proven highly effective in reducing depression.

Supplements: AuraLight.

Mineral and Nutrient Deficiencies

Magnesium, potassium, and other mineral deficiencies can contribute to insomnia and depression.

Supplements: Mineral Essence, Essential Manna, Master Formula vitamins.

Bowel Toxicity

Supplements: Megazyme, Comfortone, I.C.P.

A fasting or cleansing program is important for combating insomnia caused by excess toxins accumulating in the liver and the gastrointestinal tract. Excessive toxins may also produce frequent recurring migraine headaches, skin eruptions, discoloration, changes in pigmentation, acne, and bumpy skin.

Influenza

(See COLDS)

Irritable Bowel Syndrome

(See DIGESTIVE DISEASES)

Irritable bowel syndrome (IBS) is a common disorder of the intestines marked by the following symptoms:

- Cramps
- Gas and bloating
- Constipation
- Diarrhea and loose stools

IBS may be caused by a combination of stress and a high-fat diet. Fatty foods worsen symptoms by increasing the intensity of the contractions in the colon, thereby worsening symptoms. Chocolate and milk products in particular seem to have the most negative effect on IBS sufferers.

IBS is not the same as colitis, mucous colitis, spastic colon, and spastic bowel. Unlike colitis, IBS does not involve any inflammation and is actually called a "functional disorder" because it presents no obvious, outward signs of disease.

Single Oils: Peppermint.

Blends: Di-Tone.

Supplements: Royaldophilus, I.C.P., and ComforTone.

Take 2-3 drops Di-Tone and 2 drops peppermint in distilled water.

Supplements: Royaldolphilus, Stevia Select, and Mint Condition.

Itching

(See SKIN or FUNGAL INFECTIONS)

Jaundice

(See LIVER)

Jaundice refers to the yellowing of the skin that is a result of a stressed or damaged liver.

Single Oils: Carrot seed, Roman chamomile, German chamomile, and geranium.

Blends: JuvaFlex and Release.

Supplements: Cleansing Trio, Juva Tone, and Rehemogen.

Joint Stiffness and Pain

(See PAIN, ARTHRITIS or CONNECTIVE TISSUE)

Single Oils: Spruce, elemi, Idaho tansy, basil, rosemary cineol, oregano, fir, birch, vetiver,

Blends: PanAway, Aroma Siez, Relieve It, Ortho Sport, and Ortho Ease.

- Black pepper with rosemary, marjoram, lavender, nutmeg, or vetiver.

- Spruce with sandalwood, fir, hyssop, lemongrass, birch, helichrysum, German chamomile, Idaho tansy, or vetiver.

Recipe 1:
- 10 drops black pepper
- 2 drops rosemary
- 5 drops marjoram
- 5 drops lavender

Mix in 1/2 oz. V-6 Mixing Oil or Massage Oil Base.

Recipe 2 (Pain Relief):
- 8 drops spruce
- 8 drops sandalwood
- 7 drops fir
- 5 drops hyssop
- 4 drops lemongrass
- 5 drops helichrysum
- 4 drops birch
- 2 drops blue chamomile
- 3 drops vetiver
- 1 drop Idaho tansy

Mix in 1/2 to 1 oz. V-6 Mixing Oil or Massage Oil Base.

Supplements: Sulfurzyme, Power Meal, Ultra Young.

Juvenile Dwarfism

The essential oil *Conyza canadensis* was used by Daniel Pénoël, M.D., in his clinical practice for reversing retarded maturation. This essential oil is included in Ultra Young.

Blends: Brain Power.

Brain Power stimulates the limbic system.

Supplements: Ultra Young.

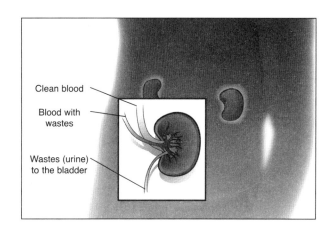

Clean blood

Blood with wastes

Wastes (urine) to the bladder

Kidney Disorders

The kidneys remove waste products from the blood, control blood pressure, and create red blood cells. The kidneys filter over 200 quarts of blood each day and remove over 2 quarts of waste products and water which flow into the bladder as urine through tubes called ureters

Strong kidneys are essential for good health. Inefficient or damaged kidneys can result in wastes accumulating in the blood and causing serious damage.

High blood pressure can be a cause and a result of chronic kidney failure, since kidneys are central to blood regulation (see BLOOD PRESSURE).

Symptoms of poor kidney function:

- Infrequent or inefficient urinations.

- Swelling, especially around the ankles.

- Labored breathing due to fluid accumulation in chest.

Impaired Kidney Function

Single Oils:

- Juniper with lemongrass (to strengthen and tone the kidneys).

A Quick Way To Strengthen the Kidneys

- Take 3 droppers K & B Tincture in 4 oz. distilled water, 3 times daily.
- Drink 8 oz. water with about 10 percent cranberry juice and the juice of 1/2 lemon.
- Drink plenty of other liquids, preferably distilled water.

Kidney Stones

A kidney stone is a solid piece of material that forms in the kidney from mineral or protein-breakdown products in the urine. Occasionally, larger stones can become trapped in a ureter, bladder, or urethra, which can block urine flow cause intense pain.

There are four types of kidney stones: Stones made from calcium (the most common type), stones made from magnesium and ammonia (a struvite stone), stones made from uric acid, and stones made from cystine (the most rare).

Some of the symptoms of kidney stones include:

- Persistent, penetrating pain in side
- A burning sensation during urination
- Blood in the urine
- Bad-smelling or cloudy urine

It is important to drink plenty of water (at least 12 eight-ounce glasses daily) to help pass or dissolve a kidney stone.

Single Oils:

- Geranium with juniper and eucalyptus.
- Helichrysum with fennel.
- Rosemary with juniper, geranium, or lemongrass.

Recipe 1:
- 1 drop rosemary
- 1 drop geranium
- 1 drop juniper
- 1 Tbsp. honey
- 1/2 lemon
- 8 oz. distilled water

Dilute in vegetable oil or soy milk. (Follow with 8 oz. distilled water.) Take 3 times daily until kidney stones pass.

Supplements: Juvatone, K & B, Megazyme, ComforTone.

Start by cleansing colon and liver with Cleansing Trio and JuvaTone. Begin with 1 tablet of JuvaTone, 3 times daily for the first week. Increase to 2-3 tablets, 3 times daily during the second week. For the next 90 days use 3-6 tablets, 3 times daily.

During this cleanse:

- Take one dropper K & B tincture every 2 hours
- Drink two quarts of Goji Tea every 2 hours.

Recipe 2:
- 10 drops juniper
- 10 drops geranium
- 10 drops lemongrass or eucalyptus

Apply as a hot compress on kidneys once a day, and massage juniper and geranium on bottom of the feet twice a day.

Recipe 3:
- 10 drops rosemary
- 10 drops juniper
- 10 drops geranium
- 1 tsp. honey
- Juice of 1 whole lemon
- 8 oz. distilled water

Recipe 4:
- Take 2 Tbsp. olive oil in 8 oz. apple juice, 2 to 3 times daily until the stone passes or take carrot seed oil.

Diuretic (To Increase Urine Flow)

Single Oils:

- Rosemary cineol, tangerine, clove, juniper, fennel, eucalyptus radiata, grapefruit, geranium, or sage.

- Lemongrass with juniper, fennel, rosemary, geranium, or marjoram.

Blends: JuvaFlex.

- Birch with EndoFlex, Di-Tone, or Acceptance.

- Lemongrass with EndoFlex.

Massage over the kidney area or apply a compress.

Supplements: K & B Tincture, Cleansing Trio, JuvaTone.

Skin Care: Cel-Lite Magic Massage Oil

NOTE: Do not use fennel longer than 10 days at a time, since it excessively increases flow through the urinary tract.

Edema (Swelling)

Swelling—particularly around the ankles—is noticeable when fluids accumulate in the tissue. This puffiness under the skin and around the ankles is more apparent at the end of the day when fluids settle to the lowest part of the body. A potassium deficiency can worsen swelling, so the first recourse is to increase potassium intake with high potassium foods and supplements such as Essential Manna and Super Cal.

Single Oils:

- Tangerine with cypress or orange.

- Cypress with tangerine, juniper, orange, lemon, fennel, geranium, or cedarwood.

Blends: Aroma Life.

- Tangerine or lavender with orange, grapefruit, lemon, cypress, juniper, basil, fennel, or marjoram.

- Cypress with fennel, juniper, helichrysum, or lemongrass, EndoFlex, or Di-Tone.

- Birch with rosemary, juniper, eucalyptus radiata, fennel, geranium, or EndoFlex.

Case History

It was reported that a man who had a heart bypass used a vein removed from his leg. The leg swelled up from fluid retention and could be moved around like jelly. The leg was first massaged from the foot up with 4 drops cypress mixed into Cel-Lite Magic Massage Oil. The massage was repeated with 4 drops each of fennel and geranium mixed into the same massage oil. After 20 minutes of massaging the swelling had dissipated.

- Sage with cypress, tangerine, lemongrass, fennel, orange, Citrus Fresh, or Cel-Lite Magic.

- Lavender with Citrus Fresh, Aroma Life, or EndoFlex.

Recipe 1:
- 10 drops tangerine
- 5 drops cypress
- 10 drops lemon or 3 drops juniper

Recipe 2:
- 10 drops birch
- 6 drops fennel
- 2 drops tansy
- 3 drops patchouly
- 10 drops tangerine

Mix in 1/2 to 1 oz. V-6 Mixing Oil or Massage Oil Base and massage into affected area. Rub on bladder Vita Flex area.

Recipe 3: alleviate fluid retention.
- 1 drop lemon
- 1 drop tangerine

Take two drops twice a day as a dietary supplement.

Recipe 4: (morning)
- 10 drops tangerine
- 10 drops cypress

Recipe 5: (evening)
- 8 drops geranium
- 5 drops cypress
- 5 drops helichrysum

Detoxifing the Kidneys

The Chinese Wolfberry has been used in China for centuries as a kidney tonic and detoxifier. Essential oils can also assist in the detoxification due to their unique lipid-soluble properties.

Blends:

- Helichrysum with juniper or fennel.

- Helichrysum with Di-Tone, JuvaFlex or EndoFlex.

Place 1-3 drops in water and take as a dietary supplement three times a day. Apply as a compress over kidneys and bladder

Supplements: K & B tincture, Cleansing Trio, JuvaTone, VitaGreen, Goji Berry Tea, and Sulfurzyme.

Mix in 1/2 oz. V-6 Mixing Oil or Massage Oil Base. Rub on legs from the feet up the legs in the morning. Seal with Cel-Lite Magic Massage Oil.

Supplements: Essential Manna, Super Cal, Super C, K & B, Master Formula vitamins.

Infection in Kidneys

Damage to the glomeruli (tiny filtering units in the kidneys) caused by bacterial infections is called *pyelonephritis*. To reduce infection, drink a gallon of water mixed with cranberry juice daily and use the following products:

Single Oils: Myrrh, cypress, juniper.

Blends: Thieves.

- Cypress or marjoram with Thieves, JuvaFlex, or Inspiration.

- Juniper with EndoFlex.

Place 1-3 drops in water and take as a dietary supplement three times a day. Apply as a compress over kidneys and bladder as well as the corresponding Vita Flex points on the feet.

Recipe 1 – Kidney Compress:
- 5 drops juniper
- 5 drops tangerine
- 3 drops geranium
- 1 drop helichrysum

Massage or apply a compress over the kidneys for one night. The following night place an ImmuPower compress over kidneys, while rubbing the kidney Vita Flex points on the feet.

Supplements: K & B tincture.

Take 3 droppers 3 times daily.

Inflammation in the Kidneys (Nephritis)

Kidney inflammation can be caused by structural components, such as poor diet, or bacterial infection from *Escherichia coli, Staphylococcus aureus, Enterobacter,* and *Klebsiellabacteri* bacteria.

Abnormal proteins trapped in the glomeruli can also cause inflammation and damage to these tiny filtering units. This is called *glomerulonephritis*. This disease can be acute (flaring up in a few days), or chronic (taking months or years to develop). The mildest forms may not show any symptoms except through a urine test. At more advanced stages, urine appears smokey (as small amounts of blood are passed) and eventually red as more blood is excreted—the signs of impending kidney failure.

Symptoms:
- Feeling of unwellness
- Drowsiness
- Nauseous
- Smokey or red-colored urine

Blends:

- Aroma Life with JuvaFlex, cypress, or juniper.

Supplements: K & B Tincture, Master Formula Vitamins, VitaGreen, ImmuneTune, Radex, Super C, and Rehemogen.

Phase I:
Perform a colon and liver cleanse

Phase II: Daily Regimen:
- 4 servings of Power Meal and 6 VitaGreen
- 3 droppers Rehemogen 3 times daily.
- 1/2 gallon Goji Tea.
- Apply Aroma Life and JuvaFlex over the kidneys, on kidney Vita Flex points of the feet, and around the navel.
- After 10 days add ImmuneTune, Radex, and Super C.

Phase III:

Drink a gallon of water mixed with cranberry juice daily.

Ureter Infections

(See KIDNEY INFECTIONS)

The ureter is the duct from the kidney to the bladder.

Single Oils: Lemon and myrtle.

Knee Cartilage Injury

(See CONNECTIVE TISSUE, SPRAINS, AND TENDONITIS)

Single Oils: Peppermint

• Lavender with lemongrass, marjoram, or ginger.

Recipe 1:
• 9 drops lemongrass
• 10 drops marjoram
• 12 drops ginger

Mix in 2 oz. V-6 Mixing Oil or Massage Oil Base. Massage 3 times daily.

For swelling, elevate and apply ice packs.

Leukemia

(See CANCER)

Leg Ulcers

(See SKIN DISORDERS)

Liver

The liver is one of the most important organs in the body, playing a major role in helping the body detoxify. When the liver is damaged due to excess alcohol consumption, viral hepatitis, or poor diet, an excess of toxins can build up in the blood and tissues that can result in degenerative disease and death.

Symptoms of stress or diseased liver include:

• Jaundice (abnormal yellow color of the skin). This may by the only visible sign of liver disease.

How to Protect Your Liver

• Avoid alcoholic beverages.

• Avoid unnecessary use of prescription drugs. Even some common over-the-counter pain relievers can have toxic effects on the liver in moderately high doses.

• Avoid mixing pharmaceutic drugs. Be especially cautious in mixing prescription drugs with alcohol.

• Avoid exposure to industrial chemicals whenever possible.

• Eat a healthy diet.

• The Chinese wolfberry (Ningxia variety) is widely used in China as a liver tonic and detoxifier.

• Nausea

• Loss of appetite

• Dark-colored urine

• Yellowish or grey-colored bowel movements

• Abdominal pain or ascites, a swelling of the abdomen caused by an accumulation of fluid

• Itching, dermatitis, or hives

• Disturbed sleep caused by the build up of unfiltered toxins in blood

• General fatigue and loss of energy

• Lack of sex drive

Detoxification of Liver and Gall Bladder

Single Oils: Helichrysum, mandarin, cardamom, geranium, and carrot seed (vegetable oil).

• Helichrysum with German chamomile, Roman chamomile, sage, geranium, Idaho tansy, blue tansy, or patchouly.

• German chamomile with cedarwood, orange, rosemary, or Roman chamomile.

• Rosemary with ravensara, geranium, German chamomile, Roman chamomile, frankincense, Idaho tansy, thyme, dill, helichrysum, or mandarin.

- Rosemary or sage with JuvaFlex or Di-Tone.

- Sage with geranium, German chamomile, Roman chamomile, frankincense, or thyme.

Take 1-3 drops daily as a dietary supplement.

Blends: JuvaFlex.

- Helichrysum with Di-Tone, JuvaFlex, EndoFlex.

Take 1-3 drops daily as a dietary supplement. Apply Acceptance topically over liver.

Supplements: JuvaTone, Rehemogen, Chelex, Sulfurzyme, Cleansing Trio, Power Meal.

Recipe 1:
- 2 drops German chamomile
- 3 drops helichrysum
- 10 drops orange
- 5 drops rosemary

Mix in 1 oz. massage oil or V-6 Mixing Oil or

French research has shown that helichrysum dilates the liver ducts and facilitates the release of toxins and poisons from the system.

JuvaTone amplifies the effect of Rehemogen and helps with liver regeneration.

Massage Oil Base. Apply over liver.

Recipe 2:
- 2 drops Roman chamomile
- 2 drops German chamomile

Massage over Vita Flex points on bottom of feet.

Hepatitis

Viral hepatitis is a serious, life-threatening disease of the liver which results in scarring (cirrhosis) and eventual organ destruction and death. There are several different kinds of hepatitis: Hepatitis A (spread by contaminated food, water, or feces) and hepatitis B and C (spread by contaminated blood or semen).

Symptoms include jaundice, weakness, loss of appetite, nausea, brownish or tea colored urine, abdominal discomfort, fever and whitish bowel movements.

Begin colon and liver cleanse with Cleaning Trio. After 3 days add JuvaTone.

Single Oils:
- Rosemary with ravensara, geranium, German chamomile, Roman chamomile, frankincense, Idaho tansy, or thyme.
- Sage with geranium, German chamomile, Roman chamomile, frankincense, thyme, clove, or myrrh.

Blends:
- Rosemary verbenon or sage with JuvaFlex, Di-Tone, Release, ImmuPower, or Thieves.

Supplements: Royaldophilus, Master Formula Vitamins, VitaGreen, JuvaTone, ImmuneTune, Super C, Radex, ImmuGel, and Rehemogen.

Daily Program:
- Super C: 6 tablets, 3 times daily.
- Radex: 3 tablets, 3 times daily.
- ImmuGel:1/2 tsp., 2 to 3 times daily.
- VitaGreen: 2 to 6 capsules, 3 times daily, according to blood type.
- Royaldophilus: 1-2 capsules at breakfast and bedtime.
- Master Formula vitamins: 2 to 6 tablets, 3 times daily, according to blood type.
- Exodus: 4 tablets, 4 times daily.

Additional treatment:

Apply a hot compress of JuvaFlex over the liver. Rub 3-4 drops of Release on the bottom of the feet and alternate once a day with JuvaFlex.

Rub ImmuPower, Exodos II, or Thieves up the spine or use Raindrop application method twice daily.

Rub Thieves on the feet, dilute in V-6 Mixing Oil or Massage Oil Base and rub on carotid arteries in the neck and behind the ears (carotid arteries are an excellent place to apply oils for fast absorption).

Ravensara is quite specific for hepatitis.

Note: Do not mix with citrus juices.

Royaldophilus is good for viral conditions.

Rehemogen cleans and fortifies the blood.

Vomiting Bile

Blends: JuvaFlex: rub around navel.

Supplements: JuvaTone and Megazyme.

Liver Cancer

(See CANCER)

Liver Spots (Senile lentigenes)

(See SKIN DISORDERS)

Single Oils: Idaho tansy.

Lou Gehrig's Disease (ALS)

(See NEUROLOGICAL DISEASES)

Supplements: JuvaTone, Chelex, Power Meal, Ultra Young, and water create a better firing of the synapse.

Lumbago (Lower Back Pain)

(See SPINE)

Lupus

Lupus is an autoimmune disease characterized by several different varieties: *Lupus vulgaris* and *Lupus erythematosus* (discoid and systemic).

- *Lupus vulgaris* is characterized by tuberculosis of the skin. Brownish lesions may form on the face and become ulcerous and form scars.

- *Lupus erythematosus* (discoid) is characterized by scaly red patches on the skin and oval or butterfly-shaped lesions on the face. It is milder than the systemic type.

- Systemic *Lupus erythematosus* is more serious than discoid lupus. It inflames the connective tissue in any part of the body, including the joints, muscles, skin, blood vessels, the membranes surrounding the lungs and heart, and sometimes the kidneys and brain.

Because lupus is an autoimmune diseaase, it has been successfully treated using MSM, a form of organic sulfur.

Single Oils: Cypress and lemongrass.

Blends: ImmuPower, Valor, EndoFlex, Joy, Acceptance, and Present Time.

Recipe:
- 30 drops cypress
- 30 drops lemongrass
- 30 drops EndoFlex

Mix in 4 oz. V-6 Mixing Oil or Massage Oil Base. Massage entire body daily.

Supplements: Sulfurzyme.

Daily Regimen:

1. EndoFlex: Add 30 drops to Bath Gel Base and use in bathwater. Soak for 30 minutes.

2. EndoFlex: Massage on bottom of the feet and follow with Thieves two hours later.

3. ImmuPower: Massage 10-15 drops on liver and feet 2-3 times daily.

4. Sulfurzyme: 1-2 Tbsp., 1-2 times daily.

5. Super Cal: 2-3 capsules, 2-3 times daily.

6. ImmuneTune: 2-4 capsules, 2-3 times daily.

7. Megazyme: 2-6 tablets, 2-3 times daily.

8. VitaGreen: 2-4 capsules, 2-3 times daily,

9. Support adrenals (See ADRENAL GLAND IMBALANCES)

Lyme Disease - Rocky Mountain Spotted Fever

Caused by the bite of an infected tick.

Blends: PanAway, Melrose, Thieves, Exodus II, and ImmuPower.

Supplements: Body Balance, Power Meal, ImmuneTune, Radex, and Exodus, Thyromin.

Colon and liver cleanse: Cleansing Trio.

Body Balance provides the minerals and enzymes necessary to fight the disease.

(See TICK BITES under INSECT BITES)

Lymphatic System

Single Oils:

- Sandalwood with helichrysum, myrtle, lemon, grapefruit, lemongrass, rosemary, lavender, or rose.

- Cypress with helichrysum, bergamot, grapefruit, lemon, orange, tangerine, rosemary, thyme, or lavender.

- Lemongrass or sage with helichrysum, lemon, grapefruit, basil, cypress, rosemary, spruce, lavender, or tangerine.

Blends:

- Helichrysum with Di-Tone, JuvaFlex, EndoFlex, Thieves, Acceptance, or Raven.

- Cypress with Citrus Fresh or Aroma Life.

- Lemongrass or sage with Citrus Fresh or En-R-Gee.

Massage oils on sore spots.

Then apply Cel-Lite Magic and essential oils, such as grapefruit and cypress. Grapefruit and cypress help to digest chemicals stored in body fat. This encourages the body to discharge chemicals and stimulate the lymphatic system.

Helichrysum is a powerful lymphatic decongestant. Others are grapefruit, myrtle, orange, tangerine, lemon, cypress, and lemongrass. Experiment by massaging other oils in the manner stated above, to find which gives the best relief.

Mix 1 or 2 drops of the oil or oil blend that works best in V-6 Mixing Oil or Massage Oil Base and massage under the arms to stimulate lymphatics. Thieves is good for this purpose but should always be diluted.

Lymphatic Cleanse:
- 3 drops cypress
- 1 drop orange
- 2 drops grapefruit

Mix in 1/2 gallon distilled water. Grade C maple syrup may be added. Drink daily.

Supplements and Skin Care: Cel-Lite Magic Massage Oil, Morning Start Bath Gel, Super C, Radex, ImmuGel, Royal Essence, VitaGreen, and Goji Berry Tea.

Colon and liver cleanse: Cleansing Trio.

Goji Berry Tea helps cleanse the lymphatic system.

Lymphoma

(See CANCER)

M.C.T. (Mixed Connective Tissue Disease)

M.C.T. is an autoimmune disease similar to lupus in which the connective tissue in the body becomes inflamed and achy. This condition is usually due to poor assimilation of protein and mineral deficiencies.

Single Oils:

- Rosemary with nutmeg and clove.

- Lemongrass with marjoram or peppermint.

- Basil with birch, cypress, or peppermint.

Blends: ImmuPower, Valor, Present Time, Joy, and Acceptance.

Recipe 1 (aches and discomfort):
- 10 drops basil
- 8 drops birch
- 6 drops cypress
- 3 drops peppermint

Apply neat on location, massage larger areas mixed with V-6 Mixing Oil or Massage Oil Base. Use Raindrop Technique.

Rub ImmuPower over the liver and on liver Vita Flex Points on the bottom of the right foot. This has been reported to help lupus, which is similar to M.C.T. (see LUPUS).

Joy and Acceptance help overcome impressions of low self-worth, low self-esteem, and self-distrust that come with disease.

Adrenal support:
- 3 drops clove
- 3 drops nutmeg
- 7 drops rosemary
- 20 drops Massage Oil or V-6 Mixing Oil.

Use as a hot compress over the adrenal glands

Supplements: ImmuGel, Master Formula, Super C, Super B, VitaGreen, ImmuneTune, ArthroTune, Super Cal, Thyromin.

Regimen:

1. Avoid acid-ash foods. Instead, use alkaline foods, such as barley or wheat sprouts.

2. VitaGreen: 2-6 capsules, 3 times daily.

3. Use Cleansing Trio to expel toxins. Avoid contact with or use of cigarettes, cleaning products, chemicals and chemical-using industries (auto garages, paint shops, etc.)

4. Build the body:

- Super C: 1-3 tablets, 2-3 times daily.
- Super Cal: 2-4 capsules, 1-2 times daily.
- ImmuneTune: 2-4 capsules, 2-3 times daily.
- Super B: 1 tablet, 3-4 times weekly.
- Master Formula: 3-6 tablets, 2-3 times daily.
- ArthroTune: 2-3 capsules, 2-3 times daily.

Malaria

Malaria is a serious disease contracted from several species of *Anopheles* mosquitos. While malaria is largely confined to the continent of Africa, an increasing number of cases have arisen in the U.S. If not treated, malaria can be fatal.

Symptoms:
- Fever
- Chills
- Anemia

The best defense against malaria is to use insect repellents effective against *Anopheles* mosquitoes. Once a person has contracted the disease, oils such as lemon can help amplify immune response.

Single Oils: Lemon.

Add lemon oil and honey to water and sip when attack is impending.

(See INSECT REPELLENT and INSECT BITES)

Measles

Single Oils:

- Lavender with Roman chamomile, melaleuca, or German chamomile.

Recipe 1:
- 15 drops lavender
- 15 drops Roman chamomile
- 5 drops melaleuca

Mix 4 drops into 1 pint of water, shake well, and sponge child down once a day.

Recipe 2:
- 5 drops lavender
- 5 drops German chamomile

Blend in 4 oz. of body lotion and dab on spots.

Recipe 3:
- 2 drops lavender
- 1 drop Roman chamomile

Add to 1 cup Epsom salts and use in bath or shower. The RainSpa shower head has a specially designed chamber that can be filled with essential oils and bath salts. As the water passes through the mixture, it disperses the oils into the spray, creating an antiseptic spa.

Memory

(See BRAIN DISORDERS)

Menopause (Premenstrual Syndrome)

PMS is one of the most common hormone-related conditions in otherwise healthy women. Women can experience a wide range of symptoms for 10 to 14 days before menstruation, and even 2 to 3 days into menstruation. These symptoms include mood swings, fatigue, headaches, breast tenderness, abdominal bloating, anxiety, depression, confusion, memory loss, sugar cravings, cramps, low back pain, irritability, weight gain, acne, and oily skin and hair. Causes include hormonal, nutritional, psychological, and stress of the Western culture.

Single Oils: Clary sage, sage, fennel, vitex

- Basil with clary sage, sage, fennel, bergamot, rosemary, rose, neroli, ylang ylang, peppermint, tarragon, spikenard, vitex, marjoram, or hyssop.

- Sage with clary sage, fennel, basil, bergamot, yarrow, German chamomile, Roman chamomile, pine, anise, or orange. Lavender and geranium are secondary.

Blends: Dragon Time, Mister, EndoFlex

- Basil or Aroma Siez with Dragon Time, Mister, EndoFlex, Acceptance, or Exodus II.

- Sage or EndoFlex with Mister.

Essential oils can be diffused or diluted in V-6 Mixing Oil or Massage Oil Base and applied topically.

Supplements: Master Formula vitamins, FemiGen, Thyromin, VitaGreen, Estro tincture, Femalin, Royal Essence, Super B, Super Cal, Mineral Essence, A.D.&E., Ultra Young, ImmuneTune, and Thyromin.

How Pollutants Contribute to Cancer

The pollutants to which we are exposed accumulate in tissues such as the breasts, thyroid, ovaries, and uterus. Some of these chemicals can mimic or imitate natural hormones, thereby activating hormone receptors that over-stimulate glands. This can increase the risk of hormone-dependent cancers, such as breast and uterine cancer.

Rub 2 to 6 drops of Dragon Time, Mister or EndoFlex on reproductive Vita Flex areas on hands and feet. Some people have had results applying to the crown of head and forehead. Also apply on the groin and across the lower back. Hot compresses can be added if needed.

Put 1 drop of EndoFlex on the tongue and roof of the mouth or apply as above. For hot flashes, apply oils on feet, solar plexus, tongue, and crown of head.

Sage, fennel, and clary sage have an estrogen-like action that helps improve estrogen, progesterone, and testosterone balance.

One drop bergamot and 1 drop geranium may help hormone balance.

Recipe 1 (Hormone Balance):
- 10 drops basil
- 10 drops marjoram
- 8 drops hyssop
- 4 drops helichrysum
- 6 drops ylang ylang

Mix in 1 oz. V-6 Mixing Oil or Massage Oil Base.

Hormone Imbalance

Femalin is designed to harmonize female hormone levels.

FemiGen can be used up to 6 times a day, particularly during menstrual periods. Vitamins B6 and B12 are important for hormonal balance, so adequate B vitamins are required. Super B is a good source of all B vitamins.

Royal Essence helps hormonal balance and increases energy. Take 1 dropper in distilled water or directly under the tongue for the fastest results.

For cramping before and during the cycle, make a blend of 10 drops Dragon Time and 4 drops basil. Rub around your ankles, lower back and stomach. A week after cycle ends, take Master HERS along with VitaGreen.

Body Balance contains soy which helps balance hormones and activate (estrogen) receptors. Take Body Balance at least once a day.

Endometriosis

This is when the uterine lining develops outside of the uterus; for example, on the outer wall of the uterus, on the ovaries, fallopian tubes, vagina, intestines, or on the abdominal wall. These fragments cannot escape like the normal uterine lining, which is shed during menstruation. Because of this, fibrous cysts often form around the misplaced uterine tissue. Symptoms can include abdominal or back pain during menstruation or pain that often increases after the period is over. Other symptoms may include heavy periods and pain during intercourse.

Single Oils: Fennel

Blends: Melrose and Thieves.

Supplements: ImmuGel, Super C, Femalin, and Protec.

Regimen:

• Douche with Femalin or Protec.

• Colon and liver cleanse: Cleansing Trio.

• Hot compress of Melrose on the stomach.

• Apply Thieves to bottom of the feet.

Menstrual Cramps - Irregular Periods

Single Oils:

• Rosemary with basil, clary sage, sage, marjoram, lavender, Roman chamomile, cypress, tarragon, vitex, or Idaho tansy.

Sage promotes menstrual discharges.

Apply oils on the abdomen or to the reproductive Vita Flex points on the hands and feet. Hot compresses may be used.

Blends: Dragon Time and EndoFlex.

Recipe 1 (Period regulator):
• 5 drops peppermint
• 9 drops *Conyza canadensis*
• 16 drops clary sage
• 11 drops sage
• 5 drops jasmine

Mix in 1/2 to 1 oz. massage oil or V-6 Mixing Oil or Massage Oil Base.

Recipe 2:
• 10 drops chamomile
• 10 drops fennel

Mix in 1 oz. V-6 Mixing Oil or Massage Oil Base.

Apply clary sage around ankles.

Recipe 3:
• 3 drops helichrysum
• 1/2 tsp. cayenne
• 6 oz. water

Mix well.

Supplements: FemiGen and Estro.

When migraine headaches accompany periods, a colon and liver cleanse may reduce symptoms.

Excessive Bleeding

• 10 drops geranium or helichrysum

Mix in 1 tsp. V-6 Mixing Oil or Massage Oil Base; rub around ankles, lower back, and stomach.

Hysterectomy

Supplements: FemiGen.

Mental Fatigue

Single Oils: Pepper, peppermint, rosemary cineol, basil, spearmint, and pine.

Blends: Clarity, En-R-Gee, Sacred Mountain, Live With Passion, Motivation, and Valor.

Supplements: Ultra Young, VitaGreen, Super B, Royal Essence, Mineral Essence, and Thyromin.

Mold

Single Oils: Cedarwood, Lemongrass, Lemon, Thyme, and Oregano

Blends: Purification and Thieves.

Mononucleosis

Single Oils:

• Ravensara with hyssop and frankincense.

Blends:

• Thyme or ravensara and mountain savory with Thieves or R.C.

Supplements: ImmuGel and Super C.

Colon and liver cleanse: Cleansing Trio.

Add ImmuGel and Super C to build the immune system.

Recipe 1:
- 3 drops Thieves
- 3 drops thyme
- 3 drops mountain savory
- 2 drops ravensara

Rub over bottom of feet.

Morning Sickness

(See NAUSEA)

Massage 1 drop of Di-Tone on outer ear or on abdomen.

Motion Sickness

Single Oils:

- Lavender, peppermint, ginger, juniper, rosemary, tarragon, spearmint.

Blends:

- Lavender, Di-Tone, Harmony, JuvaFlex.

Lavender can be combined with any other single oil or blend.

Place 1 drop on the end of the tongue or around the navel and on the thymus or rub behind the ears (on the mastoid). Diffuse or mix in water and sip slowly.

Supplements: Mint Condition and Megazyme.

Mucus (Excess)

Most oils help tissues expel mucus. Using the oils both topically and by diffusing will get them into the tissues to help rid the body of excess mucus. If congestion occurs while inhaling a diffused oil, this is the oil to help your body release and discharge mucus. An expectorant discharges mucus, soft and hard plaque, and toxins out of the body.

Single Oils: Frankincense, lavender, hyssop, helichrysum, fennel, eucalyptus, cypress, German chamomile, marjoram, mugwort, myrtle, pepper, patchouly, ravensara, rosemary, and sage.

Blends: Di-Tone, 3 Wise Men, Raven, R.C., and Purification.

Inhale or diffuse. Selected oils and blends can be take as dietary supplements. (See Appendix C)

Lavender and chamomile help to reduce the over-production of mucus. Apply on the thoracic vertebrae, T4 and T5 (at the neck-to-shoulder intersection). Also apply on bottom of the feet to slow down the parasympathetic system and thus reduce the over-production of mucus.

Multiple Sclerosis (MS)

(See NEUROLOGICAL DISEASES)

Mumps (Infectious perotitis)

Single Oils: Thyme, linalol, melissa, myrrh, cypress, and birch.

Dilute essential oils in vegetable oil for oral or topical use.

These oils can be diluted in water and absorbed in a cloth soaked in the muxture to create a compress to be placed around the face of the person with mumps.

Blends: R.C., Raven, Thieves, and Exodus II.

Supplements: ImmuGel, Dentarome Plus, Fresh Essence, Super C, and Exodus.

Muscles (Sore, Spasmed, or Pulled)

Bruised Muscles (see BRUISING)

To avoid excess blood clotting in a bruised muscle or tissue, increase circulation and slow blood clot formation by using cypress and helichrysum.

Single Oils: Myrrh, Roman chamomile, helichrysum, cypress, and lavender

- Birch with marjoram, basil, cypress, rosemary, vetiver, peppermint, spruce, fir, and oregano.

Blends: Aroma Siez, PanAway, Ortho Sport, Ortho Ease.

- Birch with Aroma Siez, PanAway, and Peace & Calming.

Apply neat or mix V-6 Mixing Oil or Massage Oil Base and massage on location.

When a bruise displays black and blue discoloration and pain, start with helichrysum,

---

For Tired, Fatigued Muscles

Tired muscles may be lacking in minerals such as calcium and magnesium. Super Cal, Essential Manna, and Mineral Essence are excellent sources of both trace and macro minerals and good for all muscle conditions. ArthroTune helps reduce stiffness from sitting for long periods.

---

birch, and oregano. Once the pain and inflammation decrease, use cypress, then basil with Aroma Siez to enhance the muscle relaxation. Follow with peppermint to stimulate the nerves and reduce inflammation. Follow with cold packs.

Supplements: ArthroTune, Super Cal, Mineral Essence, Essential Manna.

To Build Muscles

PanAway or birch with spruce, Be-Fit, or Power Meal.

Cramps and Charley Horses

Magnesium and calcium deficiency may contribute to muscle cramps and charley horses.

Single Oils:

- Rosemary with basil, clary sage, vetiver, cypress, marjoram, lavender, elemi or German chamomile.

Blends: Aroma Siez, Relieve It, Ortho Ease and Ortho Sport

- Rosemary with Aroma Siez or Relieve It.

Apply neat or mix V-6 Mixing Oil or Massage Oil Base and massage on location.

Supplements: Super Cal, ArthroTune, Mineral Essence, Essential Manna.

ArthroTune: 2-3 capsules morning and night help reduce night leg cramp.

Inflammation Due to Injury

Tissue damage is usually accompanied by inflammation. By reducing inflammation by massaging with anti-inflammatory oils, tissue damage is reduced.

Single oils (in order of activity): peppermint, German chamomile, hyssop, myrrh, birch, marjoram, ravensara, lavender, and Roman chamomile.

Recipe 1:
- 12 drops fir
- 10 drops melaleuca
- 8 drops lavender
- 6 drops marjoram
- 3 drops yarrow
- 3 drops spearmint
- 2 drops peppermint

Mix in 1 oz. V-6 Mixing Oil or Massage Oil Base and massage on location.

Inflammation Due to Infection or Virus

Single Oils: Ravensara, hyssop.

Apply neat (except oregano) or mix in V-6 Mixing Oil or Massage Oil Base and massage on location.

Pain in Muscle

Single Oils: Rosemary, nutmeg, black pepper, basil, spruce, juniper, birch, lemon, rosemary, lavender, and fir.

- Birch with basil or marjoram.

- Basil with marjoram, cypress, ginger, peppermint, spruce, vetiver, lavender or lemongrass.

- Rosemary with basil, marjoram, cypress, lemon, clary sage, lavender, German chamomile, Roman chamomile, ginger, vetiver, or elemi.

Blends: Valor, Peace & Calming, En-R-Gee, Passion, Clarity, Ortho Ease, or Ortho Sport.

- Basil with Aroma Siez, PanAway, R.C., Relieve It, or M-Grain.

- Rosemary with Aroma Siez or Clarity.

Apply Valor on bottom of feet, Peace & Calming on back of neck, and Clarity on crown of head.

Recipe 1:
- 4 drops juniper
- 5 drops birch
- 4 drops lemon
- 2 drops rosemary
- 5 drops lavender

Mix in 1 oz. V-6 Mixing Oil or Massage Oil Base.

Supplements: Arthro Plus, Super Cal, ArthroTune, Royal Essence, Mineral Essence, Power Meal, Sulfurzyme, VitaGreen, and Ultra Young.

Apply Ortho Ease Massage Oil to areas where muscles are over-exercised. This lessens the possibility of tearing or other damage.

How to Make Your Own High-Powered Massage Oil

Add these formulas to 4 oz. of V-6 Mixing Oil or Massage Oil Base to create a custom muscle-toning formula.

Recipe 1:
- 10 drops birch
- 10 drops peppermint
- 10 drops marjoram
- 8 drops elemi
- 8 drops vetiver
- 5 drops helichrysum
- 5 drops cypress

Recipe 2:
- 20 drops birch
- 15 drops marjoram
- 10 drops juniper
- 10 drops cypress
- 6 drops spruce

You can add these formulas to 4 oz. of Ortho Ease to strengthen its effects.

Sore Muscles

Blends:
- Lavender with Roman chamomile
- Birch with marjoram
- Aroma Siez

Recipe 3:
- 5 drops rosemary
- 10 drops juniper
- 10 drops lavender
- 10 drops marjoram
- 5 drops vetiver

Recipe 4:
- 9 drops cypress
- 8 drops rosemary
- 8 drops lavender
- 2 drops elemi
- 2 drops valerian

Mix in 2 oz. V-6 Mixing Oil or Massage Oil Base. Massage into the affected area and then apply a hot pack to speed the results.

Recipe 5:
- 5 drops clary sage
- 5 drops lavender
- 5 drops German chamomile
- 3 drops rosemary cineol

Mix in 1 oz. V-6 Mixing Oil or Massage Oil Base. In cold weather, add ginger and rub on knees.

Spasmed Muscles

Blends: Aroma Siez

Alternate cold packs with hot packs as you apply the essential oil. The oil can be applied neat or diluted with vegetable oil.

Tight Muscles

Single Oils: Elemi, birch, marjoram.

Blends: Aroma Siez

Recipe 6:
- 6 drops marjoram
- 4 drops cypress
- 4 drops birch
- 3 drops valerian
- 1 drop helichrysum

Recipe 7:
- 1-2 drops ravensara
- 4-5 drops Aroma Siez
- 1 drop black pepper

Mix in 1 oz. V-6 Mixing Oil or Massage Oil Base and massage on affected areas. Follow with Ortho Ease.

Torn Muscles, Ligaments, or Tendons

Blends: Marjoram, lemongrass, Ortho Sport, and Ortho Ease.

Recipe 8:
- 3 drops basil
- 5 drops Aroma Siez

Mix in 1 oz. V-6 Mixing Oil or Massage Oil Base and massage into affected areas.

General Rules

When selecting oils for injuries, think through the cause and type of injury and select oils for each segment. For instance, whiplash could encompass muscle damage, nerve damage, ligament damage, inflammation, bone injury, and possibly emotion. Select oils for each perceived problem and apply.

Weakness in Muscle

Single Oils:

- Ravensara with lemongrass, juniper, and nutmeg.

Blends: En-R-Gee

Supplements: VitaGreen, Royal Essence, and Power Meal.

To Improve Circulation

Single Oils: Cypress

Recipe 9:
- 5 drops basil
- 8 drops marjoram
- 10 drops cypress
- 3 drops peppermint

Recipe 10:
- 2-3 drops of basil
- 1-2 drops of marjoram
- 1 drop of peppermint

Recipe 11:
- 3 drops basil
- 2 drops peppermint
- 4 drops cypress
- 8 drops marjoram
- 10 drops birch

Best diluted with 1 oz. V-6 Mixing Oil or Massage Oil Base and massaged on location. Follow by massaging general area with Ortho Ease.

To Regenerate Muscle

Recipe 12:
- 8 drops spruce
- 8 drops sandalwood
- 7 drops fir
- 5 drops hyssop
- 4 drops lemongrass
- 5 drops helichrysum
- 4 drops birch
- 2 drops vetiver
- 1 drop Idaho tansy

Mix in 1/2 to 1 oz. V-6 Mixing Oil or Massage Oil Base and apply on location.

Muscular Dystrophy

Single Oils: Marjoram and lemongrass (equal parts of each), pine, and lavender.

Blends: Aroma Siez and Relieve It.

Supplements: Megazyme, Power Meal, Sulfurzyme, VitaGreen, Mineral Essence, Thyromin, Ultra Young, and Ortho Ease, and Ortho Sport Massage Oils.

Nails (brittle or weak)

Poor or weak nails, often containing ridges, indicate a sulfur deficiency.

Single Oils: Frankincense, myrrh, and lemon.

Blends: Citrus Fresh.

Supplements: Sulfurzyme, Super Cal, and Mineral Essence.

Recipe 1:
- 2 drops Wheat Germ Oil
- 2 drops frankincense
- 2 drops myrrh
- 2 drops lemon

Rub on nails twice per week to strengthen nails.

Narcolepsy

Single Oils: Mineral Essence, VitaGreen, Thyromin, BrainPower, and Ultra Young.

Nausea

Patchouli oil contains compounds that are extremely effective in preventing vomiting due to their ability to reduce the gastrointestinal muscle contractions associated with vomiting (Yang et el., 1999)

Single Oils: Peppermint, patchouly, ginger.

Blends: Di-Tone.

Nervous Fatigue

Can cause motor skill problems.

Single Oils: Juniper, geranium, and helichrysum.

- Oregano with thyme, nutmeg, jasmine, and peppermint.

Blends: Brain Power and Clarity.

Neuritis, Neuropathy, Neuralgia

(See NERVE DISORDERS)

Nerve Disorders

Nerve disorders usually involve peripheral or surface nerves and include neuritis, neuropathy, neuralgia, Bell's palsy, and carpal tunnel syndrome. In contrast, neuroligical disorders are usually associated with deep neurological disturbances in the brain, and these conditions include Lou Gehrig's disease, MS, and cerebral palsy. (See NEUROLOGICAL DISEASES)

Single Oils:

- Peppermint with lavender, cedarwood, basil, clary sage, sage, rosemary, spruce, tangerine, sandalwood, melaleuca, ravensara, marjoram, palmarosa, thyme, lemongrass, birch, cypress, and helichrysum.

Blends:

- Lavender with Valor, Peace & Calming, or Citrus Fresh.

Supplements: Sulfurzyme.

Lavender, myrrh, Roman chamomile, marjoram, German chamomile, tangerine, Valor, and Peace & Calming all have a sedative effect on the nervous system.

Recipe 1 (for nerve problems):
- 2 drops peppermint
- 10 drops juniper
- 1 drop geranium
- 8 drops marjoram
- 4 drops helichrysum

Mix neat or in 1 oz. V-6 Mixing Oil or Massage Oil Base and apply.

Supplements: Super Cal, VitaGreen, Sulfurzyme, Power Meal, Super C, and Super B.

Super Cal provides calcium necessary maintain nerve signal transmissions along neurological pathways.

Sulfur deficiency is very prevalent in nerve problems. Sulfur requires calcium and vitamin C for the body to metabolize. Super B and Sulfurzyme work well together to help repair nerve damage and the myelin sheath.

Bell's Palsy

A type of neuritis, marked by paralysis on one side of the face and inability to open or close the eyelid.

Single Oils: Peppermint with helichrysum and juniper.

Blends: Aroma Siez and Relieve It.

Supplements: Ultra Young or AuraLight.

Rub peppermint with helichrysum on the facial nerve, which is in front and behind the ear and on areas of pain.

Carpal Tunnel Syndrome

Nerves pass through a tunnel formed by wrist bones (known as carpals) and a tough membrane on the underside of the wrist that binds the bones together. The tunnel is rigid, so if the tissues within it swell for some reason, they press and pinch the nerves creating a painful condition known as carpal tunnel syndrome. This condition is primarily sports-related or due to activities that involve strenuous or repeated use of wrists. A similar condition can occur in the ankle (tarsal tunnel syndrome), or even the elbow. These two are less common.

Single Oils: Peppermint or basil.

- Birch with cypress, peppermint, marjoram, or basil.

- Helichrysum with birch, lemongrass, cypress, or peppermint.

Blends: PanAway, Relieve It, Ortho Ease, and Ortho Sport.

Best results are achieved by a layered application of PanAway and Relieve It.

Recipe 1:
- 5 drops birch
- 3 drops cypress
- 1 drop peppermint
- 2 drops marjoram
- 3 drops lemongrass

Mix neat or double quantities in 1 oz. V-6 Mixing Oil or Massage Oil Base. Also use ice pack.

Supplements: Super C, Super Cal, Mineral Essence, Essential Manna.

Neuritis, Neuropathy, Neuralgia

Neuritis is a painful inflammation of the peripheral nerves.

Neuropathy refers to actual damage to the peripheral nerves.

Neuralgia is characterized only by recurrent pain along a nerve pathway, without any nerve damage or inflammation. Carpal tunnel syndrome is an example of a neuralgia.

Neuritis is usually caused by prolonged exposure to cold, heavy-metal poisoning, diabetes, vitamin deficiencies (beriberi and pellagra), and infectious diseases such as typhoid fever and malaria.

Symptoms:
- Pain
- Burning
- Numbness or tingling
- Muscle weakness or paralysis

Neuralgia is usually caused by diabetes and vitamin deficiencies.

Symptoms:
- Temporary sharp pain in peripheral nerves

Neuropathy is permanent nerve damage resulting from an impaired blood supply to nerves, usually caused by diabetes, injuries, or bone fractures.

Symptoms:
- Tingling or numbness
- Gangrene

B vitamins and minerals such as, magnesium, calcium, potassium, and organic sulfur (MSM), are the most important minerals and vitamins for repairing nerve damage and quenching pain from inflamed nerves. Super Cal, Super B, and Essential Manna are some of the richest sources of these minerals.

Single Oils: Peppermint.

- Lavender with juniper, oregano, thyme, geranium, peppermint, blue yarrow, or clove.

Blends:

- Lavender with Valor, Aroma Siez, or Peace & Calming.

Diffuse Peace & Calming for any nervous condition. This blend helps to sedate an over-active nervous system. Valor supports the nervous system.

Supplements: Super Cal, Super B, VitaGreen, Sulfurzyme, Essential Manna, and Ultra Young.

Neuralgia

Neuralgia is pain from a damaged nerve. It can occur in the face, spine, or elsewhere.

Single Oils: Marjoram, helichrysum, peppermint, juniper, geranium, laurus nobilis, nutmeg, peppermint, and spearmint.

Nutmeg supports the nervous system to overcome neuralgia.

Blends: PanAway, Relieve It, JuvaFlex

Supplements: Ultra Young, Sulfurzyme, Super B, Chelex, Radex, JuvaTone, and Ortho Ease and Ortho Sport Massage Oils.

Sulfurzyme and Super B work well together to repair nerve damage.

Neuropathy

Damage to peripheral nerves (other than spinal or those in the brain), generally starts as tingling in hands and feet and slowly spreads along limbs to the trunk.

Numbness, sensitive skin, neuralgic pain, weakening of muscle power can all develop in varying degrees. Most common causes include complications from diabetes (diabetic neuropathy), alcoholism, vitamin B12 deficiency, tumors, too many pain killers, exposure and absorption of chemicals, metallics, pesticides and many other causes.

Single Oils:

• Juniper with geranium, helichrysum, peppermint, cypress, or lemongrass.

Blends: JuvaFlex and Brain Power.

Supplements: Super B, Royal Essence, Mineral Essence, Super C, VitaGreen, Body Balance, Master HERS/HIS.

The body should be supported with sufficient minerals and other nutrients.

Recipe 1:
• 10 drops juniper
• 10 drops geranium
• 10 drops helichrysum

Mix in 1/2 oz. V-6 Mixing Oil or Massage Oil Base. Massage on location of tingling or numbness. Also massage cypress with peppermint or lemongrass mixed with body lotion.

Recipe 2:
• 15 drops geranium
• 10 drops helichrysum
• 6 drops cypress
• 10 drops juniper
• 5 drops peppermint

Mix in 2 Tbsp. V-6 Mixing Oil or Massage Oil Base. Apply oils on location and on the feet.

If paralysis is the problem, a regeneration of up to 60 percent may be possible. If, however, the nerve damage is too severe, treatment may not help. When the damage starts to reverse, there will be pain. Apply PanAway on location and on the feet.

If the person does not have diabetes, then toxic overload may be indicated. Cleanse colon and liver with Cleansing Trio.

Nervous System (Autonomic)

The autonomic nervous system controls involuntary activities such as heartbeat, breathing, digestion, glandular activity, and contraction and dilation of blood vessels.

The autonomic nervous system is composed of two parts that balance and complement each other: the parasympathetic and sympathetic nervous systems.

The sympathetic nervous system has stimulatory effects and is responsible for secreting stress hormones such as adrenaline and noradrenaline.

The parasympathetic nervous system has relaxing effects and is responsible for secreting acetylcholine which slows the heart and speeds digestion.

To Stimulate Parasympathetic Nervous System:

Single Oils: Lavender and marjoram.

Blends: Valor and Peace & Calming.

Supplements: AuraLight

To Stimulate Sympathetic Nervous System:

Single Oils: Peppermint, ginger, and pepper.

Blends: Clarity, Magnify Your Purpose, Eucalyptus radiata, Brain Power.

Supplements: Power Meal, Super Cal, Sulfurzyme, Ultra Young, and Mineral Essence.

Neurological Diseases

Juniper promotes nerve function. Frankincense may help clear the emotions of fear and anger, which is common with people who have these neurological diseases. When these diseases are contracted, people often become suicidal.

Hope, Joy, Gathering, and Forgiveness will help work through the psychological and emotional aspects of the disease.

Vitex has been shown to reduce the symptoms of Parkinson's disease by 89 percent in animal studies.

These diseases are mainly caused by metallics in the brain, causing misfiring of neurons (see BRAIN DISORDERS).

Single Oils: Frankincense, helichrysum, oregano, sage, juniper, rosemary, clove, cardamom, and vitex.

Blends: Acceptance, Joy, Gathering, Brain Power, Clarity, and Forgiveness.

NOTE: Never use hot packs on neurological problems. Always use packs to reduce pain and inflammation. In other words, reduce temperature of the damaged site.

Recipe 1:
- 1 drop rosemary
- 1 drop helichrysum
- 1 drop ylang ylang
- 1 drop clove (clove must always be diluted in a vegetable oil)

Put the oils on as directly as is practical. It is most important to apply on the brain on reflex points on the head, forehead, temples and mastoids (the bone just behind the ear). Use direct pressure application to the brainstem along the center of the backbone on the neck at the skull and down the spine. Put the oils on a loofah brush and rub along the spine vigorously.

NOTE: Use a natural bristle brush, since the oils dissolve some plastics.

Apply oils using Raindrop Technique application on the spine.

Supplements: JuvaTone, Ultra Young, Vita-Green, Power Meal, Rehemogen, Chelex, Super Cal, Super C, and Super B.

Sulfur deficiency is very prevalent in these neurological diseases. Sulfur requires calcium and Vitamin C for the body to metabolize. Super B and Sulfurzyme work well together to help repair nerve damage and the myelin sheath.

Alzheimer's Disease

Supplements: Vitagreen (See **Above**)

Huntington's Chorea (Saint Vitus Dance)

A degenerative nerve disease that generally starts in middle age. It is marked by uncontrollable body movements, which are followed—and occasionally preceded—by mental deterioration.

Single Oils:

- Peppermint with juniper or basil.

Blends: Aroma Siez.

Recipe 1:
- 5 drops peppermint
- 10 drops juniper
- 3 drops basil
- 5 drops Aroma Siez

Mix and apply using Raindrop Technique application.

Multiple Sclerosis (MS)

Multiple sclerosis is a progressive, disabling disease of the nervous system (brain and spinal cord) in which inflammation occurs in the central nervous system. Eventually the myelin sheaths protecting the nerves are destroyed, resulting in a slowing or blocking of nerve transmission.

MS is an autoimmune disease, in which the body's own immune system attacks the nerves. Some researchers believe that MS is triggered by a virus, while others make a case that it has a strong genetic or environmental component.

Symptoms:
- Muscle weakness in extremities
- Deteriorating coordination and balance
- Numbness or prickling sensations
- Poor attention or memory
- Speech impediments
- Incontinence
- Tremors
- Dizziness
- Hearing loss

An Easy Way to Treat MS

One of the simplest ways to keep MS symptoms from worsening is by keeping the body cool and avoiding any locations or physical activities which heat the body (including hot showers or exercise). Cold baths and swimming are two of the best activities for relieving symptoms.

Applying heat is the worst thing to do for MS. If an MS patient is suffering a worsening of symptoms, lower their body temperature (by up to 3° F) by lying them on a table, covering them with a sheet, ice, shower curtain, and blankets (in that order). Work the feet with oils and watch for benefits. There have been individuals who have been able to get out of a wheel chair within a few days after treatment.

Single Oils: Juniper, helichrysum, geranium, peppermint, thyme, oregano, birch, cypress, basil, marjoram, and rosemary.

Layer helichrysum, juniper, geranium, and peppermint and apply cold packs for 30 minutes. Reapply cold packs as needed.

Blends: Valor, Aroma Siez, Acceptance, and Awaken.

Apply oils by layering or using Raindrop Technique application. Lightly massage oils in the direction of MS paralysis. For example: If it is lower down the spine, massage down. Follow massage with cold packs.

Apply Valor on spine. If MS affects the leg, rub down the spine; if it affects the neck, rub up the spine.

Juniper promotes nerve function. Apply cypress and juniper as a base layer on back of the neck, then add Aroma Siez.

Recipe 1:
- 10 drops helichrysum
- 10 drops peppermint
- 10 drops rosemary

Mix and apply neat.

To help the person emotionally with the MS symptoms, use Acceptance and Awaken. Be patient. Overcoming MS is a long-term

Risk Factors For MS

MS occurs five times more frequently in colder climates (ie., Northern United States, Canada, and Europe) than in tropical regions.

Moreover, MS almost always occurs between ages 15 and 60, with women being affected twice as often as men. MS is far more common among whites than other races.

endeavor.

Parkinson's Disease

Parkinson's disease involves the deterioration of specific nerve centers in the brain and affects more men than women by a ratio of 3:2. The main symptom is tremors, an involuntary shaking of hands, head, or both. Other symptoms include rigidity, slowed movement, gait disorder, and loss of balance. In many cases these are accompanied by a continuous rubbing together of thumb and forefinger, stooped posture, mask-like face, trouble in swallowing, depression, and difficulty performing simple tasks. These symptoms may all be seen at different stages of the disease. The tremors are most severe when the affected part of the body is not in use. There is no pain or other sensation, other than a decreased ability to move. Symptoms appear slowly, in no particular order and may elapse before they interfere with normal activities.

Single Oils: Juniper, Peppermint, and Vitex.

Blends: Peace & Calming and Valor.

Supplements: Sulfurzyme and Super B.

Juniper promotes nerve function.

Vitex has been shown to reduce Parkinson's symptoms by 89 percent in animal studies. The sulfur found in the Sulfurzyme is necessary to rebuild the myelin sheath.

Night Sweats

(See MENOPAUSE)

Single Oils: Sage, clary sage, and blue yarrow.

Blends: Mister and EndoFlex.

Supplements: Estro, FemiGen, Ultra Young, and Thyromin.

Nose

Nosebleeds

Nosebleeds are normally not serious. However, if bleeding does not stop in a short time or is excessive or frequent, consult your doctor.

Single Oils: Helichrysum and lavender.

• Lemon with cypress.

Recipe 1:
• 2 drops helichrysum or lavender
• 2 drops cypress

Apply to the nose and back of neck. Repeat as needed.

Put 1 drop helichrysum, lavender, or cypress on a tissue paper and wrap the paper around a chip of ice about the size of a thumb nail, push it up under the top lip in the center to the base of the nose. Hold from the outside with lip pressure. This helps to stop bleeding in a very short time.

Dry Nose

Single Oils:

• Lavender with lemon or peppermint.

Recipe 1:
• 2 drops lavender
• 1 drop myrrh

Dilute in 1 tsp. cold pressed olive oil and rub inside the nose when needed.

Supplements: A.D.&E..

Loss of Smell (Due to Chronic Nasal Catarrh)

Single Oils: Basil, peppermint, and frankincense.

Supplements: ImmuneTune, Exodus, and Power Meal.

Nasal wash with Epsom salts.

Polyps In The Nose

Single Oils: Citronella

Blends: Purification: dilute in 1 tsp. vegetable oil. apply neat with a cotton-tip swab.

Osteoporosis (Bone Deterioration)

Researchers have linked most degenerative diseases—such as osteoporosis—to nutritional deficiencies. Calcium, magnesium, and boron are a few of the most important minerals for bone health are are usually lacking or deficient in most modern diets. Magnesium in particular is especially important to bone health, but most American consume only a fraction of the daily 400 mg daily value needed for health.

Single Oils:

• Birch with spruce, fir, pine, cypress, peppermint, marjoram, rosemary, vetiver, or basil.

• Elemi with birch, cypress, peppermint, rosemary, marjoram, or basil.

Blends:

• Birch with Aroma Siez, Purification, Melrose, Sacred Mountain, Relieve It, or PanAway.

• Birch with PanAway or Aroma Siez.

Massage oils on location.

Supplements and Skin Care: Ortho Ease, Ortho Sport, and Relaxation Massage Oils, Super Cal, ArthroTune, Arthro Plus, Mineral Essence, Power Meal, Sulfurzyme, Thyromin, and Ultra Young.

Super Cal, AlkaLime, and Mineral Essence are all excellent sources of minerals designed to build strong bones. Super Cal not only includes calcium, but also magnesium and boron which are both vital for maintaining bone composition. Mineral Essence is an excellent source magnesium and other trace minerals. Magnesium is the second most important mineral for bone health besides calcium.

Avoid carbonated drinks which can leach calcium out of the body due to their phosphoric acid content.

Ultra Young helps stimulate growth hormone production which can result in much stronger bones.

Studies show that the majority of women that do resistance training 3-4 times a week do not develop osteoporosis.

Otitis Media

(see EAR INFECTION)

Ovarian and Uterine Cysts

(See CANCER)

Single Oils:

- Frankincense with geranium, melaleuca, oregano, or cypress.

Blends: Melrose, Dragon Time, and Mister.

Supplements: Master HERS, FemiGen, Femalin, and Protec.

Recipe 1:
- 7 drops Purification
- 2 drops frankincense

Mix with 1 tsp. V-6 Mixing Oil or add to Protec (to increase strength) and apply as a douche. Protec can be used alone as a douche.

NOTE: If irritation occurs, discontinue use for 3 days before resuming use.

Protec may also be used in a vaginal retention implant when mixed into 1 Tbsp. V-6 Mixing Oil or Massage Oil Base. Insert and retain overnight.

Recipe 2:
- 5-10 drops frankincense
- 5 drops basil

Recipe 3:
- 5-10 drops frankincense
- 5-10 drops geranium
- 5-10 drops cypress
- 1 Tbsp. V-6 Mixing Oil

Dilute in 1 Tbsp. V-6 Mixing Oil or Massage Oil and use as a vaginal retention implant. Can also be applied as compresses on location and over the lower back in conjunction with Vita Flex application or alone.

These blends can be applied on the Vita Flex points for the groin (located around the anklebone, inside and outside of the foot). Work from the ankle bone down to the arch of the foot.

Pain

One of the most effective essential oils for blocking pain is peppermint. A recent study by Gobel et al., in 1994 showed that peppermint blocks calcium channels and substance P, important factors in the transmission of pain signals. Other essential oils also have unique pain-relieving properties, including helichrysum.

MSM, a source of organic sulfur, has also been proved to be extremely effective for killing pain, especially tissue and joint pain. The subject of a best-selling book by Dr. Ronald Lawrence and Dr. Stanley Jacobs, MSM is defining the treatment of pain, especially that associated with arthritis and fibromyalgia. Sulfurzyme is an excellent source of MSM.

(See ARTHRITIS or HEADACHES)

Chronic Pain

Single Oils: Peppermint, helichrysum, spruce, birch, basil, cypress, ginger, clove, elemi, rosemary cineol, tansy, and valerian.

Blends: Relieve It and PanAway.

- Birch with clove, helichrysum, peppermint, or marjoram.
- Helichrysum with birch, clove, or peppermint.
- Spruce with helichrysum or pepper oil.

- Helichrysum with basil, cedarwood, geranium, Idaho tansy, fir, juniper, marjoram, or cypress.

- Elemi with birch and tansy equal parts

- Lavender, birch, or helichrysum with Sacred Mountain, Relieve It, Release, PanAway, or Aroma Siez.

Supplements: Sulfurzyme, Super Cal, ArthroTune.

How MSM Works to Control Pain

When fluid pressure inside cells is higher than outside, pain is experienced. The MSM found in Sulfurzyme equalizes fluid pressure inside cells by affecting the protein envelope of the cell so that water transfers freely in and out.

Skin Care: Ortho Ease, Ortho Sport.

To pinpoint the most effective essential oil for quenching pain, it may be necessary to try each of the essential oils in these categories in order to find the most effective oil.

Bone-Related Pain (hips, shoulder, etc)

Single Oils: Birch, cypress, fir, spruce, pine, peppermint, and helichrysum

Massage the oil on location or apply on Vita Flex points on feet. Repeat as needed.

Supplements: Sulfurzyme, Super Cal

Skin Care: Ortho Ease, Ortho Sport

Muscle-related Pain

Single Oils: Basil, peppermint rosemary verbenon, or marjoram.

Blends: Pain Away, Relieve It.

Massage the oil on location or apply on Vita Flex points on feet. Repeat as needed.

Supplements: Sulfurzyme, Super Cal.

Skin Care: Ortho Ease, Ortho Sport.

Muscle or nerve pain related to injury or inflammation.

Single Oils: Peppermint, lavender, nutmeg, and black pepper.

Blends: PanAway, Relieve It.

Massage the oil on location or apply on Vita Flex points on feet. Repeat as needed.

Supplements: Sulfurzyme, Super Cal.

Skin Care: Ortho Ease, Ortho Sport.

For Inflammation

Single Oils: German chamomile, basil, helichrysum, melissa, vetiver, patchouly, spruce, and geranium.

Massage the oil on location or apply on Vita Flex points on feet. Repeat as needed.

Supplements: Sulfurzyme.

Skin Care: Ortho Ease, Ortho Sport

For pain associated with traumas and accidents

Single Oils: Sandalwood, geranium

Massage around hairline of the head and tips of the toes.

Recipe 1 (pain relief):
- 12 drops fir
- 10 drops melaleuca
- 8 drops lavender
- 6 drops marjoram
- 3 drops spearmint
- 2 drops peppermint

Mix in 1 ounce V-6 Mixing Oil or Massage Oil.

Supplements: Sulfurzyme, Super Cal.

Skin Care: Ortho Ease, Ortho Sport.

Joint Pain:

Single Oils: Birch, cypress, fir, spruce, pine, peppermint, and helichrysum.

Massage the oil on location or apply on Vita Flex points on feet. Repeat as needed.

How to Use Essential Oils for Pain Control

Any single oil can be added to a blend, such as PanAway, to increase the effect.

Hot compresses drive the oils faster and deeper when applied on location.

PanAway is powerful for pain reduction. When applied on location or to the Vita Flex points on the feet, it can act within seconds. Alternate with Relieve It. These 2 blends are a powerful combination for deep-tissue pain that is not bone-related.

Supplements: Sulfurzyme, Super Cal.

Skin Care: Ortho Ease, Ortho Sport, ArthroTune.

Pancreatitis

Pancreatitis is an inflammation of the pancreas that can be either acute or chronic. Acute pancreatitis can be caused by a sudden blockage in the main pancreatic duct, which results in enzymes becoming backed-up and literally digesting the pancreas unless remedied. Chronic pancreatitis occurs more gradually, with attacks recurring over weeks or months.

Symptoms:

• Abdominal pain, muscle aches, vomiting, abdominal swelling and gas, sudden hypertension, jaundice, rapid weight loss, and fever.

In the case of acute pancreatitis, a total fast for at least 4-5 days is one of the safest and most effective methods of treatment. In the case of infection, fasting should be combined with immune stimulation (by using Exodus) combined with vitamin C and B-complex vitamins.

Single Oils: Vetiver, peppermint, mountain savory, and oregano.

Blends: Exodus II, ImmuPower, and Thieves.

Supplements: Exodus, ImmuGel, VitaGreen, Super B, Super C, and Megazyme.

Parasympathetic Nervous System

(See NERVOUS SYSTEM-AUTONOMIC)

Parasites, Intestinal

Many types of parasites use up nutrients, while giving off toxins. This can leave the body depleted, nutritionally deficient, and susceptible to infectious disease.

Occasionally parasites can lie dormant in the body and then become active due to ingestion of a particular food or drink. This can result in the appearance and disappearance of symptoms even though parasite are still present.

Symptoms:
• Fatigue
• Weakness
• Diarrhea
• Gas and bloating
• Cramping
• Nausea
• Irregular bowel movements.

The first step to controlling parasites is beginning a fasting or cleansing program. A colon cleanse is particularly important.

Single Oils: Tarragon, basil, peppermint, ginger, lemongrass, nutmeg, fennel, juniper, rosewood.

• Basil with tarragon, peppermint, ginger, spearmint, hyssop, fennel, or Roman chamomile.

• Cypress with tarragon, ginger, rosemary, anise, clove, lemongrass, nutmeg, caraway seed, fennel, lemon, juniper, rosewood, or mountain savory.

• Thyme with melaleuca, oregano, tarragon, peppermint, myrrh, or mugwort.

Blends: Di-Tone, JuvaFlex

• Basil with Di-Tone.

• Cypress or thyme with Di-Tone or JuvaFlex.

Internal Application:
Take 1-3 drops of essential oil diluted in vegetable oil or soy milk. (Only use essential oils and blends that are listed in Appendix C).

Topical Application:

Place 10-15 drops of essential oil in 100° F water. Lay a cloth on water, then place on stomach. Cover with plastic wrap, then with a heavy towel to keep in the heat.

Direct application:

Place up to 15 drops in palm and rub over stomach and navel. Apply a hot compress.

Retention Enema:

Dilute a blend of ginger and Di-Tone with V-6 Mixing Oil and implant in enema. Use each night for 7 nights. Take 7 days off. Repeat this cycle 3 times to eliminate all stages of parasite development.

Vita Flex application:

Apply up to 6 drops to instep area on both feet (small intestine and colon Vita Flex points).

Using Di-Tone For Parasite Control

The essential oil blend Di-Tone is excellent for parasite removal. Add 6 drops to vegetable oil or soy milk and take as a dietary supplement twice a day. Di-Tone can also be diluted in massage oil and applied over abdomen.

Supplements: Megazyme, ComforTone, I.C.P., and ParaFree.

The parasite *Cryptosporidium parrum* may be present in many municipal or tap waters. To remove, water must be distilled or filtered using a .3 micron filter.

Periodontal Disease

Periodontal disease is an infection of the gum and bone that hold the teeth in place. In advanced stages, they lead to painful chewing problems and even tooth loss. Like any infection, gum disease can make it hard to keep your blood sugar under control.

Gum infection

Single Oils: Clove, cinnamon, and peppermint.

Blends: Thieves

- Helichrysum with PanAway.
- Birch with sage or myrrh.
- Birch or sage with Melrose or Thieves.

Recipe 1:
- 2 to 5 drops of clove
- 2 drops of thyme
- Thieves
- Exodus

Dilute in vegetable oil and rub on gums. Melrose (diluted if necessary) can also be used on gums.

Place ImmuGel on a piece of gauze. Roll like a piece of rope and place along the gum. This works particularly well for leukemia patients because their gums tend to inflame, swell, and become infected.

Brush with Dentarome or Dentarome Plus toothpaste.

Gargle with Fresh Essence Mouthwash.

Bleeding

Single Oils: Mountain savory, clove, and cistus.

Supplements: Dentarome, Dentarome Plus, and Fresh Essence Mouthwash.

For infection use mountain savory, clove and cistus.

Gingivitis and Pyorrhea

Single Oils: Helichrysum, mountain savory, cistus, and clove.

Blends: Exodus II and Thieves.

Supplements: Super C, Dentarome, Dentarome Plus, and Fresh Essence Mouthwash.

Super C: 14 tablets taken at intervas throughout the day.

Mouth Ulcers

Single Oils: Myrrh with Oregano.

Blends: Thieves with Exodus II.

Apply 1-2 drops on location neat or dilute in V6 Mixing oil.

Brush with Dentarome or Dentarome Plus Toothpaste.

Gargle with Fresh Essence Mouth Wash. Add 1-2 drops of Thieves, clove, and Exodus II to make stronger.

Brush with Thieves and Dentarome. If infection is due to leukemia, saturate gauze with ImmuGel and Thieves. Lay over gums and change morning and night. Massage abscessed area with Thieves. Irrigate mouth with Fresh Essence.

Perspiration (Excess)

Excessive perspiration may indicate adrenal and thyroid problems, or diabetes.

Single Oils: Geranium, rosewood.

- Sage with nutmeg, rosemary, or basil.

Blends: Purification.

- Sage with EndoFlex or En-R-Gee.

Sage helps regulate sweating.

pH Balance

(See FUNGAL INFECTIONS)

Phlebitis - Thrombosis

(See CARDIOVASCULAR CONDITIONS)

Single Oils: Helichrysum, and Idaho tansy followed with lavender: 5-10 drops each, layered 3 times directly towards the heart.

Supplements: Megazyme, Super Cal, and Power Meal.

Rehemogen: 3 droppers in water, 3 times daily.

Pinkeye

(See EYE DISORDERS)

Diffuse: Purification, 3 Wise Men, or Immu-Power while sleeping.

Plaque

(See CARDIOVASCULAR CONDITIONS)

Pleurisy

Single Oils: Ravensara, mountain savory, and thyme.

Blends: Raven, R.C., ImmuPower, and Exodus II.

Supplements: Exodus, ImmuneTune, Super C, Ultra Young, Mineral Essence, and Sulfurzyme.

Pneumonia - Emphysema

(See INFECTION)

Single Oils:

- Frankincense with cypress, ravensara, sandalwood, eucalyptus (globulus and radiata), mountain savory, thyme, birch, or hyssop.

- Lavender with lemon, lemongrass, ginger, tarragon, peppermint, oregano, frankincense, thyme, clove, fennel, or spearmint.

- Melaleuca with fir, spruce, Idaho tansy, oregano, helichrysum, thyme, cinnamon, or cedarwood.

Blends:

- R.C., Raven, Sacred Mountain, Inspiration, or Exodus II.

- Lavender with Melrose, ImmuPower, Di-Tone, or Thieves.

- Melaleuca with Melrose, Aroma Siez, Purification, R.C., Di-Tone, or Christmas Spirit.

Massage on the Vita Flex points on the feet and hands. Apply 4 drops oregano and 4 drops thyme using Raindrop Technique.

Other oils and blends may be substituted for oregano and thyme (See Raindrop Technique).

Diffuse Purification, ImmuPower, Melrose, R.C., to kill airborne germs and bacteria. Both Sacred Mountain and Inspiration are powerful antiseptics for the respiratory tract.

Mix R.C., frankincense, and lemon for congestion.

Peppermint removes mucous and reduces fever and throat infection.

Myrrh is very effective on throat troubles and phlegm.

Myrtle is good for chronic coughs.

Cedarwood for congestion and coughs.

Recipe 1 (For lung congestion):
• 2 drops sage
• 4 drops myrrh
• 5 drops clove
• 6 drops ravensara
• 15 drops frankincense

Mix in 1/2 oz. V-6 Mixing Oil or Massage Oil Base. Use in a rectal implant, and retain throughout the night.

Recipe 1 (For relief of pneumonia, emphysema, and pleurisy symptoms):
• 10 drops rosemary
• 8 drops ravensara
• 8 drops frankincense
• 2 drops oregano
• 2 drops peppermint

Mix oils and gargle 4 times daily.

Recipe 2:
• 2 drops ravensara
• 1 drop thyme
• 3 drops frankincense
• 3 drops lemon
• 3 drops rosemary

Mix in 1/2 teaspoon honey. First week gargle 4 times daily, 2nd week 2 times daily, 3rd week 3 times daily, and 4th week 1 time daily. Stop for 1 month and repeat if necessary.

ImmuGel helps strengthen resistance to infection (do not mix with citrus juices). Royal-dophilus is good for any viral condition and should be taken up to 4 times a day.

Exodus is proving to be a powerful body defense and immune builder that speeds the body's healing process. Exodus II is the companion product to Exodus.

Rosemary is good for colds, flu, and pneumonia. Anise and clove aid in strengthening the respiratory system. Clary sage relieves respiratory complaints. Fennel stimulates the respiratory system. Peppermint stimulates respiratory system, helps remove mucous, and reduces fever. Marjoram is calming to the respiratory system.

Chest Congestion:
• Ravensara
• Eucalyptus
• Frankincense
• Lemon

Congestion:
• ImmuPower
• Aroma Siez
• Exodus II

Apply on throat and chest to help release mucous.

Compress:
• Aroma Siez
• Birch
• Spruce

For long-term chest congestion from welding, smoking, etc., use R.C. and myrtle in hot packs or compresses on chest and back and intense inhalation.

The antibacterial and antiviral oils, which are very powerful prophylactic agents for protection against colds, flu, etc., are basil, lavender, hyssop, frankincense, rosemary, bergamot, eucalyptus, melaleuca, clove, oregano, cistus, thyme, and mountain savory.

Recipe 1 (Bath for flu and colds):
• 2 oz. Evening Peace Bath Gel
• 2 drops eucalyptus
• 6 drops frankincense
• 3 drops helichrysum
• 6 drops spruce
• 15 drops ravensara
• 1 drop birch

Mix in bath and soak until cool.

Cough

Recipe 1:
- 2 drops cypress
- 1 drop eucalyptus

Mix in 6 ounces of water, shake well and sip. Keep covered and shake before use.

Recipe 2:
- 2 drops eucalyptus
- 2 drops lemon
- 2 Tbsp. honey.

Put 1 tsp. in glass of warm water and sip slowly.

Heavy, deep cough:
- 3 drops frankincense (known to alleviate coughs)
- 3 drops lemon
- 2 drops ravensara
- 1 drop thyme

Mix in 1/2 teaspoon honey and sip slowly.

Congestion and Coughing

- Mix Raven or R.C. with 2 drops eucalyptus.
- Massage or apply hot compress over chest and back.
- Hold saturated wash cloth or towel over nose, on throat and neck glands.
- Diffuse.
- Mix in water and gargle.

Dry Cough

Recipe 1:
- 2 drops lemon
- 3 drops eucalyptus

Mix in 2 Tbsp. honey and dissolve 1 tsp. in 4 oz. of warm distilled water and sip slowly.

Sore Throat

Recipe 1:
- 2 drops thyme
- 2 drops cypress
- 1 drop eucalyptus
- 1 drop peppermint
- 1 drop myrrh

Dilute in juice or soy milk, mix well, and gargle.

Recipe 2:
- 2 drops eucalyptus
- 5 drops lemon
- 2 drops birch

Mix in 2 Tbsp. honey, dissolve in warm water, shake well, and gargle

Rub sage or Purification on throat area.

Strep Throat

Single Oils: Oregano, thyme, frankincense, myrrh, and mountain savory.

Apply 1-2 drops on tongue.

Blends: Thieves, Exodus II.

Dilute with vegetable oil or soy milk, apply 1-2 drops on tongue.

Supplements: ImmuneTune, Super C, Immu-Gel, and Royal Essence, Radex, Super C, Royal Essence, VitaGreen, Royaldophilus, Rehemogen, Exodus, and Cleansing Trio.

- ImmuneTune: 2 to 4 capsules, 3 times daily.
- Super C: 2 to 3 tablets, 3 times daily.
- Radex: 2 to 4 tablets, 3 times daily.
- Use Raindrop Technique with ImmuPower and/or Exodus II on spine and back.
- Gargle every hour with Royal Essence.

Polio

Single Oils:

- Lemon with ylang ylang, frankincense, birch, myrtle, cypress, myrrh, tarragon, or sage.

Recipe:
- 2 drops lemon
- 10 drops ylang ylang
- 7 drops frankincense
- 10 drops birch
- 7 drops myrtle
- 8 drops cypress
- 15 drops myrrh
- 10 drops tarragon
- 6 drops sage

Mix in 1 ounce V-6 Mixing Oil or Massage Oil.

Pregnancy and Postpartum

Essential oils can be invaluable companions during pregnancy. Oils like lavender and myrrh may help reduce stretch marks and improve the elasticity of the skin. Geranium and the blend Gentle Baby have similar effects and can be massaged on the perineum (tissue between vagina and rectum) to lower the risk of tearing or the need for an episiotomy (an incision in the perineum) during birth.

Single Oils: Lavender, myrrh, geranium.

• Jasmine with lavender, myrrh, or geranium.

• Helichrysum with fennel, peppermint, ylang ylang, or clary sage.

Blends: Gentle Baby, Joy, Magnify Your Purpose, Envision, and Valor.

To use during labor:
• 4 drops helichrysum
• 4 drops fennel
• 2 drops peppermint
• 5 drops ylang ylang
• 3 drops clary sage

Mix in 1 ounce of V-6 Mixing Oil or Massage Oil Base. Apply only after labor starts. Massage on reproductive Vita Flex areas on the ankles. Also rub on lower stomach and lower back.

Diffuse Gentle Baby to reduce stress before and after the birth. Expectant fathers may also wear Gentle Baby to reduce anxiety while waiting for delivery.

Constipation

Constipation can be a major problem for some women during pregnancy, contributing to hemorrhoids and varicose veins. It can also affect the child. Many babies are born with weak immune function. This may be due in part from mothers having accumulated waste build up in their colons.

• Cleanse colon and liver with Cleansing Trio. It might also be helpful to take ComforTone for maintenance of the colon and liver during pregnancy.

(See HEMORRHOIDS, VARICOSE VEINS)

Lactation

Single Oils: Fennel, and sage. Massage into breast.

Supplements: VitaGreen, Power Meal, and Essential Manna.

Mix 20 drops fennel in 1 oz. V-6 Mixing Oil or Massage Oil Base and massage over breast and on Vita flex points of the feet. Geranium helps restore and increase milk.

NOTE: *Do not use fennel longer than 10 days at a time, as it will excessively increase flow through the urinary tract.*

Mastitis (Infected Breast)

Single Oils: Tangerine with lavender.

Blends: Citrus Fresh with lavender and Exodus II.

Supplements: ImmuGel and Exodus.

Recipe 1:
• 10 drops tangerine
• 10 drops lavender

Mix in 1 ounce of V-6 Mixing Oil or Massage Oil. Rub on the breasts and under armpits twice daily.

Morning Sickness

Single Oils: Spearmint, peppermint.

Blends: Di-Tone.

Supplements: Mint Condition, Megazyme.

Apply 1 drop of Di-Tone on the mastoid bone under and behind each ear and a couple of drops around the navel.

Postpartum Depression

Single Oils: Vetiver.

Blends: Trauma Life.

Supplements: AuraLight.

Food: Essential Mann (all flavors).

Uterine tonic

Single Oils: Thyme.

Prostate Problems

(See BENIGN PROSTATE HYPERPLASIA)

Due to research conducted by Jerilynn Prior, M.D., an endocrinologist at the University of British Columbia, it was discovered that ovarian, prostate, and other types of reproductive cancer are directly related to petrochemicals ingested and stored in the reproductive organs. These petrochemicals interfere with hormone receptors, rendering them unable to function properly, eventually leading to cancer.

Single Oils: Cypress with helichrysum, frankincense, myrtle, peppermint, myrrh, sage, juniper, yarrow, or spruce.

Blends: Protec.

- Cypress with Mister, Dragon Time, or EndoFlex.

Supplements: ProGen, Master Formula vitamins, Royal Essence, Protec, Dragon Time Bath and Shower Gel.

Mix 3-5 drops of oil in 1 tsp. V-6 Mixing Oil or Massage Oil Base. Apply as a rectal implant at bed time and retain all night.

Protec may be used as a rectal implant. Start with 2 Tbsp. for 7 consecutive days and nights. Rest for 3 nights and then repeat until you have used it for 21 nights. Then rest 4 days. If irritation occurs, discontinue use for 3 days before restarting.

Oils may be applied topically in the region between the rectum and the scrotum. Mister works well here.

You can also rub oils on reproductive Vita Flex areas.

Recipe 1:
- 10 drops frankincense
- 5 drops myrrh
- 3 drops sage

Mix in 1 Tbsp. V-6 Mixing Oil or Massage Oil Base.

Zinc helps reduce prostate swelling. Royal Essence and Master HIS are good sources of zinc (and all minerals).

Adding natural progesterone to the body helps normalize levels of zinc, copper, and hormones, which in turn helps prostate problems.

Peppermint acts as an anti-inflammatory to the prostate.

Prostate Cancer

(See CANCER, PROSTATE)

Prostatitis

Prostatitis is an inflammation of the prostate that can present similar symptoms as benign prostate hyperplasia: frequent urinations etc.

Single Oils:

- Rosemary with myrtle, clary sage, sage, mountain savory, fennel, bergamot, sandalwood, ylang ylang, geranium, yarrow, or peppermint.

- Thyme with rosemary, tarragon, lavender, eucalyptus, spruce, clove, or cinnamon.

Blends: Mister, Dragon Time.

- Aroma Siez with Mister or Dragon Time.

- Thyme with Melrose, Purification, R.C., or Di-Tone.

Mix 3 or 5 drops of oil in 1 tsp. V-6 Mixing Oil in a rectal implant at bed time. Apply oils topically on area between rectum and scrutom and on reproductive Vita Flex areas on the feet.

Psoriasis

(See SKIN DISORDERS)

Radiation Damage

Many cancer treatments use radiation therapy that can severely damage both the skin and vital organs. Using antioxidant essential oils topically, as well as proper nutrients internally, is critical for minimizing radiation damage.

Single Oils: Melaleuca.

Blends: Melrose.

- Melaleuca or neroli with Melrose.

Supplements: Radex, A.D.&E., Super C, Power Meal, ImmuneTune, and Essential Manna.

For external damage:

• Apply A.D.&E. topically.

Mix Melrose with melaleuca and apply neat or mix in 1 oz. V-6 Mixing Oil or Massage Oil Base. Rub on location.

For internal damage:

• Take Super C, Power Meal, A.D.&E..

Raynaud's Disease

Raynaud's disease is characterized by chronic constriction in the peripheral blood vessels whenever a part of the body is exposed to cold. This can cause extreme pain, and eventually gangrene if not treated. It occurs most often in the extremities such as feet and hands.

Raynaud's disease can also be triggered by emotional trauma.

Slowly rewarming the effected part or sedating the patient is the quickest way to restore circulation. Use nutrients or oils which increase circulation or dilate blood vessels.

Single Oils: Helichrysum, clover, and cypress.

Blends: PanAway.

Supplements: Super B, PanAway.

Give a full body massage with helichrysum, cypress, or PanAway diluted with V-6 Mixing Oil or Massage Oil Base.

Restless Leg Syndrome

Single Oils: Oregano, basil, marjoram, lavender, cypress, Roman chamomile, and peppermint.

Blends: Peace & Calming and Aroma Siez

Supplements: Mineral Essence, Thyromin, and VitaGreen.

Use Raindrop Technique with the essential oils of oregano, basil, marjoram, lavender, cypress, and peppermint.

Rheumatic Fever

Rheumatic fever results from a *Streptococcus* infection that primarily strikes children (usually before age 14). It can lead to inflammation that damages the heart muscle and valve.

Rheumatic fever is caused by the same genus of bacteria that causes strep throat and scarlet fever. Diffusing essential oils can help reduce the likelihood of contracting the disease. Essential oils like mountain savory, rosemary, melaleuca, and oregano, have powerful antimicrobial effects.

In cases where a child is already infected, the use of essential oils in the Raindrop Technique may be appropriate.

Single Oils: Mountain savory, peppermint, thyme, rosemary verbenon, melaleuca, and oregano

Blends: Thieves, Exodus II, and ImmuPower.

Supplements: Exodus, ImmuneTune, Super C, Sulfurzyme, A.D.&E., HRT, and Goji Berry Tea.

Diffuse as needed to kill airborne microbes. In cases of infection, apply essential oils using the Raindrop Technique.

Rheumatoid Arthritis

(See ARTHRITIS)

Rheumatoid arthritis is a painful inflammatory condition of the joints marked by swelling, thickening, and inflammation of the synovial membrane lining the joint. (In contrast, osteo-arthritis is characterized by a breakdown of the joint cartilage without any swelling or inflammation.)

Rheumatoid arthritis is classified as an autoimmune disease because it is caused by the body's own immune system attacking the joints.

Other factors can aggravate arthritis such as:

• Deficiencies of minerals and other nutrients

• Microbes and toxins

• Lack of water intake

Essential oils constitute some of the most effective treatments for combating arthritis pain and combating infection (in cases where it is present). Peppermint has been studied for its ability to kill pain by blocking substance P and calcium channels (Gobel et al., 1994).

In cases where arthritis is caused by infections organisms, such as *Borrelia burgdorferi*, *Chlamydia*, and *Salmonella*, essential oils may counteract and prevent infection, especially when diffused or applied topically. Highly antimicrobial essential oils include: mountain savory, rosemary, melaleuca, and oregano. Of particular benefit is the fact that the oils can pass into the bloodstream when applied topically.

MSM has been documented to be one of the most effective natural supplements for reducing the pain associated with rheumatism and arthritis. The subject of a number of clinical studies, MSM was used extensively by Ronald Lawrence, M.D., in his clinical practice to dramatically reduce rheumatism and arthritis symptoms. (MSM is the key ingredient in the supplement Sulfurzyme.)

Single Oils: Peppermint, birch, oregano, spruce.

- Birch with spruce, fir, pine, cypress, peppermint, vetiver, mountain savory, marjoram, rosemary, basil, oregano, or vitex.

- Lavender with birch, cypress, peppermint, rosemary, marjoram, basil, ginger, pepper, or tarragon.

- Cypress with spruce, fir, pine, cedarwood, juniper, rosemary, peppermint, helichrysum, birch, basil, lemon, Idaho tansy, or nutmeg.

- Thyme with birch, basil, rosemary, cypress, melaleuca, spruce, peppermint, or oregano.

Blends: Aroma Siez, PanAway, Relieve It, Ortho Ease, and Ortho Sport.

- Birch with Aroma Siez, PanAway, Relieve It, or Peace & Calming.

- Lavender or thyme with PanAway or Aroma Siez.

- Cypress with Aroma Life, PanAway, Purification, Melrose, Aroma Siez, or Sacred Mountain.

Supplements: Sulfurzyme, Super Cal, ArthroTune, Royal Essence, Mineral Essence, Goji Berry Tea, and Exodus.

Essential Oils For Rheumatoid Arthritis

- Birch and oregano work well together to reduce rheumatic pain.

- For sharp rheumatic pain, use lavender with marjoram.

- Vetiver is rubefacient (induces local warming)

- PanAway and Relieve It have cortisone-like action without the cortisone side effects.

- ArthroTune increases circulation, helps alleviate arthritis, rheumatic conditions.

Massage oils on location neat or dilute 1-2 drops in 1 tsp. of V6 Mixing Oil or Massage Oil Base.

Rhinopharyngitis

Single Oils: Eucalyptus radiata, thyme, and ravensara.

Blends: Raven, R.C., Thieves, and Exodus II.

Supplements: Exodus, ImmuGel, Dentarome, and Fresh Essence.

Ringworm

(See FUNGAL INFECTIONS)

Scabies

Scabies are caused by arachnids known as itch mites—tiny parasites the burrow into the skin, usually in the fingers and genital areas. The most common variety, *Sarcoptes scabiei,* can quickly infest other people. Although it only lives six weeks, it continually lays eggs which are burrowed into the skin.

Essential oils have been studied for their ability to not only repel insects, but also kill them and their eggs as well. Because many oils are nontoxic to humans, they make excellent treatments to combat scabies infestations.

Single Oils: Citronella, peppermint, palmarosa, lavandin, Roman chamomile, eucalyptus globulus, black pepper, and ginger.

Blends: Di-Tone, Purification, and Peace & Calming.

Skin Care: Lavender Hair and Scalp Wash.

Apply neat on location, or dilute in 1 Tbsp. V6 Mixing oil if necessary. To treat hair or scalp, add 2-4 drops of essential oil to 1 Tbsp. of Lavender Hair and Scalp Wash.

Scar Tissue

Some essential oils may be valuable for reducing or minimizing the formation of scar tissue:

Single Oils: Helichrysum, lavender, cypress, elemi, blue yarrow, rose, cistus, frankincense, myrrh, and sandalwood.

Blends: 3 Wise Men and Inspiration.

Supplements: A.D.&E., Super C, Radex, Sulferzyme, Power Meal, and Essential Manna.

Sciatica

Sciatica is a type of lower back pain that radiates from the lumbar spine area (above the hips) down the back side of the leg. Sciatica is caused from neuralgia (nerve pain) or neuritis (nerve inflammation) originating from the sciatic nerve, which travels from the lower leg to lower back and is the longest nerve in the human body.

Acute sciatica has a sudden onset and is usually triggered by a misaligned vertebra pressing against the sciatic nerve due to accident, injury, pregnancy, or inflammation.

Symptoms:
• Lower back pain
• Swelling or stiffness in a leg
• Loss of sensation in a leg
• Muscle wasting in a leg

(See SPINE INJURIES and PAIN)

Schizophrenia

Single Oils: Cardamom, melissa, frankincense, rosemary, basil, and peppermint.

Blends: Brain Power, Clarity, and M-Grain.

Supplements: Mineral Essence and Ultra Young.

Scleroderma

Also known as systemic sclerosis, scleroderma is a non-infectious, chronic, autoimmune disease of the connective tissue. Caused by an over-production of collagen, the disease can involve either the skin or internal organs and can be life-threatening. Scleroderma is far more common among women than men.

Single Oils: Frankincense, Roman chamomile, lavender, patchouly, sandalwood, and myrrh

Blends: Melrose.

Supplements: Cleansing Trio, JuvaTone, Thyromin, Mineral Essence, Power Meal, and Sulfurzyme.

For scar tissue in advanced stages: R.C. diffused and in a rectal implant with frankincense.

Topical application: Roman chamomile, lavender, and patchouly in equal portions over location with V-6 Mixing Oil to eliminate dryness. Alternate with equal portions of sandalwood and myrrh with V-6 Mixing Oil or Massage Oil Base.

Scoliosis

(See SPINE or RAINDROP TECHNIQUE)

Scoliosis is an abnormal lateral or side-to-side curvature or twist in the spine. It is different from hyperkyphosis (roundback) or hyperlordosis (swayback) which involve excessive front-to-back accentuation of existing spine curvatures.

While a few cases of scoliosis can be attributed to congenital deformities (such as MS, cerebral palsy, Down's syndrome, or Marfan's syndrome), the vast majority of scoliosis are of unknown origin.

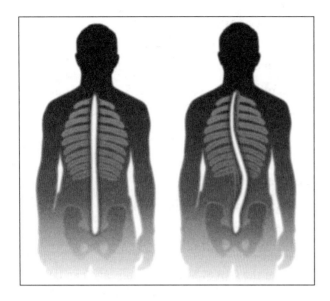

Some medical professionals believe that many cases of scoliosis begin with hard-to-detect inflammation along the spine caused by latent viruses. Others believe that it may be due to persistent muscle spasms that have pulled the vertebrae off the spine out of alignment.

Symptoms:

- When bending forward, the left side of the back is higher or lower than the right side (the patient must be viewed from the rear).

- One hip may appear to be higher or more prominent than the other.

- Uneven shoulders or scapulas (shoulder blades)

- When the arms are hanging loosely, the distance between the left arm and left side is different than the distance between the right arm and right side.

The Raindrop Technique is one of the most effective therapies for straightening spines misaligned due to scoliosis.

Single Oils: Oregano, thyme, basil, birch, cypress, marjoram, and peppermint

Blends: Aroma Siez and PanAway.

Supplements: Mineral Essence, Super Cal, Essential Manna, Power Meal, Sulfurzyme, and Ortho Ease Massage Oil.

Scurvy

Supplements: Super C and Power Meal.

Seizures

(See BRAIN FUNCTION or EPILEPSY)

Single Oils: Frankincense, sandalwood, melissa, and basil.

Blends: Valor, Aroma Siez, and Exodus II.

Supplements: Mineral Essence, A.D.&E., and Goji Berry Tea.

Remove all forms of sugar from diet.

Grand Mal Seizures

Blends: Brain Power, Clarity, Valor, Peace & Calming, Joy, Sacred Mountain, and Aroma Siez.

- Valor: Massage on bottom of feet.

- Diffuse: Brain Power, Peace & Calming.

- Joy: Rub over heart.

- Sacred Mountain: 2-3 drops on back of neck and on crown.

- Aroma Siez: Raindrop Technique on Spine. (See RAINDROP TECHNIQUE)

Supplements: Master Formula, VitaGreen, Super B, Mineral Essence, Royal Essence, Power Meal, Sulfurzyme, Body Balance, and Ultra Young.

Sexually Transmitted Diseases

Herpes Simplex Type II

The herpes simplex virus type 2, herpes is transmitted by sexual contact and results in sores or lesions. Four to seven days after contact with an infected partner, tingling, burning, or persistent itching usually heralds an outbreak. One or two days later, small pimple-like bumps appear over reddened skin. The itching and tingling continue, and the pimples turn into painful blisters, which burst, bleeding with a yellowish pus. Five to seven days after the first tingling, scabs form, and healing begins.

Antiviral essential oils have generally been very effective in treating herpes lesions and reducing their onset. Oils like melaleuca, melissa, and rosemary (verbenon) have been successfully used by Daniel Penoel, M.D. in his clinical practice.

Those with herpes should avoid diets high in the amino acid L-arginine, instead substituting with L-lysine. Lysine interferes with the growth of the virus. Foods such as amaranth are very high in lysine. (Amaranth is used in Wolfberry Bars and Essential Manna).

Single Oils: Melissa, ravensara, melaleuca, Idaho tansy, lemon, oregano, thyme, cumin, mountain savory, clove, and cinnamon.

• Lavender with peppermint, melaleuca, Idaho tansy, melissa, ravensara, bergamot, clary sage, or lemon.

Blends: Melrose, Thieves, Exodus II, Immu-Power, or Purification.

• Lavender with Melrose, Thieves, Exodus II, ImmuPower, or Purification.

Regimen:

As soon as a lesion is noticed, apply neat:
• 1 drop lavender
• 1 drop Melaleuca alternifolia or Melrose

This formula can also be diluting in 1 tsp. V-6 Mixing Oil or Massage Oil Base.

To facilitate healing, alternate with Melrose, Hope, or Melissa.

Recipe 1:
• 2 drops sage
• 2 drops neroli
• 4 drops ravensara
• 2 drops lavender

For Vaginal Application:

Inject 10-15 drops with ear bulb syringe (or insert an oil-saturated tampon). If burning sensation lasts longer than 3-5 minutes, dilute with V-6 Mixing Oil or Massage Oil Base.

For Topical Application:

Mix in 1 oz. V-6 Mixing Oil or Massage Oil Base. Apply around lesions. For body massage, use 10 drops frankincense in 1/2 oz. V-6 Mixing Oil or Massage Oil Base once a day.

Supplements: Exodus, ImmuGel, Immune-Tune, Sulfurzyme, Power Meal, Essential Manna, Super C, Super B, VitaGreen, Master Formula, Cleansing Trio, and Mineral Essence.

AVOID using Ultra Young, since this supplement is high in L-arginine.

Genital Warts

Single Oils: Melissa, thyme, Idaho tansy, melaleuca alternifolia, melaleuca ericifola, and lavender.

Blends: Melrose, Thieves, and ImmuPower.

Supplements: A.D.&E., ImmuGel, ImmuneTune, and JuvaTone.

Gonorrhea and Syphilis

Single Oils: Oregano, melissa, thyme, mountain savory, and cinnamon.

Blends: Thieves and Exodus II.

Supplements: Exodus, ImmuGel, Essential Manna, Mineral Essence, and Radex.

Sexual Dysfunctions

Lack of Libido

Single Oils:

FOR WOMEN: Geranium, ylang ylang, clary sage, nutmeg, and rose. Jasmine (an absolute) can also be used in inhalation therapy or topical use, but must never be ingested.

FOR MEN: Cinnamon, myrrh, black pepper, pine, ylang ylang, ginger, nutmeg, and rose.

Blends: Joy, Passion, Sensation, Mister, and Dragon Time.

Supplements: Ultra Young, Sensation Moisture Cream, VitaGreen, FemiGen, ProGen, FemiGen, and Sulfurzyme.

• Ylang Ylang helps balance sexual emotion and sex drive problems. Its aromatic influence elevates sexual energy and enhances relationships.

• Clary sage helps with lack of sexual desire, regulates and balances hormones.

- Nutmeg supports the nervous system to overcome frigidity.

- Sulfurzyme provides MSM (sulfur), which can help the libido.

NOTE: When diffusing cinnamon, be aware that it can irritate nasal passages. Always dilute cinnamon in V-6 Mixing Oil or Massage Oil Base or blend with 20 parts or more of lavender to 1 part cinnamon.

Excessive Sexual Desire

Single Oils: Marjoram.

Shingles (Herpes Zoster)

Shingles is an active (generally short-lived) viral infection of the central nervous system that affects certain areas of the skin. This usually starts with fatigue, fever, chills, and at times intestinal upset. On the third to fourth day, th3e affected skin area becomes excessively sensitive. On the fourth or fifth day, small painful blisters erupt along the nerve pathway and crust over. Normally these heal in about 5 days without further problems. One attack usually gives immunity for life. However, with some, particularly the elderly, pain can persist for months, even years.

The virus that causes shingles is *Varicella zoster*, which also causes chicken pox. A childhood bout with chicken pox leaves some viruses dormant in sensory (skin) nerves. If the immune system is compromised from things such as severe emotional stress, illness, or long-term use of corticosteroids, the dormant viruses may start to infect the pathway of the skin nerves.

Essential Oils vs. Shingles

Equal amounts of Ravensara and *Calophyllum inophyllum* applied to a shingles outbreak have produced dramatic improvement and complete remission within 7 days (*Alternative Medicine, The Definitive Guide*, p. 56, 971).

NOTE: Occurrences of shingles around the eyes or on the forehead can cause blindness. Consult an ophthalmologist (eye doctor) immediately if such outbreaks occur.

Single Oils: Elemi, tansy, clove, oregano, mountain savory, thyme, juniper, geranium, and peppermint.

- Ravensara with *Calophyllum inophyllum* (a fatty acid oil).

- Melaleuca with lemon, geranium, bergamot, eucalyptus, lavender, peppermint, or chamomile.

Supplements: ArthroTune, Super Cal,.

Raindrop Technique (layer in order): Oregano, mountain savory, and thyme (warm pack for 30 minutes between each oil application). Be sure to place a towel between the skin and hot pack. Continue with juniper, geranium, and peppermint with an ice pack for 30 minutes between each oil application.

Recipe 1:
- 5 drops elemi
- 5 drops tansy
- 2 drops clove

Recipe 2:
- 10 drops chamomile
- 5 drops lavender
- 4 drops bergamot
- 2 drops geranium

Mix in 1 oz. V-6 Mixing Oil or Massage Oil Base. Apply on location and also apply a cold or body temperature compress.

Shock

Shock is usually caused by the sudden loss of a large volume of bodily fluids and is characterized by extremely low arterial blood pressure.

Symptoms or signs:
- Irregular breathing
- Low blood pressure
- Dilated pupils
- Cold and sweaty skin
- Weak and rapid pulse
- Dry mouth

Any injury that results in the sudden loss of substantial amounts of fluids can trigger shock.

Shock can also be caused by allergic reactions (anaphylactic shock), infections in the blood (septic shock), or emotional trauma (neurogenic shock).

Shock should be treated by covering the victim with a blanket and elevating the victim's feet. Inhaling essential oils can also help—especially in cases of emotional shock.

Single Oils: Helichrysum, peppermint.

- Melaleuca with frankincense, lavender, sandalwood, or rosemary cineol.

- Helichrysum with basil or peppermint.

Blends:

- Melaleuca with Trauma Life, Clarity, 3 Wise Men, Valor, Harmony, or Present Time.

- Helichrysum with Clarity.

Rub 1-2 drops of essential oil on temples, back of neck, and under nose. Put 1-2 drops in hands and then cup over nose and breathe deeply.

Sinusitis

Essential oils such as ravensara strengthen the respiratory system, open the pulmonary tract, and fight respiratory infection.

Single Oils: Ravensara, myrtle, eucalyptus radiata, Eucalyptus globulus, thyme linalol, rosemary verbenon.

- Ravensara with eucalyptus, frankincense, and lemon (for congestion).

- Spruce or peppermint (to open the sinuses)

Rub essential oils over the nose and sinus cavities and inhale.

Blends:

- Helichrysum with R.C., Raven, or Thieves, ImmuPower, and Purification.

- Melaleuca and helichrysum with ravensara, lemongrass, myrtle, spruce, frankincense, cedarwood, hyssop, or pine.

- Ravensara with eucalyptus (globulus or radiata), rosemary, peppermint, frankincense, lemon, clove, fir, birch, or cypress.

- Mountain savory on Sinus, Vita Flex on points

Swab nasal cavity with Purification.

Recipe 1:
- 3 drops *Melaleuca ericifolia*
- 3 drops R.C.

Use cotton swab to apply on inside of nostrils. Keep away from eyes.

Recipe 2:
- 10 drops peppermint
- 5 drops *Eucalyptus radiata*
- 2-3 drops melaleuca

Put in a capsule and take internally.

Recipe 3:
- 1 drop lemon
- 2 drops eucalyptus
- 3 drops rosemary
- 2 drops peppermint

Mix in 1 tsp. V-6 Mixing Oil or Massage Oil Base. Massage on sinuses (forehead, nose, under cheekbones) and on chest and upper back.

Psoriasis, eczema, dermatitis, dry skin, allergies, and similar problems indicate an excessive acid pH of the body. The more acid in the blood and skin, the less effect the oils will have. People who have a strong reaction to oils are usually highly acidic. We must maintain an alkaline balance in our blood and skin for the oils to work the best. AlkaLime and VitaGreen are both helpful for this balancing. (See FUNGUS)

Skin Disorders

(See BURNS)

Our skin is our armor and the largest absorbent organ of the body. Protecting its environment is most important. Many chemical molecules are too large to absorb and lay on the surface of the skin, causing irritation, resulting in rashes, itching, blemishes, flaky and dry skin, dandruff, and allergies. Essential oils are soluble with the lipids in the skin and are easily absorbed.

319

Many skin conditions may be related to the liver. So, it may be necessary to cleanse, stimulate, and condition the liver and cleanse the colon for 30 to 90 days before the skin begins to improve.

Skin abscesses are small pockets of pus that collect under the skin. They are usually caused by a bacterial or fungal infection.

A number of essential oils may help reduce inflammation and combat infection.

Single Oils: Melaleuca, frankincense, helichrysum, peppermint, lavender, lemon, German chamomile, eucalyptus radiata, rosemary verbenon, thyme, mountain savory, palmarosa, patchouly, rosewood, ravensara, oregano.

Blends: Melrose, Purification, Exodus II, ImmuPower, Thieves, Melrose, Sacred Mountain.

Supplements: JuvaTone, Cleansing Trio, Goji Berry Tea.

Bring to Head:

Single Oils: Lavender, Thieves, frankincense, helichrysum, lemon, chamomile, or rosemary.

For Closing Abscesses:

Single Oils: Thyme, myrrh, frankincense, or birch.

Acne

Acne results from an excess accumulation of dirt and sebum around the hair follicle and the pores of the skin. This accumulation may be due to an over-production of sebum, an oily substance that is secreted by the sebaceous glands in the hair follicles. As the pores and hair follicles become blocked, bacteria begins to feed on the sebum. This leads to inflammation and infection around the hair follicle and the formation of a pimple or a puss-filled blackhead.

Lemongrass helps clears acne and balances oily skin conditions. Lemongrass is the predominant ingredient in Morning Start Bath and Shower Gel, which can be used to balance the pH of the skin, decongest the lymphatics and stimulate circulation.

Tips for Clearing Up Acne

- Eliminate dairy products, fried foods, chemical additives, and sugar from diet.

- Avoid use of makeup or chlorinated water.

- Avoid contact with plastics which may exude estrogenic chemicals.

- Topically apply essential oils such as melaleuca alternifolia to problem areas. Melaleuca was shown to be equal to benzoyl peroxide in the treatment of acne, according research published in the *Medical Journal of Australia* (Basset et al., 1990)

- Begin a cleansing program with the Cleansing Trio and Sulfurzyme.

One of the most common forms of acne, *Acne vulgaris,* occurs primarily in adolescents due to hormone imbalances which stimulate the creation of sebum.

Acne in adults can be also be caused by hormone balances, as well as use of chlorinated compounds, endocrine system imbalances, or poor dietary practices. Heavy or greasy makeup can also contribute to acne.

Stress may also play a role. According to research conducted by Dr. Asawa in Japan, acne and other skin problems are a direct result of the physical and emotional stress.

Essential oils constitute outstanding treatments of acne because of the ability to dissolve sebum, kill bacteria, and preserve the acid mantle of the skin. Because essential oils may be slightly drying to the skin when applied undiluted, it may be necessary to dilute them with grapeseed oil or massage oil base to keep the skin hydrated.

Single Oils: Melaleuca, geranium, vetiver, lavender, patchouly, Roman chamomile, rosewood, cedarwood, eucalyptus radiata, clove.

- Frankincense with melaleuca.

- Melaleuca with lemon, lemongrass, thyme, basil, rosemary, lavender, eucalyptus, geranium, neroli, and spikenard.

- Lavender with Roman chamomile, geranium, rosewood, cypress, palmarosa, myrrh, patchouly, melaleuca, mountain savory, rose, rosemary, sandalwood, cedarwood, sage, tarragon, or ylang ylang.
- Helichrysum or thyme with rosewood, patchouly, geranium, lavender, juniper, mountain savory, jasmine, myrrh, peppermint, Roman chamomile.

Blends: Melrose, Gentle Baby.

Apply topically undiluted at night. Alternate every other night.

- Lavender with Purification, Sensation, Melrose, or Gentle Baby.
- Lemongrass with Purification, Melrose, or Gentle Baby.
- Helichrysum with Gentle Baby.
- Thyme with JuvaFlex, Gentle Baby, or Forgiveness.
- Frankincense with JuvaFlex or EndoFlex.

Apply 1-3 drops on location to help remove sebum, cleanse pores, and kill bacteria.

Supplements: Master Formula, Power Meal, Mineral Essence, Exodus, Stevia, Rehemogen, and VitaGreen.

To resolve acne caused by hormonal imbalance: Estro Tincture, Ultra Young.

Skin care products: Rose Ointment, Mint Facial Scrub, Orange Blossom Facial Wash, Sandalwood or Sensation Moisturizing cream, Morning Start Bath and Shower Gel, Rawhide and Pharaoh Aftershaves, Dragon Time Bath and Shower Gel, Evening Peace Bath and Shower Gel, and Lavender Hair and Scalp Wash.

Burns

(See BURNS)

Chapped, Dry, or Cracked Skin

Single Oils: Roman chamomile, neroli, rose, palmarosa, sandalwood, jasmine, lavender, spikenard, and myrrh.

- Rosewood with patchouly, geranium, Roman chamomile, rose, sandalwood, or helichrysum.

Skin Care Products: Sandalwood Moisturizer Cream, AromaSilk Satin Body Lotion, and Rose Ointment.

Body lotions combined with essential oils are very effective for rehydrating the skin of chapped hands and maintaining the natural pH balance of the skin.

Recipe 1:
- 1 drop rosewood
- 1 drop patchouly
- 1 drop geranium

Alternate oils of rose, chamomile, or sandalwood to body lotion.

Bath and shower gels, such as Dragon Time, Evening Peace, Morning Start, and Sensation, are formulated to help balance the acid mantle of the skin.

Clogged Pores

Single Oils: Lemon, orange, geranium.

Blends: Purification.

Personal Care: AromaSilk, Orange Blossom Face Wash, Sandalwood Toner.

Mint Facial Scrub contains oat bran and corn flower, which are mild abrasives to help remove dirt, black heads, and old pimple cores, and stimulate cell regeneration. If the texture is too abrasive, mix with Orange Blossom Facial Wash. This is excellent for those with severe or mild acne.

Spread over face and let dry for perhaps 5 minutes to draw out impurities, pulling and toning the skin at the same time. Put a hot towel over face for greater penetration. Wash off with warm water by gently patting skin with warm face cloth. If you do not have time to let the mask dry, gently massage in a circular motion for 30 seconds, then rinse.

Afterwards, apply Sandalwood Moisture Cream or AromaSilk Satin Body Lotion. This also works well underneath foundation makeup.

Diaper Rash (See PSORIASIS/ECZEMA)

Single Oils: lavender, helichrysum, patchouly, and cypress.

Skin Care Products: Lavaderm Cooling Mist.

Freckles

Single Oils: Idaho tansy.

Apply 2-4 drops and spread over face. Mix with lotion if it is too drying or stings. Use 2-3 times a week.

Fungal Infection

Single Oils: Oregano, melaleuca alternifolia, melaleuca ericifolia.

Blends: Melrose.

Apply 1-2 drops 3-4 times daily. If there is any skin irritation, dilute with 1/2 to 1 ounce of V-6 Mixing Oil or Massage Oil Base.

Recipe 4:
• 3 drops rosemary
• 6 drops lavender

Recipe 5:
• 10 drops patchouly
• 4 drops lavender
• 2 drops blue chamomile
• 5 drops lemon

Mix with 1/2 to 1 ounce of V-6 Mixing Oil or Massage Oil Base.

• Melrose 2-4 drops with lotion

Skin Care: Sandalwood Moisturizer Cream and Rose Ointment.

How Essential Oils Help the Skin

To rejuvenate and heal skin:
• Rosewood

To prevent and retard wrinkles:
• Sage, lavender, spikenard, myrrh

To regenerate the skin
• Geranium, helichrysum, spikenard

To restore skin elasticity
• Rosewood, lavender
• Ylang ylang with lavender

To combat premature aging of the skin
Apply frankincense, helichrysum or patchouly on location, neat or diluted in 1 oz. V-6 Mixing Oil or Massage Oil Base (depending on skin sensitivity).

• 6 drops rosewood
• 4 drops geranium
• 3 drops lavender
• 2 drops frankincense

Itching and Dermatitis

Itching (or dermatitis) can be due to allergies, damaged liver function, allergies, or over exposure to chemicals or sunlight.

Single Oils: Peppermint, oregano, lavender, helichrysum, valerian, and patchouly.

Blends: Aroma Siez.

Supplements: Super B, JuvaTone, and Comfor-Tone.

Melanoma (See CANCER)

Moles

To remove moles: Apply one or two drops of oregano neat, directly on the mole, one or two times a day.

Single Oils: Frankincense, geranium, birch, lavender, and oregano.

Blends: Melrose

Skin care products: Rose Ointment.

Poison Oak - Poison Ivy

Single Oils: Peppermint, eucalyptus dives, melaleuca, rosemary verbenon, or basil.

- Melaleuca with lemon, lemongrass, thyme, basil, rosemary verbenon, lavender, eucalyptus dives, or geranium.

- Lavender with German chamomile, Roman chamomile, geranium, Idaho tansy, fennel, rosewood, lemongrass, patchouly, rosewood and myrtle.

- Frankincense with melaleuca, lemongrass, or vetiver.

Blends:

- Melaleuca with Thieves.

- Lavender or lemongrass with Purification, Sensation, Melrose, Gentle Baby, or Raven.

- Frankincense with Release, JuvaFlex, Endo-Flex, or Purification.

Apply on location neat or diluted in V6 Mixing Oil.

Supplements: Master Formula.

Skin Care Products: Rose Ointment, Stevia, AromaSilk Satin Body Lotion, Morning Start Bath and Shower Gel.

Psoriasis/Eczema

Psoriasis is a non-infectious skin disorder that is marked by skin lesions that can occur in limited areas (such as the scalp) or that can cover up to 80-90 percent of the body.

The overly rapid growth of skin cells is the primary cause of the lesions associated with psoriasis. In some cases, skin cells grow four times faster than normal, resulting in the formation of silvery layers that flake off.

Symptoms:
- Occurs on elbows, chest, knees, and scalp
- Slightly elevated reddish lesions covered with silver-white scales
- Coverage can range from one small patch to e covering the entire body
- Rashes subside after exposure to sunlight
- Rashes recur over a period of years

Single Oils: Roman chamomile, melaleuca, patchouly, helichrysum, and lavender

Blends: Melrose, JuvaFlex - compress 3 times a week.

Dilute 1-2 drops of essential oil in 1 tsp. of vegetable oil.

Recipe:
- 2 drops patchouly
- 2 drops Roman chamomile
- 2 drops lavender
- 2 drops Melrose

Add to Rose Ointment or body lotion and apply on affected area.

Supplements: Cleansing Trio, JuvaTone, Sulfurzyme, and Rehemogen.

Use JuvaTone at least 120 days. To soften cracking skin, cover with Rose Ointment.

Sagging Skin

Single Oils: Lavender, helichrysum, patchouly, and cypress.

Skin Care Products: Cel-Lite Magic and Massage Oil

Recipe 1 (morning):
- 10 drops tangerine
- 10 drops cypress

Mix with 1/2 oz. V-6 Mixing Oil or Massage Oil Base and begin massaging on location.

Recipe 2 (night):
- 8 drops geranium
- 5 drops cypress
- 5 drops helichrysum
- 1 drop peppermint

Mix with 1/2 oz. V-6 Mixing Oil or Massage Oil Base and massage starting at the feet and legs. Seal with Cel-Lite Magic.

Thyromin may help reduce wrinkles and rehydrate dry skin. This supplement strengthens the thyroid, which is important to many body functions that affect the skin.

Stretch Marks

Stretch marks are most commonly associated with pregnancy, but can also occur during growth spurts and periods of rapid weight gain.

Single Oils: Lavender, frankincense, spikenard, geranium, and myrrh.

Blends: Gentle Baby.

Supplements: Sulfurzyme.

Ulcers, Skin

Single Oils: Rosewood, clove, helichrysum, Roman chamomile, patchouly, myrrh, and lavender.

• Lavender with both Roman and German chamomile, geranium, rosewood, or patchouly.

Blends: Melrose, Purification, Relieve It, 3 Wise Men, and Gentle Baby.

• Lavender with Purification, Thieves, or Gentle Baby.

Supplements and Skin Care: Super C, Radex, Exodus, Cleansing Trio, AromaSilk Satin Body Lotion, and Boswellia Wrinkle Cream.

Vitilgo

Single Oils: Vetiver, sandalwood, and myhr

Blends: Purification and Melrose

Wrinkled or Rough Skin

Single Oils: Frankincense, helichrysum, cypress, rose, lavender, ylang ylang, patchouly, sage, geranium, clary sage, rosewood, sandalwood, jasmine, neroli, palmarosa, spikenard.

Blends:

• Frankincense with Gentle Baby or lavender with Sensation.

Add 10 drops of frankincense to the Sandalwood Moisture Cream and apply.

Recipe 1:
• 5 drops sandalwood
• 5 drops helichrysum
• 5 drops geranium
• 5 drops lavender
• 5 drops frankincense

Mix with lotion and apply to skin

Supplements: Ultra Young, Master Formula, Thyromin, Stevia, and Exodus.

Skin Care Products: AromaSilk Satin Body Lotion, Rose Ointment, Mint Scrub, and Sandalwood Moisture Cream.

Sandalwood Moisture Cream is excellent for dry or prematurely aging skin.

Rose Ointment was developed to feed and rehydrate the skin and to supply nutrients necessary to slow down the aging process. Moreover, it contains no synthetic chemicals to cause irritation.

Sleep Disorders

(See APNEA or INSOMNIA)

Single Oils: Lavender, valerian, marjoram, Roman chamomile, and orange.

Blends: Peace & Calming, Surrender, Inspiration, Hope, and Humility.

Take 1-3 drops as dietary supplements, or inhale.

Supplements: AuraLight, Megazyme, and Mineral Essence.

Sores

Single Oils: Roman chamomile, lavender, patchouly, and vetiver.

Blends: Melrose, Gentle Baby, Valor, and Harmony.

Supplements: Super C and Ultra Young.

Sore Throat

(See COLDS)

Spina Bifida

Spina bifida (SB) is a defect in which the spinal cord of the fetus fails to close during the first month of pregnancy. This results in varying degrees of permanent nerve damage, paralysis in lower limbs, and incomplete brain development.

SB has three different variations:

- The most severe form is Myelomeningocele. The spinal cord and its protective sheath (known as the meninges) protrude from an opening in the spine.

- The next most severe form is Meningocele. Only the meninges protrude from the opening in the spine

- The mildest form is Occulta. It is characterized by malformed vertebrae. Symptoms of this disease range from bowel and bladder dysfunctions to excess build up in the brain of cerebrospinal fluid.

The easiest way to prevent SB is through folic acid supplementation (at least 400 mcg daily) by all women of child-bearing age.

TO PREVENT:

Supplements: Master Formula HERS, Super B

TO REDUCE SYMPTOMS:

Single Oils: Mountain savory, helichrysum, thyme, and melaleuca.

Blends: Melrose, Thieves, and Exodus II.

Supplements: ImmuGel, Super C, and Radex.

Sprain

Single Oils: Lemon, birch, basil, pine, spruce, cypress, and peppermint.

Blends: PanAway or Relieve It with lemongrass.

Supplements: Ortho Sport Massage Oil, Sulfurzyme, and Mineral Essence.

(See CONECTIVE TISSUES AND MUSCLES)

Stress

Single Oils: Lavender, chamomile, Blue Tansy, marjoram, rose, sandalwood, frankincense, and cedarwood.

Blends: Humility, Harmony, Valor, and Joy .

Supplements: Super B, Ultra Young, Super C, Radex, VitaGreen, and Master Formula.

Smoking Cessation

Single Oils: Cinnamon, clove, nutmeg.

Blends: Harmony, Peace & Calming, Thieves, Exodus II.

Supplements: Cleansing Trio, Rehemogen, JuvaTone, and Stevia.

Application of Harmony: Put 1 drop on each foot; have another person cross his/her arms and pull slightly on the heels for 2-3 minutes or until it "feels right". Anoint the crown of the head with 1 drop. Rub 1 drop over the heart. Rub 1 drop around the navel.

Alternate with Peace & Calming.

Cleanse colon and liver with Cleansing Trio and JuvaTone.

The liver cleanse detoxifies the liver and helps to remove the cravings for nicotine, caffeine, sugar, chocolate, etc. It may be necessary to take 3 tablets of JuvaTone up to 3 times daily.

Rehemogen cleans and detoxifies the blood and works synergistically with JuvaTone, rebuilding the liver and erasing the addiction blueprint in the liver (see ADDICTIONS).

Stevia has been reported to decrease cravings for tobacco and alcohol.

Spastic Colon

(See IRRITABLE BOWEL SYNDROME)

Spine Injuries and Pain

According to numerous chiropractors, the Raindrop Technique using therapeutic-grade essential oils is revolutionizing the treatment of many types of back pain, spine inflammation, and vertebral misalignments. (See RAINDROP TECHNIQUE)

All of the essential oils described in this chapter can be used effectively in a Raindrop application as well as in more traditional massage therapy.

> Chiropractors have found that by applying Valor on the bottom of the feet, spinal manipulations take 60 percent less time and work, and the results last 75 percent longer.

The following include some essential oils and supplements for supporting the structural integrity of the spine and reducing discomfort:

Single Oils: Birch, spruce, peppermint, marjoram, and basil.

Blends: Valor, Aroma Siez, Thieves, Immu-Power, and PanAway.

Supplements: Super C, Mineral Essence, Royal Essence, and ArthroTune.

Aching Back

Single Oils: Clary sage with lavender and chamomile, basil, peppermint, geranium, or elemi.

Recipe 1:
- 5 drops clary sage
- 5 drops lavender
- 5 drops chamomile

Mix in 1 oz. V-6 Mixing Oil or Massage Oil Base

(See MUSCLES)

Calcification of Spine

Single Oils: Geranium with rosemary, eucalyptus radiata, ravensara, oregano, vetiver, or elemi.

Single Oils: R.C.

Supplements: ArthroTune, Sulfurzyme, Super Cal, and Ortho Ease Massage Oil.

Apply oils directly on the spine and on the spinal Vita Flex areas on bottom of the feet by massage and Raindrop Technique.

Herniated Disk and Deterioration

For this situation, it is best to consult a specialist. It is not likely that this situation may be helped with oils, although with continued use, there would mostly likely be some relief.

For temporary relief until medical attention can be given:

Single Oils: Helichrysum, pine, basil, thyme, melissa (Use with cold compress).

Blends: Relieve It, PanAway, Aroma Siez.

- Basil with Aroma Siez, or spruce with Relieve It.

Supplements: Sulfurzyme, ArthroTune, Super Cal, Ortho Sport and Ortho Ease Massage Oils.

Apply oils to back with Raindrop Technique, then apply basil along the sides of the spine. Stimulate with the "pointer technique" as described under Nerve Damage. This has been very effective for disk problems.

Lumbago (Lower back pain)

Chronic lower back pain can have many causes, including a damaged or pinched nerve (neuralgia) or congested colon.

Single Oils: For neuralgia: Marjoram, nutmeg, basil, Roman chamomile, elemi, and peppermint.

Blends: Di-Tone, Ortho Sport and Ortho Ease Massage Oils.

- Lavender with spruce, fir, birch, helichrysum, basil, peppermint, cypress, sandalwood, Relieve It or PanAway.

Apply using Raindrop Technique. Also apply on colon, stomach, and small intestine Vita Flex areas on the feet. Also apply around the navel. In severe cases use compresses or hot packs.

Supplements: Cleansing Trio, Sulfurzyme, Super C, and Super Cal.

Pointer Technique for Nerve Damage

The "pointer technique" may also be used on the foot Vita Flex points.

If there is nerve damage, apply about 6 drops of peppermint starting at the hips and finishing at the neck, using Raindrop Technique. Starting at the bottom of the spine, use a small-nosed pointer (about the size of a pencil but with a round end). Stimulate each vertebra between each rib on the vertebra knuckles all the way up on each side of the spine. Use medium pressure and a rocking motion for 1-10 seconds at each location. Then follow the same procedure once more up the center of the spine directly on each vertebra.

Neck Pain and Stiffness

Single Oils:

- Basil with marjoram and lavender or helichrysum with birch, nutmeg, pine, spruce, elemi, cypress, basil, or peppermint.

Recipe 1:
- 5 drops basil
- 5 drops marjoram
- 3 drops lavender

Recipe 2:
- 2 drops helichrysum
- 10 drops birch
- 8 drops cypress
- 15 drops basil
- 4 drops peppermint

Mix in 1 oz. V-6 Mixing Oil or Massage Oil Base.

Sciatica

Characterized by pain in the buttocks and down the back of the thigh. The pain worsens when coughing and sneezing or bending the back. The pain is caused by pressure on the sciatic nerve as it leaves the spine in the lower pelvic region. This nerve is the largest in the body, with branches throughout the lower body and legs.

Single Oils: Pine, helichrysum, peppermint, and nutmeg.

- Thyme with birch, basil, rosemary, cypress, spruce, peppermint, sandalwood, or oregano.
- Helichrysum with birch, clove, peppermint, or tarragon.
- Hyssop with birch, Roman chamomile, or Idaho tansy.

Blends:

- Thyme with Aroma Siez or PanAway.
- Helichrysum with PanAway or Aroma Siez.

Supplements: Ortho Ease or Ortho Sport Massage Oils, ArthroTune, Sulfurzyme, and Super B.

Birch with oregano is very powerful for bruised and damaged sciatica.

Use 2 drops of oil in left palm; circulate clockwise with right hand thumb. Rub on low end of spine and on sciatica Vita Flex points on feet. Always do both feet.

Sulfurzyme and Super B work well together to help rebuild nerve damage and the myelin sheath.

Stomach

(See DIGESTIVE DISORDERS)

Stretch Marks

(See PREGNANCY)

Stroke

(See BRAIN DISORDERS)

Sunburn

(See SKIN DISORDERS)

Sympathetic Nervous System

(See NERVOUS SYSTEM-AUTONOMIC)

Tachycardia

(See CARDIOVASCULAR CONDITIONS)

Tendonitis

(See CONNECTIVE TISSUE)

Testicular Regulation

Single Oils:

- Rosemary with clary sage, sage, fennel, bergamot, sandalwood, ylang ylang, geranium, yarrow, or pine.

Blends:

- Aroma Siez with Mister or Dragon Time.

Supplements: Progen, Mineral Essence, Master Formula vitamins, Ultra Young Plus.

Teeth Grinding

Single Oils: Lavender

Blends: Peace & Calming

Diffuse Peace & Calming or rub lavender on the feet.

Tooth Ache

(See PERIODONTAL DISEASE)

Single Oils: Clove.

Blends: Thieves.

Other: Fresh Essence Mouthwash.

Thyroid

Located at the base of the neck just below the Adam's apple, the thyroid is the energy gland of the human body. It produces T3 and T4 thyroid hormones that control the body's metabolism. The thyroid also controls other vital functions such as digestion, circulation, immune function, hormone balance, and emotions.

The thyroid gland is actually controlled by the pituitary gland which signals the thyroid when to produce thyroid hormone. The pituitary gland, in turn, is directed by chemical signals sent by the hypothalamus gland.

A lack of thyroid hormone does not necessarily mean that the thyroid is not functioning properly (although in many cases, this may be the case). In some instances, the pituitary may be malfunctioning because of its failure to release sufficient TSH (thyroid stimulating hormone) to spur the thyroid to make thyroid hormone.

Other cases of thyroid hormone deficiency may be due to the hypothalamus failing to release sufficient TRH (thyrotropin releasing hormone).

In cases where thyroid hormone deficiency is caused by a malfunctioning pituitary or hypothalamus, better results may be achieved by using supplements or essential oils that stimulate the pituitary or hypothalamus.

How to Measure Thyroid Function

To check your thyroid function, use the Barnes Basal Temperature Test:

- Shake a thermometer and leave on the bedside table just prior to going to sleep.

- Immediately upon awakening in the morning, insert the thermometer snugly in the armpit and lie quietly for ten minutes.

- Repeat test for two consecutive days and once more after a week.

- The temperature should range between 97.8° to 98.2° F (36.5 to 36.7° C). Temperatures below 97.8° indicate hypothyroidism (low thyroid function) and temperatures above 98.2 indicate hyperthyroidism (overactive thyroid function) which is far rarer.

NOTE: Women will obtain the most accurate readings when not menstruating or on the

People with type A blood have more of a tendency to have weak thyroid function.

Watch Out for Chlorine

Since chlorine shuts down thyroid function by preventing absorption of iodine and the amino acid tyrosine, drink chlorine-free water.

To remove chlorine from water, it should either be distilled or passed through activated carbon filters. As an alternative, you can let tap water stand unsealed and add a drop of lemon, peppermint, or spearmint.

Hyperthyroid (Graves Disease)

When the thyroid becomes overactive and produces excess thyroid hormone, the following symptoms occur:

Symptoms of hyperthyroidism:
- Anxiety
- Restlessness
- Insomnia
- Premature gray hair
- Diabetes mellitus
- Arthritis
- Vitilego (loss of skin pigment)

Graves disease, like Hashimoto's disease, is an autoimmune disease which results in an excess of thyroid hormone production.

MSM has been studied for its ability to reverse many kinds of autoimmune diseases. MSM is a key component of Sulfurzyme.

Single Oils: Myrryh, spruce, blue tansy.
- Lemongrass with myrrh
- Spruce with myrrh

Blends: EndoFlex.

Supplements: Sulfurzyme, Thyromin, VitaGreen, and Mineral Essence.

Hypothyroid

Those who do not produce enough thyroid hormone have a condition known as hypothyroidism. Approximately 40 percent of the U.S. population suffers from this disorder, and these people tend to also suffer hypoglycemia (low blood sugar).

Symptoms: Fatigue, yeast infections, candida, lack of energy, reduced immune function, poor resistance to disease, and recurring infections. (see HYPOGLYCEMIA).

Single Oils:
- Lemongrass with myrtle, peppermint, spearmint, myrrh, or clove.

Blends: EndoFlex
- Lemongrass with EndoFlex.

Place 1 drop of EndoFlex on back (top) of large toes.

Supplements: Thyromin and VitaGreen.

How to Use Thyromin

Thyromin is a supplement designed to feed and help rebuild the thyroid.

Thyromin is best taken at bedtime. Start with 1 capsule *immediately* before going to sleep. Check your temperature in the morning. If the Basal Temperature indicates no improvement, add 1 capsule in the morning.

If still no significant change, go to 2 capsules at night and 1 in the morning. Use this stepped approach until temperature is in correct range. VitaGreen enhances the effect of the Thyromin and may be helpful to take along with it.

NOTE: Take half of the total amount of Thyromin at night and half in the morning.

Hashimoto's Thyroiditis

This is an autoimmune disease in which the body's own immune system attacks the thyroid gland. In these cases, MSM may help mitigate some of the effects of this disease.

Supplements: Sulfurzyme, Thyromin and VitaGreen.

Tinnititis (Ringing in Ears)

(See HEARING IMPAIRMENT)

Toothache

(See PERIODONTAL DISEASE)

Single Oils: Clove, birch, Blue Tansy, melaleuca, and Idaho tansy.

Blends: Thieves and Exodus.

Supplements: Dentarome, Dentarome Plus, and Fresh Essence.

Rub oil on gums at location of pain or dental infection. Dentists have used clove for many years. German chamomile can be used for teething pains.

NOTE: *For small children, dilute oils in V-6 Mixing Oil or Massage Oil Base.*

Tonsillitis

(See COLDS)

The tonsils are a collection of infection-fighting lymphatic tissues (immune cells) that surround the throat. When these become infected due to streptococcal infection, they become inflamed, causing a condition known as tonsillitis.

It become popular in the 1960's and 1970's to have the tonsils removed when they became infected. However, tonsillectomies have become much less frequent as researchers have begun to appreciate the important role that the tonsils play in protecting and fighting infectious diseases and optimizing immune response.

The pharyngeal tonsils located at the back of the throat (known as the adenoids) can also become infected—a condition known as adenitis.

Single Oils: Clove, oregano, mountain savory, ravensara, and thyme.

Blends: Exodus II (massage outside of throat and put in water for a mouth wash) and Fresh Essence (gargle).

Supplements: ImmuGel and Super C.

Toxemia

(See INFECTION)

When toxins or bacteria begin to accumulate in the bloodstream, a condition called toxemia is created. When toxemia occurs during late pregnancy, it is referred to as "preeclampsia."

Single Oils: Fennel, tangerine, orange, and cypress.

Blends: Citrus Fresh, Inner Child, and Purification.

Supplements: I.C.P., ComforTone, Exodus, Super C, and Essential Manna (high in potassium, which is extremely important).

Tuberculosis

(See INFECTION)

Tuberculosis (TB) is a highly contagious lung disease caused by *Mycobacterium tuberculosis*. It passes readily between people through coughs, sneezes, and airborne bacteria. The most worrisome aspect of this disease is it latency. People may harbor the germ for years, yet display no outward or visible signs of infection. However, when their immune systems become challenged or downregulated due to stress, candida, diabetes, corticosteroid use, or other factors, the bacteria can become reactivated and develop into a full-blown case of TB.

Prior to the 1940's, tuberculosis was one of the leading causes of the death in the United States. After the introduction of anti-TB drugs following World War II, the disease largely disappeared. However, the incidence of TB has recently staged a surprising resurgence, with the number of TB cases increasing dramatically since 1984. In fact, in 1993 over 25,000 cases of TB were reported.

Because many essential oils have broad-spectrum antimicrobial properties, they can be diffused to prevent the spread of airborne bacteria like *Mycobacterium tuberculosis*. Essential oils and blends such as Thieves, Purification, Raven, R.C, and Sacred Mountain are extremely effective for killing germs.

Some essential oils have also been shown to immune-stimulating. Lemon oil has been shown increase lymphocyte production—a pivotal part of the immune system (Valnet, 1990).

Herbs like *Echinacea purpurea* have also been documented to enhance immune function. (Echinacea is included in Exodus).

Single Oils: Ravensara, rosemary verbenon, lemon, cinnamon, thyme linalol, sandalwood, or eucalyptus radiata.

- Cypress with ravensara, rosemary verbenon, lemon, cinnamon, sandalwood, or eucalyptus (all varieties).

- Frankincense with ravensara, thyme, eucalyptus, cypress, rosemary, birch, rose, myrtle and Idaho tansy.

- Thyme with eucalyptus, ravensara, birch, chamomile, lemon, lemongrass, cinnamon, clove, oregano, peppermint, or spearmint.

- Sage with mountain savory or spruce.

Blends:

- Cypress with Raven, R.C., or Sacred Mountain.

- Thyme with R.C., Raven, or Thieves.

- Frankincense with R.C., ImmuPower, Raven, or Inspiration.

Diffuse or massage on the chest after diluting with V6 Mixing Oil or Massage Oil Base. Apply on the lung Vita Flex points on the feet and hands.

Regimen:

1. Alternate diffusing Raven and R.C.

2. Dilute 1-2 drops myrtle, mountain savory, eucalyptus radiata, and ravensara in 1 Tbsp. of V-6 Mixing Oil. Apply as a rectal implants:

   - 2 drops sage
   - 4 drops myrrh
   - 5 drops clove
   - 6 drops ravensara
   - 15 drops frankincense

Mix in 1/2 oz. V-6 Mixing Oil or Massage Oil Base. Apply as rectal implant.

3. Put 2 drops Raven in a capsule and swallow 3 times daily.

4. Dilute 1-2 drops of Raven in V-6 Mixing Oil and use as a nightly rectal implant.

5. Apply a hot compress of Exodus II on the spine and Raven on the back.

6. Rub Thieves on the bottom of the feet.

7. Rub ImmuPower up the spine daily and apply as a compress on back and chest twice a day. Use Raindrop Technique.

Supplements: ImmuGel, Radex, Super C, Royal Essence, VitaGreen, ImmuneTune, and Rehemogen.

Exodus: 3-4 capsules 3 times daily for 21 days and rest for 7 days.

Cleanse colon and liver with Cleansing Trio and JuvaTone.

Trauma (Emotional)

(See SHOCK)

Emotional trauma can be generated from life events that involve loss, bereavement, accidents, or misfortunes. Esential oils, through their ability to tap the emotional and memory center of the brain, may facilitate the release and management of emotional trauma in a way that minimizes psychological turmoil.

Blends: Trauma Life, Hope, Forgiveness, Release, Envision, and Valor.

Supplements: Super C and Mineral Essence.

Tumors

(See CANCER)

Typhoid Fever

Typhoid fever is an infectious disease caused by a bacteria known as *Salmonella typhi*. Usually contracted through infected food or water, typhoid is common in lesser-developed countries.

Some people infected with typhoid fever display no visible symptoms of disease, while others become seriously ill. Both people who recover from typhoid fever and those who remain symptomless are carriers for the disease, and can infect others through the bacteria they shed in their feces.

To avoid contracting typhoid fever—especially when traveling overseas—it is essential to drink purified or distilled water and thoroughly cooked foods. Fresh vegetables can be carriers of the bacteria, especially if they have been irrigated with water that has come into contact with human waste.

Symptoms:
- Sustained, high fever (101° to 104° F).
- Stomach pains
- Headache
- Rash of reddish spots
- Impaired appetite
- Weakness

Single Oils: Ravensara, cinnamon, peppermint, black pepper, or mountain savory.

Add oils to water for purification.

Dilute in massage oil and apply on location.

Ulcers

Ulcers may be caused by *Helicobacter pylori* (bacteria). Several gastroduodenal diseases include gastritis and gastric or peptic ulcers.

Single Oils: Clove, cinnamon, oregano, thyme, and vetiver

Blends: Thieves.

Urinary Tract/Bladder Infection

Infections and inflammation of the urinary tract are caused by bacteria that travel up the urethra. This disorder is more common in women than men because of the woman's shorter urethra. If the infection travels up the ureters and reaches the kidneys, kidney infection can result.

(See KIDNEY DISORDERS)

Symptoms:
- Frequent urge to urinate with only a small amount of urine coming out
- Strong smelling urine
- Blood in urine
- Burning or stinging during urination

Bladder infection (known as cystitis or interstitial cystitis) is marked by the following symptoms:

- Tenderness or chronic pain in bladder and pelvic area
- Frequent urge to urinate
- Pain intensity fluctuates as bladder fills or empties
- Symptoms worsen during menstruation

Single Oils: Oregano, mountain savory, or melaleuca.

- Sage with mountain savory, juniper, cedarwood, fennel, rosemary, melaleuca, lavender, sandalwood, hyssop, German chamomile, or lemongrass.
- Thyme with oregano, rosemary verbenon, tarragon, lavender, spruce, eucalyptus (all varieties), clove, cinnamon, German chamomile, frankincense, Roman chamomile, melaleuca, lemongrass, geranium, helichrysum, fennel, peppermint, patchouly, spearmint, and tangerine.

Blends: Di-Tone, EndoFlex, Inspiration.

- Sage with Purification, Inspiration, or Melrose.
- Thyme with Melrose, Purification.
- Oregano with Thieves.
- R.C. or Di-Tone.
- Juniper with EndoFlex.

Inspiration may help clear up bladder infections. Rub 2-3 drops over bladder or apply in compress over bladder.

Supplements: K&B tincture, AlkaLime

Use K&B tincture (2-3 droppers in distilled water) 3-6 times daily. K & B Tincture helps strengthen and tone weak bladder, kidneys, and urinary tract (see KIDNEY DISORDERS).

Bladder Infection Blends

- 3 drops thyme
- 4 drops blue chamomile
- 8 drops frankincense
- 6 drops Roman chamomile
- 9 drops melaleuca
- 13 drops lemongrass
- 10 drops geranium
- 4 drops helichrysum
- 10 drops fennel
- 8 drops lavender
- 6 drops peppermint
- 6 drops patchouly
- 11 drops spearmint
- 10 drops tangerine

Mix in 2 oz. V-6 Mixing Oil or Massage Oil Base.

OR

- 3 droppers of K & B Tincture
- 1 drop mountain savory

Mix in water and drink every 2 hours.

Use cistus, ImmuPower, Inspiration in Raindrop Technique application or massage along lower back and pubic area.

Take 1 tsp. of AlkaLime daily, in water only, 1 hour before or after meal.

Juniper with EndoFlex may be applied as a hot compress.

Vaginal Infection

Single Oils: Myrrh, mountain savory, oregano, melaleuca, and thyme.

Blends: Melrose, 3 Wise Men, and Inspiration.

- Oregano and Thyme with Melrose.

Use Raindrop Technique with Thyme and Oregano. Douche with a mixture of 2 drops Oregano, 1 drop Thyme and 5 drops Melrose in 1 Tbsp. V-6 Mixing Oil or Massage Oil Base. Shake well and douche, or mix into 1 Tbsp. of V-6 Mixing Oil or Massage Oil Base and do a vaginal retention implant.

Vaginal Yeast Infection

Vaginal yeast infections are usually caused from overgrowth of fungi like *Candida albicans*. These naturally-occurring intestinal yeast and fungi are normally kept under control by the immune system, but when excess sucrose is consumed or antibiotics are used, these organisms convert from relatively harmless yeast into an invasive, harmful fungus that secretes toxins as part of its life cycle.

Vaginal yeast infections are just one symptom of systemic fungal infestation. While the yeast infection can be treated locally, the underlying problem of systemic candidiasis may still remain unless specific dietary and health practices are used.

(See FUNGAL INFECTIONS)

Uterine Cancer

(See CANCER)

Varicose Veins (Spider Veins)

The blue color of varicose veins is congealed blood in the surrounding tissue from hemorrhaging of capillaries around the veins. This blood has to be dissolved and re-absorbed.

Helichrysum helps dissolve the coagulated blood in the surrounding tissue.

Cypress helps strengthen capillary walls.

Idaho tansy helps weak veins.

Single Oils: Helichrysum

- Basil with cypress, birch, helichrysum, peppermint, or Idaho tansy.

- Cypress with helichrysum, lemongrass, tangerine, lavender, bergamot, or lemon.

Blends:

- Basil with Citrus Fresh, Aroma Life, or Aroma Siez.

- Cypress or lemongrass with Aroma Life.

Supplements: Cel-Lite Magic, VitaGreen, Super B, and Royal Essence.

Recipe 1:
- 3-4 drops basil
- 1 drop birch
- 1 drop cypress
- 1 drop helichrysum

Apply neat on location. Rub very gently towards heart with smooth strokes along the vein, then up and over the vein until dry. Do this twice.

Follow with a soft massage of the whole leg using Citrus Fresh, Aroma Life, or Cel-Lite Magic Massage Oil. This activates the entire vascular and limbic systems. Wrap the leg to hold and support it. Elevate the leg to allow the vein and capillary walls time to regenerate. It is best to do this at night and to elevate the foot off the bed, an inch at a time, until it is 4 inches higher than the head. Wear support hose during daytime. Be patient. It may take up to a year to regenerate the cellular wall and prevent further hemorrhaging.

If at home, use 6 drops of tangerine with 6 drops of cypress over the area. Then do lymphatic pump (see under LYMPHATIC SYSTEM).

You may also use 2 drops helichrysum with 2 drops of cypress. Apply twice, followed by Cel-Lite Magic Massage Oil. Follow the directions above or apply by layering. For example, massage 1-3 drops of helichrysum on location, followed by 1-3 drops of cypress and Cel-Lite Magic. Follow directions above.

Recipe: 2
- 2 drops basil
- 2 drops Idaho tansy
- 8 drops sage
- 3 drops sandalwood

Mix in 1/2 oz. V-6 Mixing Oil or Massage Oil Base and apply as above.

If a clot develops in a vein, rub cypress and helichrysum neat on location to dissolve it.

Vascular Cleansing

We absorb heavy metals from air, water, food, skin care products, mercury fillings in teeth, etc. These chemicals lodge in the fatty tissues of the body, which in turn give off toxic gases that may cause allergic symptoms. Ridding our bodies of

Amalgam fillings in teeth contain mercury. People who are sensitive to these metals may want to consider amalgam removal. However, the process is expensive, and the replacement is not always without problems, since the compounds in the new fillings can still cause reactions.

these heavy metals is extremely important in order to have healthy immune function, especially if we have amalgam fillings.

Single Oils: Helichrysum, cypress, frankincense.

- Helichrysum with German chamomile, Roman chamomile, frankincense, cypress, lemongrass, geranium, or cardamom.v

Blends: Arom Life

Supplements: JuvaTone, VitaGreen, Radex, Super C, ImmuneTune, ImmuGel, Royal Essence, Chelex, K&B Tincture, HRT tincture, Rehemogen, A.D.&E., or Megazyme.

Helichrysum is a powerful chelator and anticoagulant.

Frankincense, cypress, helichrysum, and lemongrass strengthen the vascular walls.

For cleansing the vascular system, chelating heavy metals, and removing plaque, use JuvaTone, VitaGreen, and Radex.

Rehemogen cleans and fortifies the blood.

Chelex: 1 dropperful in 4 ounces of water 2 times daily, helps to remove metallics from the system. Cardamom and VitaGreen enhance the action. Massage the body with Aroma Life and 1-2 drops of helichrysum, followed by Cel-Lite Magic Massage oil. These oils are dilators and help with the chelation of metallics.

Recipe:
- 10 drops juniper
- 10 drops cypress
- 10 drops lemongrass

Mix in 1 oz. V-6 Mixing Oil or Massage Oil Base and rub under arms, on skin above kidneys, and bottoms of feet.

Intravenous chelation causes scar tissue on the vascular walls. The following supplements provide a natural method:

- A.D.&E. liquid vitamins
- Megazyme
- Rehemogen
- Cleansing Trio

This method takes longer than standard chelation therapy, but has minimal side effects.

To help pull dental mercury out of gum tissue, mix 3 drops helichrysum and 4 drops Thieves and put on a rolled gauze and place next to the gums. Only apply to one area at a time; for example, apply on lower left gum on the first night, the upper left the second night and so on.

NOTE: For very sensitive gums or on children, dilute with V-6 Mixing Oil or Massage Oil Base.

(See CIRCULATION PROBLEMS)

Drink at least 64 ounces of distilled water daily to flush toxins and chemicals out of the body.

Vitiligo

(See SKIN DISORDERS)

Warts (Genital)

Warts are a form of viral infection caused by the human papillomavirus (HPV), of which there are more than 60 different types.

One type of HPV virus is among the most common causes of sexually transmitted disease. Up to 24 million Americans may be currently infected with HPV, usually spread through sexual contact. HPV lives only in genital tissue.

Single Oils: Oregano, thyme, melaleuca, frankincense, and hyssop

Blends: Thieves, and Melrose.

Supplements: A.D.&E..

Dilute 1-2 drops in vegetable oil and apply on location. Use frankincense for stubborn warts.

Whooping Cough

(See COLDS, INFECTION)

Wounds, Scrapes, Cuts

When selecting oils to for surface injuries, try treat the whole person, not just the cut itself. This means thinking through the cause and type of injury and selecting oils for each aspect of the trauma. For instance, a wound could encompass muscle damage, nerve damage, ligament damage, inflammation, infection, bone injury, fever, and possibly an emotion. Therefore, select an oil or blend that treats each of these.

Single Oils:

- Lavender with melaleuca, neroli, rosemary, Idaho tansy, eucalyptus (globulus and radiata), German chamomile, Roman chamomile, helichrysum, peppermint, clove, sandalwood, rose hip seed oil, ravensara, patchouly, geranium, rose, or palmarosa.

- Birch with melaleuca, neroli, lavender, lemon, frankincense, grapefruit, rosemary, thyme, or Roman chamomile.

- Thyme with melaleuca, rosemary, oregano, Roman chamomile, German chamomile, patchouly, lavandin, cedarwood, or lemon.

- Sage with hyssop, melaleuca, rosemary, Roman chamomile, German chamomile, mountain savory, myrrh, or patchouly.

- Lemongrass with peppermint, melaleuca, or bergamot.

The Essential Ingredient

Rose Ointment makes an ideal sealing and penetrating ointment for all wounds, cuts, and abrasions. It reduces the evaporation of the essential oils, thereby allowing them to keep in contact with the skin longer and potentiate their antimicrobial and tissue-regenerating benefits. The ointment also seals and protects the wound from dirt, debris, and reinfection.

Blends:

- Lavender or birch with Purification, Raven, or Melrose.

- Thyme with Melrose, Purification, Thieves, or 3 Wise Men.

- Any blend is beneficial and can be used in an emergency.

Supplements, skin care: Rose Ointment, and Stevia.

First-Aid Spray

In a sterile spray bottle, mix 5 drops lavender, 3 drops melaleuca, and 2 drops cypress in 8 ounces of saline water. Clean wound thoroughly. Shake well, spray the area, and cover with sterile gauze on which 1-3 drops of lavender have been placed. This should be repeated 2 times daily as necessary. After 3 days expose the cut or abrasion to the air if possible. A drop of oil 1-2 times daily will complete the healing process.

Bleeding from Open Wounds

Compress:
- 1 drop geranium
- 1 drop lemon
- 1 drop chamomile.

An Example of How to Use Essential Oils to Treat Cuts

A patient's finger was bleeding badly from a deep cut, apparently needing stitches. The application of 3 drops of helichrysum and 1 drop of clove staunched the bleeding and blocked the pain. Next, 1 drop each of lavender, Melrose, and lemongrass were applied. The wound was covered with Rose Ointment and a band-aid. The dressing was changed twice a day (morning and night), with myrrh and patchouly added each time.

The wound began healing well but became infected several days later. The application of Thieves on the infected area reduced the redness and infection. Within 2 weeks the cut had healed and 2 months later there was no trace of a scar.

Alternate with hyssop, cypress, rose, and palmarosa.

Neat or direct application: 2 or more times daily for 3 or 4 days. Afterwards this can be reduced to 1-2 times daily until wound is healed.

For both children and adults:

Lavender can be used undiluted to disinfect wounds, scrapes, and cuts. Roman chamomile is also very mild and non-toxic; it is an excellent pain reliever and remedy for scratches, chapped and dry skin. Add Roman chamomile to Rose Ointment for a wonderful first aid salve.

Bruises and wounds: (may be used on infants and children):
- 3 drops helichrysum
- 3 drops lavender

Mix in 1/8 oz. V-6 Mixing Oil or Massage Oil Base.

Infected or fresh cuts:
- 7 drops geranium
- 5 drops peppermint
- 10 drops melaleuca
- 8 drops orange

Dilute in vegetable oil and apply.

NOTE: *Both helichrysum and peppermint sting when applied to an open wound. To reduce discomfort, dilute these oils with lavender oil or mix in Rose Ointment before applying. When applied to a wound or cut that has sealed-over, peppermint will soothe, cool, and reduce inflammation in damaged tissue.*

To reduce bleeding and prevent hemorrhaging: Rose hip seed oil, essential oils of rose, helichrysum, and lemon,

To reduce scar-formation: Rose hip seed oil, stevia extract, rose, frankincense, hyssop, helichrysum, and myrrh.

Recipe 1:
• 10 drops helichrysum
• 6 drops lavender
• 8 drops lemongrass
• 4 drops patchouly

Mix in 1/2 to 1 oz. V-6 Mixing Oil or Massage Base and apply.

• Mix lavender, lemongrass, and geranium.

• Mix lecithin with 1-2 drops each of lavender and helichrysum.

To promote healing and cell regeneration: patchouly, lavender, neroli, myrrh, helichrysum, sandalwood, and Idaho tansy.

To disinfect: Thyme (linalol and thymol), Idaho tansy, hyssop, melaleuca, mountain savory

To reduce inflammation: German chamomile.

For surgical wounds:
• 24 drops lavender
• 18 drops helichrysum
• 18 drops frankincense

Apply with 2 Tbsp. V-6 Mixing Oil or Massage Base.

Worms

(See PARASITES)

Wrinkles

(See SKIN DISORDERS)

Yeast Infection

(See HORMONES, VAGINAL YEAST INFECTION)

Melaleuca alternifolia

During World War II, melaleuca was found to have very strong antibacterial properties and worked well in preventing infection in open wounds. Melrose is a blend containing two types of melaleuca oil, making it an exceptional antiseptic and tissue regenerator. An excellent combination to disinfect and promote healing is Melrose and Rose Ointment.

References

Al-Awadi FM, et al. "Studies on the activity of individual plants of an antidiabetic plant mixture." *Acta Diabetol Lat*. 1987;24(1):37-41.

Aqel MB. "Relaxant effect of the volatile oil of *Rosmarinus officinalis* on tracheal smooth muscle." *J Ethnopharmacol*. 1991;33(1-2):57-62.

Aruna, K. and V.M. Sivaramakrishnan. "Anticarcinogenic Effects of the Essential Oils from Cumin, Poppy and Basil." Food Chem Toxicol. 1992;30(11):953-56.

Azizan A, et al. "Mutagenicity and antimutagenicity testing of six chemicals associated with the pungent properties of specific spices as revealed by the Ames Salmonella/microsomal assay." *Arch Environ Contam Toxicol*. 1995;28(2):248-58.

Bassett IB, et al. "A comparative study of tea-tree oil versus benzoylperoxide in the treatment of acne." *Med J Aust*. 1990;153(8):455-8.

Benencia F, et al. "Antiviral activity of sandalwood oil against herpes simplex viruses-1 and -2." *Phytomedicine*. 1999;6(2):119-23

Bernardis LL, et al. "The lateral hypothalamic area revisited: ingestive behavior." *Neurosci Biobehav Rev*. 20(2):189-287 (1996).

Bilgrami KS, et al. "Inhibition of aflatoxin production & growth of *Aspergillus flavus* by eugenol & onion & garlic extracts." *Indian J Med Res*. 1992;96:171-5.

Bradshaw RH, et al. "Effects of lavender straw on stress and travel sickness in pigs." *J Altern Complement Med*. 1998;4(3):271-5.

Brodal A. Neurological Anatomy in Relation to Clinical Medicine. New York: Oxford University Press, 1981.

Buchbauer G, et al. "Aromatherapy: evidence for sedative effects of the essential oil of lavender after inhalation." *Z Naturforsch* [C]. 1991;46(11-12):1067-72.

Carson CF, et al. "Antimicrobial activity of the major components of the essential oil of *Melaleuca alternifolia*." *J Appl Bacteriol*. 1995;78(3):264-9.

Compendium of Olfactory Research. Edited by Avery N. Gilbert. Dubuque, IA: Kendall Hunt Publishing, 1995.

Concha JM, et al. 1998 William J. Stickel Bronze Award. "Antifungal activity of *Melaleuca alternifolia* (tea-tree) oil against various pathogenic organisms." *J Am Podiatr Med Assoc*. 1998;88(10): 489-92

Cornwell S, et al. "Lavender oil and perineal repair." *Mod Midwife* 1995;5(3):31-3.

Delaveau P, et al. "Neuro-depressive properties of essential oil of lavender." *C R Seances Soc Biol Fil*. 1989;183(4):342-8.

Didry N, et al. "Activity of thymol, carvacrol, cinnamaldehyde and eugenol on oral bacteria." *Pharm Acta Helv*. 1994;69(1):25-8.

Diego MA, et al. "Aromatherapy positively affects mood, EEG patterns of alertness and math computations." *Int J Neurosci*. 1998 Dec;96(3-4):217-24.

Dolara P, et al. "Analgesic effects of myrrh." *Nature*. 1996 Jan 4;379(6560):29.

Dunn C, et al. "Sensing an improvement: an experimental study to evaluate the use of aromatherapy, massage and periods of rest in an intensive care unit." *J Adv Nurs*. 1995;21(1):34-40.

Dwivedi C, et al. "Chemopreventive effects of sandalwood oil on skin papillomas in mice." *Eur J Cancer Prev*. 1997;6(4):399-401.

Elson CE, et al. "Impact of lemongrass oil, an essential oil, on serum cholesterol." *Lipids*. 1989;24(8):677-9.

Fang, H.J., et al. "Studies on the chemical components and anti-tumour action of the volatile oils from Pelargonium graveoleus." *Yao Hsueh Hsueh Pao*. 1989;24(5):366-71.

Faoagali JL, et al. "Antimicrobial effects of melaleuca oil." *Burns*. 1998;24(4):383. No abstract available.

Fleming, T., Ed. PDR for Herbal Medicines, Medical Economics Company, Inc., Montvale, NJ (1998).

Fyfe L, et al. "Inhibition of *Listeria monocytogenes* and *Salmonella enteriditis* by combinations of plant oils and derivatives of benzoic acid: the development of synergistic antimicrobial combinations." *Int J Antimicrob Agents.* 1997;9(3):195-9.

Gattefossé, René-Maurice. Gattefossé's Aromatherapy. Saffron Walden, UK: C.W. Daniel & Co., 1993.

Gobel H, et al. "Effect of peppermint and eucalyptus oil preparations on neurophysiological and experimental algesimetric headache parameters." *Cephalalgia.* 1994; 14(3):228-34.

Guillemain J, et al. "Neurodepressive effects of the essential oil of Lavandula angustifolia Mill." *Ann Pharm Fr.* 1989;47(6):337-43.

Gumbel, D. Principles of Holistic Therapy with Herbal Essences, Haug International, Brussels, Belgium (1993)

Hammer KA, et al. "In vitro susceptibilities of lactobacilli and organisms associated with bacterial vaginosis to *Melaleuca alternifolia* (tea tree) oil." Antimicrob Agents Chemother. 1999;43(1):196.

Hammer KA, et al. "Susceptibility of transient and commensal skin flora to the essential oil of *Melaleuca alternifolia* (tea tree oil)." *Am J Infect Control.* 1996;24(3):186-9.

Hasan HA, et al. "Inhibitory effect of spice oils on lipase and mycotoxin production." *Zentralbl Mikrobiol.* 1993;148(8):543-8.

Hausen BM, et al. "Comparative studies of the sensitizing capacity of drugs used in herpes simplex." *Derm Beruf Umwelt.* 1986;34(6):163-70.

Hay IC, et al. "Randomized trial of aromatherapy. Successful treatment for alopecia areata." *Arch Dermatol.* 1998; 134(11):1349-52.

Hirsch, Alan. "Inhalation of 2 acetylpyridine for weight reduction." *Chemical Senses* 18:570 (1993).

Hirsch, Alan. A Scentsational Guide to Weight Loss. Rockport, MA: Element, 1997.

Inouye S, et al. "Antisporulating and respiration-inhibitory effects of essential oils on filamentous fungi." Mycoses. 1998;41(9-10):403-10.

Jayashree T, et al. "Antiaflatoxigenic activity of eugenol is due to inhibition of lipid peroxidation." *Lett Appl Microbiol.* 1999; 28(3):179-83.

Juergens UR, et al. "The anti-inflammatory activity of L-menthol compared to mint oil in human monocytes in vitro: a novel perspective for its therapeutic use in inflammatory diseases." *Eur J Med Res.* 1998; 3(12):539-45.

Kim HM, et al. "Lavender oil inhibits immediate-type allergic reaction in mice and rats." *J Pharm Pharmacol.* 1999;51(2):221-6.

Kucera LS, et al. "Antiviral activities of extracts of the lemon balm plant." *Ann NY Acad Sci.* 1965 Jul 30;130(1):474-82.

Kulieva ZT. "Analgesic, hypotensive and cardiotonic action of the essential oil of the thyme growing in Azerbaijan." *Vestn Akad Med Nauk SSSR.* 1980;(9):61-3.

Lachowicz KJ, et al. "The synergistic preservative effects of the essential oils of sweet basil (*Ocimum basilicum* L.) against acid-tolerant food microflora." *Lett Appl Microbiol.* 1998;26(3):209-14.

Lantry LE, et al. "Chemopreventive effect of perillyl alcohol on 4-(methylnitrosamino)-1-(3-pyridyl)-1-butanone induced tumorigenesis in (C3H/HeJ X A/J)F1 mouse lung." *J Cell Biochem Suppl.* 1997;27:20-5.

Larrondo JV, et al. "Antimicrobial activity of essences from labiates." *Microbios.* 1995; 82(332): 171-2.

Lis-Balchin, M., et al. "Antimicrobial activity of Pelargonium essential oils added to a quiche filling as a model food system." *Lett Appl Microbiol.* 1998;27(4):207-10.

Lis-Balchin, M., et al. "Comparative antibacterial effects of novel Pelargonium essential oils and solvent extracts." *Lett Appl Microbiol.* 1998;27(3): 135-41.

Lorenzetti BB, et al. "Myrcene mimics the peripheral analgesic activity of lemongrass tea." *J Ethnopharmacol.* 1991;34(1):43-8.

Mahmood N, et al. "The anti-HIV activity and mechanisms of action of pure compounds isolated from Rosa damascena." *Biochem Biophys Res Commun.* 1996;229(1):73-9.

Mangena T, et al. "Comparative evaluation of the antimicrobial activities of essential oils of *Artemisia afra, Pteronia incana* and *Rosmarinus officinalis* on selected bacteria and yeast strains." *Lett Appl Microbiol.* 1999;28(4):291-6.

Maury, Marguerite. The Secret and Life of Youth. Saffon Waldon, UK: C.W. Daniels & Co., 1995.

McGuffin, M., et al. Botanical Safety Handbook, CRC Press, Boca Raton, FL (1997)

Meeker HG, et al. "The antibacterial action of eugenol, thyme oil, and related essential oils used in dentistry." *Compendium*. 1988;9(1):32, 34-5, 38 passim.

Michie, C.A., et al. "Frankincense and myrrh as remedies in children." *J R Soc Med*. 1991;84(10): 602-5.

Modgil R, et al. "Efficacy of mint and eucalyptus leaves on the physicochemical characteristics of stored wheat against insect infestation." *Nahrung*. 1998;42(5):304-8.

Moleyar V, et al. "Antibacterial activity of essential oil components." *Int J Food Microbiol*. 1992;16(4): 337-42.

Montagna, F. J. HDR Herbal Desk Reference Kendall/Hunt Publishing Company, Dubuque, IA (1979).

Murray, M. Encyclopedia of Nutritional Supplements, Prima Publishing, Rocklin, CA (1996).

Nagababu E, et al. "The protective effects of eugenol on carbon tetrachloride induced hepatotoxicity in rats." *Free Radic Res*. 1995;23(6):617-27.

Naidu KA. "Eugenol--an inhibitor of lipoxygenase-dependent lipid peroxidation." *Prostaglandins Leukot Essent Fatty Acids*. 1995;53(5):381-3.

Nakamoto K, et al. "In vitro effectiveness of mouthrinses against *Candida albicans*." *Int J Prosthodont*. 1995;8(5):486-9.

Nasel, C. et al. "Functional imaging of effects of fragrances on the human brain after prolonged inhalation." *Chemical Senses*. 1994;19(4):359-64

Nenoff P, et al. "Antifungal activity of the essential oil of *Melaleuca alternifolia* (tea tree oil) against pathogenic fungi in vitro." *Skin Pharmacol*. 1996;9(6):388-94.

Nikolaevskii VV, et al. "Effect of essential oils on the course of experimental atherosclerosis." *Patol Fiziol Eksp Ter*. 1990; (5):52-3.

Nishijima H, et al. "Mechanisms mediating the vasorelaxing action of eugenol, a pungent oil, on rabbit arterial tissue." *Jpn J Pharmacol*. 1999 Mar;79(3):327-34.

Panizzi L, et al. "Composition and antimicrobial properties of essential oils of four Mediterranean Lamiaceae." *J Ethnopharmacol*. 1993;39(3):167-70.

Pattnaik S, et al. "Antibacterial and antifungal activity of ten essential oils in vitro." *Microbios*. 1996;86(349):237-46.

Pedersen, M. Nutritional Herbology, A Reference Guide to Herbs, Wendell W. Whitman Company, Warsaw, IN (1998)

Pénoël, Daniel and P. Franchomme. L'aromatherapie exactment. France, 1990: Roger Jallois

Pénoël, Daniel. Natural Home Health Care Using Essential Oils. Salem, UT: Essential Science Publishing, 1998.

Privitera, James. Silent Clots. Covina, CA: 1996

Reddy BS, et al. "Chemoprevention of colon carcinogenesis by dietary perillyl alcohol." *Cancer Res*. 1997;57(3):420-5.

Reddy AC, et al. "Effect of curcumin and eugenol on iron-induced hepatic toxicity in rats." *Toxicology* 1996;107(1):39-45.

Reddy AC, et al. "Studies on anti-inflammatory activity of spice principles and dietary n-3 polyunsaturated fatty acids on carrageenan-induced inflammation in rats." *Ann Nutr Metab*. 1994;38(6): 349-58.

Rompelberg CJ, et al. "Antimutagenicity of eugenol in the rodent bone marrow micronucleus test." *Mutat Res*. 1995;346(2):69-75.

Rompelberg CJ, et al. "Effect of short-term dietary administration of eugenol in humans" *Hum Exp Toxicol*. 1996;15(2):129-35.

Saeed SA, et al. "Antithrombotic activity of clove oil." *JPMA J Pak Med Assoc*. 1994;44(5):112-5.

Samman MA, et al. "Mint prevents shamma-induced carcinogenesis in hamster cheek pouch." *Carcinogenesis*. 1998;19(10):1795-801.

Shapiro S, et al. "The antimicrobial activity of essential oils and essential oil components towards oral bacteria." *Oral Microbiol Immunol*. 1994;9(4): 202-8.

Sharma JN, et al. "Suppressive effects of eugenol and ginger oil on arthritic rats." *Pharmacology*. 1994;49(5):314-8.

Shirota S, et al. "Tyrosinase inhibitors from crude drugs." *Biol Pharm Bull*. 1994; 17(2):266-9.

Srivastava KC. "Antiplatelet principles from a food spice clove." *Prostaglandins Leukot Essent Fatty Acids*. 1993;48(5):363-72.

Steinman, David and Samuel S. Epstein. "The Safe Shopper's Bible: A Consumer's Guide to Nontoxic Household Products, Cosmetics, and Food." Macmillan, New York, NY (1995).

Sukumaran K, et al. "Inhibition of tumour promotion in mice by eugenol." *Indian J Physiol Pharmacol*. 1994;38(4):306-8.

Syed TA, et al. "Treatment of toenail onychomycosis with 2% butenafine and 5% *Melaleuca alternifolia* (tea tree) oil in cream." *Trop Med Int Health*. 1999;4(4):284-7.

Sysoev NP. "The effect of waxes from essential-oil plants on the dehydrogenase activity of the blood neutrophils in mucosal trauma of the mouth." *Stomatologiia* 1991;70(1):12-3.

Takacsova M, et al. "Study of the antioxidative effects of thyme, sage, juniper and oregano." *Nahrung*. 1995;39(3):241-3.

Tantaoui-Elaraki A, et al. "Inhibition of growth and aflatoxin production in *Aspergillus parasiticus* by essential oils of selected plant materials." *J Environ Pathol Toxicol Oncol*. 1994;13(1):67-72.

Tisserand, R. and T. Balacs Essential Oil Safety, Churchill Livingstone, New York, NY (1996).

Tiwari BK, et al. "Evaluation of insecticidal, fumigant and repellent properties of lemongrass oil." *Indian J Exp Biol*. 1966;4(2):128-9.

Tovey ER, et al. "A simple washing procedure with eucalyptus oil for controlling house dust mites and their allergens in clothing and bedding." *J Allergy Clin Immunol*. 1997; 100(4):464-6.

Tyler, V. E. Herbs of Choice Pharmaceutical Products Press, Binghamton, NY (1994).

Tyler, V. E. The Honest Herbal, Lubrect & Cramer, Ltd., Port Jervis, NY (1995).

Unnikrishnan MC, et al. "Tumour reducing and anticarcinogenic activity of selected spices." *Cancer Lett*. 1990;51(1):85-9.

Valnet, Jean. Robert Tisserand, ed. "The Practice of Aromatherapy." Healing Arts Press, Rochester, VT (1990).

Veal L. "The potential effectiveness of essential oils as a treatment for headlice, *Pediculus humanus capitis*." *Complement Ther Nurs Midwifery*. 1996;2(4):97-101.

Vernet-Maury E, et al. "Basic emotions induced by odorants: a new approach based on autonomic pattern results." *J Auton Nerv Syst*. 1999;75(2-3):176-83.

Wagner J, et al. "Beyond benzodiazepines: alternative pharmacologic agents for the treatment of insomnia." *Ann Pharmacother*. 1998;32(6):680-91.

Wan J, et al. "The effect of essential oils of basil on the growth of *Aeromonas hydrophila* and *Pseudomonas fluorescens*." *J Appl Microbiol*. 1998;84(2):152-8.

Wang, L.G., et al. "Determination of DNA topoisomerase II activity from L1210 cells--a target for screening antitumor agents." Chung Kuo Yao Li Hsueh Pao. 1991;12(2):108-14.

Weyers W, et al. "Skin absorption of volatile oils. Pharmacokinetics." *Pharm Unserer Zeit*. 1989; 18(3):82-6.

Wie MB, et al. "Eugenol protects neuronal cells from excitotoxic and oxidative injury in primary cortical cultures." *Neurosci Lett*. 1997: 4;225(2):93-6.

Yamada K, et al. "Anticonvulsive effects of inhaling lavender oil vapour." B*iol Pharm Bull*. 1994;17(2):359-60.

Yamasaki K, et al. "Anti-HIV-1 activity of herbs in Labiatae." *Biol Pharm Bull*. 1998;21(8):829-33.

Yang, K.K. et al., "Antiemetic principles of Pogostemon cablin (Blanco) Benth." Phytomedicine 1999, 6(2): 89-93. Youdim KA, et al. "Beneficial effects of thyme oil on age-related changes in the phospholipid C20 and C22 polyunsaturated fatty acid composition of various rat tissues." *Biochim Biophys Acta*. 1999;1438(1): 140-6.

Young, Robert O. Sick and Tired. Alpine, UT, 1977.

Yousef, R.T. and G.G. Tawil. "Antimicrobial activity of volatile oils." *Pharmazie* 1980; 35(11);798-701

Zanker KS, et al. "Evaluation of surfactant-like effects of commonly used remedies for colds." *Respiration*. 1980;39(3):150-7.

Appendix A - AFNOR Standards

AFNOR/ISO Standards for Therapeutic-Grade
Chamaemelum nobilis
Gas Chromatograph profile 4.10

CONSTITUENTS	Min %	Max %
Isobutyl angelate + Isoamyl methacrylate	30	45
Isoamyl angelate	12	22
Methyl allyl angelate	6	10
2-methyl butyl angelate	3	7
Isoamyl isobutyrate	3	5
Trans-pino-carveol	2	5
Isobutyl n-butyrate	2	9
α-pinene	1.5	5
Pinocarvone	1.3	4
Isobutyl methacrylate	1	3
2-methyl butyl methacrylate	.5	1.5

AFNOR/ISO Standards for Therapeutic-Grade
Lavandula angustifolia
Gas Chromatograph profile 4.10

CONSTITUENTS	Min %	Max %
Linalol	25	38
Linalyl acetate	25	45
cis-β-ocimene	4	10
trans-β-ocimene	1.5	6
terpinen-4-ol	2	6
Lavendulyl acetate	2	—
Lavendulol	.3	—
β-phellandrene	traces	.5
α-terpineol	—	1
Octanone-3	traces	2
Camphor	traces	.5
Limonene	—	.5
1,8 cineole	—	1

AFNOR/ISO European and World Standards
for Therapeutic-Grade
Eucalyptus globulus
Gas Chromatograph profile 4.11

CONSTITUENTS	Pure Essential Oil		Rectified Essential Oil	
	crushed raw	traditional	70%-75%	80%-85%
1,8 cineol min %	48	58	70	80
α-Pinene min % max %	10 20	20 22	Traces 20	Traces 12
Aromadendrene min % max %	6 10	1 5	— traces	— traces
Limonene min % max %	2 4	1 8	2 15	2 15
p-cymene min % max %	1 3	1 5	1 6	1 10
trans-pinocarveol min % max %	1 4	1 5	traces 10	traces 6
Globulol min % max %	.5 2.5	.5 1.5	— traces	— traces

343

AFNOR/ISO European and World Standards for Therapeutic-Grade
Salvia sclarea
Gas Chromatograph profile 4.10

CONSTITUENTS	Traditional	Crushed Green
Linalyl acetate		
min %	62	56
max %	78	70.5
Linalol		
min %	6.5	13
max %	13.5	24
Sclareol		
min %	.4	.4
max %	2.6	2.6
d-germacrene		
min %	1.5	1.2
max %	12	7.5
α-terpineol		
min %	traces	1
max %	1.2	5

AFNOR/ISO Standards for Therapeutic-Grade
Basilicum ocimum
Gas Chromatograph profile 4.8

CONSTITUENTS	Min %	Max %
Methyl chavicol	75	85
1,8 cineol	1	3.5
Trans-beta ocimene	.9	2.8
Linalol	.50	.30
Methyl eugenol	.3	2.5
Terpinen-4-ol	.20	.60
Camphor	.15	.50

AFNOR/ISO Standards for Therapeutic-Grade
Syzygium aromaticum
Gas Chromatograph profile 4.8

CONSTITUENTS	Min %	Max %
Eugenol	80	92
B-caryophyllene	4	17
Eugenyl acetate	.2	4

AFNOR/ISO Standards for Therapeutic-Grade
Cupressus sempervirens
Gas Chromatograph profile 4.11

CONSTITUENTS	Min %	Max %
α-pinene	40	65
δ-3-carene	12	25
limonene	1.8	5
α-Terpenyl acetate	1	4
Myrcene	1	3.5
Cedrol	.8	7
β-pinene	.5	3
D-germacrene	.5	3
Terpinen-4-ol	.2	2

Appendix B - Food "Ash" pH

The following is a list of common foods with an approximate, relative potential of acidity (-) or alkalinity (+), as present in 1 ounce of food.

Food	Value	Food	Value	Food	Value
Alfalfa Grass	+29.3	Celery	+13.3	Ketchup	-12.4
Almond	+3.6	Cheese, Hard	-18.1	Kohlrabi	+5.1
Apricot	-9.5	Cherry, Sour	+3.5	Lecithin, pure (soy)	+38.0
Artichokes	+1.3	Cherry, Sweet	-3.6	Leeks (bulbs)	+7.2
Asparagus	+1.1	Chia, sprouted	+28.5	Lemon, fresh	+9.9
Avocado (protein)	+15.6	Chicken	-18.0 to -22.0	Lentils	+0.6
Banana, Ripe	-10.1	Chives	+8.3	Lettuce	+2.2
Banana, Unripe	+4.8	Coconut, fresh	+0.5	Lettuce, Fresh cabbage	+14.1
Barley Grass	+28.7	Coffee	-25.1	Lettuce, Lamb's	+4.8
Barley malt syrup	-9.3	Comfrey	+1.5	Limes	+8.2
Beans, French cut	+11.2	Corn oil	-6.5	Liquor	-28.6 to -38.7
Beans, Lima	+12.0	Cranberry	-7.0	Liver	-3.0
Beans, White	+12.1	Cream	-3.9	Macadamia Nuts	-11.7
Beef	-34.5	Cucumber, fresh	+31.5	Mandarin Orange	-11.5
Beer	-26.8	Cumin	+1.1	Mango	-8.7
Beet sugar	-15.1	Currant	-8.2	Margarine	-7.5
Beet, fresh red	+11.3	Currant, Black	-6.1	Marine Lipids	+4.7
Biscuit, White	-6.5	Currant, Red	-2.4	Mayonnaise	-12.5
Blueberry	-5.3	Dandelion	+22.7	Meats, Organ	-3.0
Borage	+3.2	Date	-4.7	Milk sugar	-9.4
Brazil Nuts	-0.5	Dog grass	+22.6	Milk, Homogenized	-1.0
Bread, Rye	-2.5	Eggs	-18.0 to -22.0	Millet	+0.5
Bread, White	-10.0	Endive, fresh	+14.5	Molasses	-14.6
Bread, whole-grain	-4.5	Fennel	+1.3	Mustard	-19.2
Bread, whole-meal	-6.5	Fig juice powder	-2.4	Nut soy (Soaked, then air dried)	+26.5
Brussels Sprouts	-1.5	Filbert	-2.0	Olive Oil	+1.0
Buckwheat groats	+0.5	Fish, Fresh Water	-11.8	Onion	+3.0
Butter	-3.9	Fish, Ocean	-20.0	Orange	-9.2
Buttermilk	+1.3	Flax seed oil	-1.3	Oysters	-5.0
Cabbage, Green, December harvest	+4.0	Flax seed	+3.5	Papaya	-9.4
Cabbage, Green, March harvest	+2.0	Fructose	-9.5	Peach	-9.7
Cabbage, Red	+6.3	Garlic	+13.2	Peanuts	-12.8
Cabbage, Savoy	+4.5	Gooseberry, Ripe	-7.7	Pear	-9.9
Cabbage, White	+3.3	Grapefruit	-1.7	Peas, fresh	+5.1
Cantaloupe	-2.5	Grapes, Ripe	-7.6	Peas, ripe	+0.5
Caraway	+2.3	Hazelnut	-2.0	Pineapple	-12.6
Carrot	+9.5	Honey	-7.6	Pistachios	-16.6
Cashews	-9.3	Horseradish	+6.8	Plum, Italian	-4.9
Cauliflower	+3.1	Juice, natural fruit	-8.7	Plum, yellow	-4.9
Cayenne Pepper	+18.8	Juice, white sugar sweetened fruit	-33.4	Pork	-38.0
		Kamut Grass	+27.6	Potatoes, stored	+2.0

Primrose	+4.1	Soy Flour	+2.5	Tofu	+3.2
Pumpkin	-5.6	Soy Sprouts	+29.5	Tomato	+13.6
Quark	-17.3	Soybeans, fresh	+12.0	Turbinado	-9.5
Radish, Sprouted	+28.4	Spelt	+0.5	Turnip	+8.0
Radish, Summer black	+39.4	Spinach		Veal	-35.0
Radish, White (spring)	+3.1	(other than March)	+13.1	Walnuts	-8.0
Raspberry	-5.1	Spinach, March harvest	+8.0	Watercress	+7.7
Red radish	+16.7	Straw grass	+21.4	Watermelon	-1.0
Rhubarb stalks	+6.3	Strawberry	-5.4	Wheat Germ	-11.4
Rice syrup, brown	-8.7	Sugar cane juice,		Wheat Grass	+33.8
Rice, brown	-12.5	dried (Sucanat)	-9.6	Wheat	-10.1
Rose Hips	-15.5	Sugar Cane, Refined		Wine	-16.4
Rutabaga	+3.1	(white)	-17.6	Zucchini	+5.7
Sesame seeds	+.5	Sunflower Oil	-6.7		
Shave grass	+21.7	Sunflower Seeds	-5.4		
Sorrel	+11.5	Sweeteners, artificial	-26.5		
Soy beans, (cooked,		Tangerine	-8.5		
then ground)	+12.8	Tea (Black)	-27.1		

Reference:
Young, Robert O. Sick and Tired.
Alpine, UT, 1977.

Appendix C - Essential Oils Certified as GRAS

Angelica		GRAS	FA	Melissa (lemonbalm)		GRAS	FA
Basil		GRAS	FA	Mandarin		GRAS	FA
Bergamot		GRAS	FA	Marjoram		GRAS	FA
Celery Seed		GRAS	FA	Myrrh	(FL)	GRAS	FA
Cedarwood			FA	Myrtle		GRAS	FA
Chamomile, Roman		GRAS	FA	Neroli		GRAS	FA
Chamomile, German		GRAS	FA	Nutmeg		GRAS	FA
Cinnamon Bark		GRAS	FA	Orange		GRAS	FA
Cistus			FA	Oregano		GRAS	FA
Citrus rinds (all)		GRAS	FA	Palmarosa		GRAS	FA
Citronella		GRAS	FA	Patchouly	(FL)	GRAS	FA
Clary Sage		GRAS	FA	Pepper		GRAS	FA
Clove		GRAS	FA	Peppermint		GRAS	FA
Coriander		GRAS	FA	Petitgrain		GRAS	FA
Cumin		GRAS	FA	Pine	(FL)	GRAS	FA
Dill		GRAS	FA	Rosemary		GRAS	FA
Eucalyptus	(FL)	GRAS	FA	Rose		GRAS	FA
Elemi			FA	Rosewood			FA
Fennel			FA	Savory		GRAS	FA
Fir			FA	Sage		GRAS	FA
Frankincense	(FL)	GRAS	FA	Sandalwood	(FL)	GRAS	FA
Galbanum	(FL)	GRAS	FA	Spearmint		GRAS	FA
Geranium		GRAS	FA	Spikenard			FA
Ginger		GRAS	FA	Spruce	(FL)	GRAS	FA
Grapefruit		GRAS	FA	Tarragon		GRAS	FA
Helichrysum			FA	Tangerine		GRAS	FA
Hyssop		GRAS	FA	Thyme		GRAS	FA
Juniper		GRAS	FA	Valerian	(FL)	GRAS	FA
Jasmine		GRAS	FA	Vetiver		GRAS	FA
Laurus nobilis		GRAS	FA	Ylang ylang		GRAS	FA
Lavandin		GRAS	FA				
Lavender		GRAS	FA				
Lemon		GRAS	FA				
Lemongrass		GRAS	FA				
Lime		GRAS	FA				
Melaleuca alternifolia			FA				

CODE:

FA = FDA-approved food additive
(FL) = Flavoring agent
GRAS = Generally regarded as safe

Appendix D - Bible References

Cedarwood

Leviticus 14:51—"And he shall take the cedar wood, and the hyssop, and the scarlet, and the living bird, and dip them in the blood of the slain bird, and in the running water, and sprinkle the house seven times:"

Leviticus 14:52—"And he shall cleanse the house with the blood of the bird, and with the running water, and with the living bird, and with the cedar wood, and with the hyssop, and with the scarlet."

Numbers 19:6—"And the priest shall take cedar wood, and hyssop, and scarlet, and cast [it] into the midst of the burning of the heifer."

Numbers 24:6—"As the valleys are they spread forth, as gardens by the river's side, as the trees of lign aloes which the Lord hath planted, [and] as cedar trees beside the waters."

2 Samuel 5:11—"And Hiram king of Tyre sent messengers to David, and cedar trees, and carpenters, and masons: and they built David an house."

2 Samuel 7:2—"That the king said unto Nathan the prophet, See now, I dwell in an house of cedar, but the ark of God dwelleth within curtains."

2 Samuel 7:7—"In all [the places] wherein I have walked with all the children of Israel spake I a word with any of the tribes of Israel, whom I commanded to feed my people Israel, saying, Why build ye not me an house of cedar?"

1 Kings 4:33—"And he spake of trees, from the cedar tree that [is] in Lebanon even unto the hyssop that springeth out of the wall: he spake also of beasts, and of fowl, and of creeping things, and of fishes."

1 Kings 5:6—"Now therefore command thou that they hew me cedar trees out of Lebanon; and my servants shall be with thy servants: and unto thee will I give hire for thy servants according to all that thou shalt appoint: for thou knowest that [there is] not among us any that can skill to hew timber like unto the Sidonians."

1 Kings 5:8—"And Hiram sent to Solomon, saying, I have considered the things which thou sentest to me for: [and] I will do all thy desire concerning timber of cedar, and concerning timber of fir."

1 Kings 5:10—"So Hiram gave Solomon cedar trees and fir trees [according to] all his desire."

1 Kings 6:9—"So he built the house, and finished it; and covered the house with beams and boards of cedar."

1 Kings 9:11—"([Now] Hiram the king of Tyre had furnished Solomon with cedar trees and fir trees, and with gold, according to all his desire,) that then king Solomon gave Hiram twenty cities in the land of Galilee."

2 Kings 19:23—"By thy messengers thou hast reproached the Lord, and hast said, With the multitude of my chariots I am come up to the height of the mountains, to the sides of Lebanon, and will cut down the tall cedar trees thereof, [and] the choice fir trees thereof: and I will enter into the lodgings of his borders, [and into] the forest of his Carmel."

1 Chronicles 22:4—"Also cedar trees in abundance: for the Zidonians and they of Tyre brought much cedar wood to David."

2 Chronicles 1:15—"And the king made silver and gold at Jerusalem [as plenteous] as stones, and cedar trees made he as the sycomore trees that [are] in the vale for abundance."

2 Chronicles 2:8—"Send me also cedar trees, fir trees, and algum trees, out of Lebanon: for I know that thy servants can skill to cut timber in Lebanon; and, behold, my servants [shall be] with thy servants,"

2 Chronicles 9:27—"And the king made silver in Jerusalem as stones, and cedar trees made he as the sycomore trees that [are] in the low plains in abundance."

Ezra 3:7—"They gave money also unto the masons, and to the carpenters; and meat, and drink, and oil, unto them of Zidon, and to them of Tyre, to bring cedar trees from Lebanon to the sea of Joppa, according to the grant that they had of Cyrus king of Persia."

Isaiah 41:19—"I will plant in the wilderness the cedar, the shittah tree, and the myrtle, and the oil tree; I will set in the desert the fir tree, [and] the pine, and the box tree together:"

Ezekiel 17:3—"And say, Thus saith the Lord God; A great eagle with great wings, longwinged, full of feathers, which had divers colours, came unto Lebanon, and took the highest branch of the cedar:"

Ezekiel 17:22—"Thus saith the Lord God; I will also take of the highest branch of the high cedar, and will set [it]; I will crop off from the top of his young twigs a tender one, and will plant [it] upon an high mountain and eminent:"

Ezekiel 17:23—"In the mountain of the height of Israel will I plant it: and it shall bring forth boughs, and bear fruit, and be a goodly cedar: and under it shall dwell all fowl of every wing; in the shadow of the branches thereof shall they dwell."

Zechariah 11:2—"Howl, fir tree; for the cedar is fallen; because the mighty are spoiled: howl, O ye oaks of Bashan; for the forest of the vintage is come down."

Cinnamon

Revelation 18:13—"And cinnamon, and odours, and ointments, and frankincense, and wine, and oil, and fine flour, and wheat, and beasts, and sheep, and horses, and chariots, and slaves, and souls of men."

Fir

1 Kings 6:15—"And he built the walls of the house within with boards of cedar, both the floor of the house, and the walls of the ceiling: [and] he covered [them] on the inside with wood, and covered the floor of the house with planks of fir."

1 Kings 6:34—"And the two doors [were of] fir tree: the two leaves of the one door [were] folding, and the two leaves of the other door [were] folding."

1 Kings 9:11—"([Now] Hiram the king of Tyre had furnished Solomon with cedar trees and fir trees, and with gold, according to all his desire,) that then king Solomon gave Hiram twenty cities in the land of Galilee."

2 Kings 19:23—"By thy messengers thou hast reproached the Lord, and hast said, With the multitude of my chariots I am come up to the height of the mountains, to the sides of Lebanon, and will cut down the tall cedar trees thereof, [and] the choice fir trees thereof: and I will enter into the lodgings of his borders, [and into] the forest of his Carmel."

2 Chronicles 2:8—"Send me also cedar trees, fir trees, and algum trees, out of Lebanon: for I know that thy servants can skill to cut timber in Lebanon; and, behold, my servants [shall be] with thy servants."

2 Chronicles 3:5—"And the greater house he cieled with fir tree, which he overlaid with fine gold, and set thereon palm trees and chains."

Psalms 104:17—"Where the birds make their nests: [as for] the stork, the fir trees [are] her house."

Song Of Solomon 1:17—"The beams of our house [are] cedar, [and] our rafters of fir."

Isaiah 14:8—"Yea, the fir trees rejoice at thee, [and] the cedars of Lebanon, [saying], Since thou art laid down, no feller is come up against us."

Isaiah 37:24—"By thy servants hast thou reproached the Lord, and hast said, By the multitude of my chariots am I come up to the height of the mountains, to the sides of Lebanon; and I will cut down the tall cedars thereof, [and] the choice fir trees thereof: and I will enter into the height of his border, [and] the forest of his Carmel."

Isaiah 41:19—"I will plant in the wilderness the cedar, the shittah tree, and the myrtle, and the oil tree; I will set in the desert the fir tree, [and] the pine, and the box tree together:"

Isaiah 55:13—"Instead of the thorn shall come up the fir tree, and instead of the brier shall come up the myrtle tree: and it shall be to the Lord for a name, for an everlasting sign [that] shall not be cut off."

Isaiah 60:13—"The glory of Lebanon shall come unto thee, the fir tree, the pine tree, and the box together, to beautify the place of my sanctuary; and I will make the place of my feet glorious."

Ezekiel 27:5—"They have made all thy [ship] boards of fir trees of Senir: they have taken cedars from Lebanon to make masts for thee."

Ezekiel 31:8—"The cedars in the garden of God could not hide him: the fir trees were not like his boughs, and the chestnut trees were not like his branches; nor any tree in the garden of God was like unto him in his beauty."

Hosea 14:8—"Ephraim [shall say], What have I to do any more with idols? I have heard [him], and observed him: I [am] like a green fir tree. From me is thy fruit found."

Nahum 2:3—"The shield of his mighty men is made red, the valiant men [are] in scarlet: the chariots [shall be] with flaming torches in the day of his preparation, and the fir trees shall be terribly shaken."

Zechariah 11:2—"Howl, fir tree; for the cedar is fallen; because the mighty are spoiled: howl, O ye oaks of Bashan; for the forest of the vintage is come down."

Frankincense

Leviticus 2:15—"And thou shalt put oil upon it, and lay frankincense thereon: it [is] a meat offering."

Leviticus 2:16—"And the priest shall burn the memorial of it, [part] of the beaten corn thereof, and [part] of the oil thereof, with all the frankincense thereof: [it is] an offering made by fire unto the Lord."

Leviticus 5:11—"But if he be not able to bring two turtledoves, or two young pigeons, then he that sinned shall bring for his offering the tenth part of an ephah of fine flour for a sin offering; he shall put no oil upon it, neither shall he put [any] frankincense thereon: for it [is] a sin offering"

Leviticus 6:15—"And he shall take of it his handful, of the flour of the meat offering, and of the oil thereof, and all the frankincense which [is] upon the meat offering, and shall burn [it] upon the altar [for] a sweet savour, [even] the memorial of it, unto the Lord."

Leviticus 24:7—"And thou shalt put pure frankincense upon [each] row, that it may be on the bread for a memorial, [even] an offering made by fire unto the Lord."

Numbers 5:15—"Then shall the man bring his wife unto the priest, and he shall bring her offering for her, the tenth [part] of an ephah of barley meal; he shall pour no oil upon it, nor put frankincense thereon; for it [is] an offering of jealousy, an offering of memorial, bringing iniquity to remembrance."

1 Chronicles 9:29—"[Some] of them also [were] appointed to oversee the vessels, and all the instruments of the sanctuary, and the fine flour, and the wine, and the oil, and the frankincense, and the spices."

Nehemiah 13:5—"And he had prepared for him a great chamber, where aforetime they laid the meat offerings, the frankincense, and the vessels, and the tithes of the corn, the new wine, and the oil, which was commanded [to be given] to the Levites, and the singers, and the porters; and the offerings of the priests."

Nehemiah 13:9—"Then I commanded, and they cleansed the chambers: and thither brought I again the vessels of the house of God, with the meat offering and the frankincense."

Song Of Solomon 3:6—"Who [is] this that cometh out of the wilderness like pillars of smoke, perfumed with myrrh and frankincense, with all powders of the merchant?"

Song Of Solomon 4:6—"Until the day break, and the shadows flee away, I will get me to the mountain of myrrh, and to the hill of frankincense."

Song Of Solomon 4:14—"Spikenard and saffron; calamus and cinnamon, with all trees of frankincense; myrrh and aloes, with all the chief spices:"

Matthew 2:11—"And when they were come into the house, they saw the young child with Mary his mother, and fell down, and worshiped him: and when they had opened their treasures, they presented unto him gifts; gold, and frankincense, and myrrh."

Revelation 18:13—"And cinnamon, and odours, and ointments, and frankincense, and wine, and oil, and fine flour, and wheat, and beasts, and sheep, and horses, and chariots, and slaves, and souls of men."

Hyssop

Leviticus 14:49—"And he shall take to cleanse the house two birds, and cedar wood, and scarlet, and hyssop:"

Leviticus 14:51—"And he shall take the cedar wood, and the hyssop, and the scarlet, and the living bird, and dip them in the blood of the slain bird, and in the running water, and sprinkle the house seven times:"

Leviticus 14:52—"And he shall cleanse the house with the blood of the bird, and with running water, and with the living bird, and with the cedar wood, and with the hyssop, and with the scarlet:"

Numbers 19:6—"And the priest shall take cedar wood, and hyssop, and scarlet, and cast [it] into the midst of the burning of the heifer."

Numbers 19:18—"And a clean person shall take hyssop, and dip [it] in the water, and sprinkle [it] upon the tent, and upon all the vessels, and upon the persons that were there, and upon him that touched a bone, or one slain, or one dead, or a grave:"

1 Kings 4:33—"And he spake of trees, from the cedar tree that [is] in Lebanon even unto the hyssop that springeth out of the wall: he spake also of beasts, and of fowl, and of creeping things, and of fishes."

Psalms 51:7—"Purge me with hyssop, and I shall be clean: wash me, and I shall be whiter than snow."

John 19:29—"Now there was set a vessel full of vinegar: and they filled a spunge with vinegar, and put [it] upon hyssop, and put [it] to his mouth."

Hebrews 9:19—"For when Moses had spoken every precept to all the people according to the law, he took the blood of calves and of goats, with water, and scarlet wool, and hyssop, and sprinkled both the book, and all the people."

Myrrh

Esther 2:12—"Now when every maid's turn was come to go in to king Ahasuerus, after that she had been twelve months, according to the manner of the women, (for so were the days of their purifications accomplished, [to wit], six months with oil of myrrh, and six months with sweet odours, and with [other] things for the purifying of the women;)"

Psalms 45:8—"All thy garments [smell] of myrrh, and aloes, [and] cassia, out of the ivory palaces, whereby they have made thee glad."

Proverbs 7:17—"I have perfumed my bed with myrrh, aloes, and cinnamon."

Song Of Solomon 1:13—"A bundle of myrrh [is] my wellbeloved unto me; he shall lie all night betwixt my breasts."

Song Of Solomon 3:6—"Who [is] this that cometh out of the wilderness like pillars of smoke, perfumed with myrrh and frankincense, with all powders of the merchant?"

Song Of Solomon 4:6—"Until the day break, and the shadows flee away, I will get me to the mountain of myrrh, and to the hill of frankincense."

Song Of Solomon 4:14—"Spikenard and saffron; calamus and cinnamon, with all trees of frankincense; myrrh and aloes, with all the chief spices:"

Song Of Solomon 5:1—"I am come into my garden, my sister, [my] spouse: I have gathered my myrrh with my spice; I have eaten my honeycomb with my honey; I have drunk my wine with my milk: eat, O friends; drink, yea, drink abundantly, O beloved."

Song Of Solomon 5:5—"I rose up to open to my beloved; and my hands dropped [with] myrrh, and my fingers [with] sweet smelling myrrh, upon the handles of the lock."

Song Of Solomon 5:13—"His cheeks [are] as a bed of spices, [as] sweet flowers: his lips [like] lilies, dropping sweet smelling myrrh."

Matthew 2:11—"And when they were come into the house, they saw the young child with Mary his mother, and fell down, and worshiped him: and when they had opened their treasures, they presented unto him gifts; gold, and frankincense, and myrrh."

Mark 15:23—"And they gave him to drink wine mingled with myrrh: but he received [it] not."

John 19:39—"And there came also Nicodemus, which at the first came to Jesus by night, and brought a mixture of myrrh and aloes, about an hundred pound [weight]."

Myrtle

Zechariah 1:8—"I saw by night, and behold a man riding upon a red horse, and he stood among the myrtle trees that [were] in the bottom; and behind him [were there] red horses, speckled, and white."

Zechariah 1:10—"And the man that stood among the myrtle trees answered and said, These [are they] whom the Lord hath sent to walk to and fro through the earth."

Zechariah 1:11—"And they answered the angel of the Lord that stood among the myrtle trees, and said, We have walked to and fro through the earth, and, behold, all the earth sitteth still, and is at rest."

Spikenard

Mark 14:3—"And being in Bethany in the house of Simon the leper, as he sat at meat, there came a woman having an alabaster box of ointment of spikenard very precious; and she brake the box, and poured [it] on his head."

John 12:3—"Then took Mary a pound of ointment of spikenard, very costly, and anointed the feet of Jesus, and wiped his feet with her hair: and the house was filled with the odour of the ointment."

Appendix E - Classification of Essential Oil Constituents

Carbohydrates
Monosaccharides
Oligosaccharides
Sugar Alcohols & Cyclitols

Lipids
Organic Acids
Fatty Acids
Lipids

Hydrocarbons & Derivatives
Acetylenes
Thiophenes

Nitrogen-containing constituents
Amino Acids
Amines
Cyanogenic Glucosides
Glucosinates
Purines
Pyrinidines
Proteins
Peptides
Alkaloids
Amaryllidaceae Alkaloids
Betain Alkalydes
Di-Terpinoid Alkalides
Indul Alkaloids
Monoterpene Alkaloids
Sesquiterpene Alkaloids
Peptide Alkalides
Phenolics
Anthocylines
Benzofurans
Chromones
Coumarins
Flavonoids
Flavonones
Isoflavonoids
Neoflavonoids
Phenolics
    Phenolic Acids
    Phenolic Ketones
    Phenolproponoids

Terpenoids
Monoterpenoids
Sesquiterpenoids
Sesquiterpene Lactones
Di-terpenoids
Triterpenoids
Saponin
Steroid Saponins
Phytosterols
Carotenoids

Appendix F - Scientific Research: Essential Oils

Scientific Research List

1. "Effect of a Diffused Essential Oil Blend on Bacterial Bioaerosols"

2. "Screening for Inhibitory Activity of Essential Oils on Selected Bacteria, Fungi, and Viruses"

3. "Antibacterial Properties of Plant Essential Oils"

4. "Influence of Some Spice Essential Oils on *Aspergillus parasiticus* Growth and Production of Aflatoxins in a Synthetic Medium"

5. "Antioxidant Activity of Some Spice Essential Oils on Linoleic Acid Oxidation in Aqueous Media"

6. "Antimicrobial Activity of Some Egyptian Spice Essential Oils"

7. "Antimicrobial Properties of Spices and Their Essential Oils"

8. "The Antimicrobial Activity of Essential Oils and Essential Oil Components Towards Oral Bacteria"

9. "Anticarcinogenic Effects of the Essential Oils From Cumin, Poppy and Basil"

10. "Effects of Essential Oil on Lipid Peroxidation and Lipid Metabolism in Patients with Chronic Bronchitis"

11. "Effect of Essential Oils on the Course of Experimental Atherosclerosis"

12. "Inhibition of Growth and Aflatoxin Production in *Aspergillus parasiticus* by Essential Oils of Selected Plant Materials"

13. "Odors and Learning"

14. "Weight Reduction through Inhalation of Odorants"

15. "Anti-inflammatory Activity of *Passiflora incarnata* L. in Rats"

16. "Medroxyprogesterone Interferes with Ovarian Steroid Protection Against Coronary Vasospasm"

17. "Methyl-Sulfonyl-Methane (M.S.M.): A Double-Blind Study of Its Use in Degenerative Arthritis"

18. "Chemopreventive Effect of Perillyl Alcohol on 4-(methylnitrosamino)-1-(3-pyridyl)-1-butanone Induced Tumorigenesis in (C3H/HeJ X A/J)F1 Mouse Lung"

19. "Chemoprevention of Colon Carcinogenesis by Dietary Perillyl Alcohol"

1. Effect of a Diffused Essential Oil Blend on Bacterial Bioaerosols

Author: S. C. Chao, D. G. Young, and C. J. Oberg

Journal: Journal of Essential Oil Research 10, 517-523 (Sept/Oct 1998)

Location: Weber State University, Ogden, UT

Conclusion: Diffusion of the oil blend, Thieves, can significantly reduce the number of aerosol-borne bacteria.

Abstract: A proprietary blend of oils (named Thieves) containing cinnamon, rosemary, clove, eucalyptus, and lemon was tested for its antibacterial activity against airborne *Micrococcus luteus*, *Pseudomonas aeruginosa,* and *Staphylococcus aureu*s. The bacteria cultures were sprayed in an enclosed area, and Thieves was diffused for a given amount of time. There was an 82 percent reduction in *M. luteus* bioaerosol, a 96 percent reduction in the *P. aeruginosa* bioaerosol, and a 44 percent reduction in the *S. aureus* bioaerosol following 10 minutes of exposure.

2. Screening for Inhibitory Activity of Essential Oils on Selected Bacteria, Fungi, and Viruses

Author: S.C. Chao, D.G. Young, and C.J. Oberg

Journal: Journal of Essential Oil Research

Location: Weber State University, Ogden, UT

Conclusion: Many essential oils were demonstrated to have antimicrobial.

Abstract: 45 essential oils were tested for their inhibitory effect against bacteria, yeast, molds, and two bacteriophage. Of the oils tested, all oils showed inhibition compared to controls. Cinnamon bark and tea tree essential oils showed an inhibitory effect against all the test organisms and phage. Other oils with broad ranges of inhibition included lemongrass, mountain savory, Roman chamomile, rosewood, and spearmint.

3. Antibacterial properties of plant essential oils

Author: S. G. Deans, G. Ritchie

Journal: International Journal of Food Microbiology 5, 165-180 (1987)

Location: Scotland Agricultural College

Conclusion: Many essential oils have antibacterial properties.

Abstract: Fifty plant essential oils were tested in different concentrations for antibacterial activity against 25 genera of bacteria. The ten most antibacterial oils were: angelica, bay, cinnamon, clove, thyme, almond, marjoram, pimento, geranium, and lovage.

4. Influence of Some Spice Essential Oils on Aspergillus parasiticus Growth and Production of Aflatoxins in a Synthetic Medium

Author: R. S. Farag, Z. Y. Daw, S. H. Abo-Raya

Journal: Journal of Food Science, Vol 54, No. 1, 74-76 (1989)

Location: Cairo University, Giza, Egypt

Conclusion: Essential oils of thyme, cumin, clove, caraway, rosemary, and sage all possess antifungal properties.

Abstract: The essential oils of thyme, cumin, clove, caraway, rosemary, and sage were tested for antifungal properties. The essential oils completely inhibited growth of fungal mycelium and aflatoxin production. The oils from most effective to least effective were: thyme > cumin > clove > caraway > rosemary > sage. The basic components of these oils were determined by gas-liquid chromatography to be: thyme—thymol, cumin—cumin aldehyde, clove—eugenol, caraway—carvone, rosemary—borneol, and sage—thujone.

5. Antioxidant Activity of Some Spice Essential Oils on Linoleic Acid Oxidation in Aqueous Media

Author: R. S. Farag, A.Z.M.A. Badei, F. M. Hewedi, G.S.A. El-Baroty

Journal: JAOCS, Vol. 66, No. 6 (June 1989)

Location: Cairo University, Giza, Egypt

Conclusion: Essential oils of caraway, clove, cumin, rosemary, sage, thyme possess antioxidant activity on linoleic acid oxidation.

Abstract: Essential oils of caraway, clove, cumin, rosemary, sage and thyme were examined for antioxidant activity in linoleic acid. These oils were all found to have an antioxidant effect which increased when their concentrations were increased. The effectiveness of these essential oils on linoleic acid oxidation was in the following order: caraway, sage, cumin, rosemary, thyme, clove.

6. Antimicrobial Activity of Some Egyptian Spice Essential Oils

Author: R.S. Farag, Z. Y. Daw, F. M. Hewedi, G.S.A. El-Baroty

Journal: Journal of Food Protection, Vol. 52 (September 1989)

Location: Cairo University, Giza, Egypt

Conclusion: Essential oils of sage, rosemary, caraway, cumin, clove, and thyme were shown to have antimicrobial properties.

Abstract: Essential oils of sage, rosemary, caraway, cumin, clove, and thyme were studied for their antibacterial effects. The minimum inhibitory concentration for each essential oil was also determined. Various essential oils were inhibitory at extremely low concentrations (0.25-12 mg/ml). Gram-positive bacteria were shown to be more sensitive to the essential oils than were gram-negative. Thyme and cumin oils had stronger antimicrobial activity than the other oils. The chemical structures of compounds in the essential oils were related to the antimicrobial activity.

7. Antimicrobial Properties of Spices and Their Essential Oils

Author: L. R. Beuchat

Journal: Nat. Antimicrob. Syst. Food Preserv. 167-79 (1994)

Location: University of Georgia, Griffin, Georgia

Conclusion: Many spices and herbs possess antimicrobial properties against various bacteria, yeasts, and molds.

Abstract: Many spices and herbs possess antimicrobial actions. These include plants of the genus *Allium*, such as onions and garlic; spices such as thyme, oregano, savory, sage, cinnamon, clove, vanilla, and others. Microbes inhibited by these herbs and spices include gram-positive and gram-negative bacteria, yeasts, and molds.

8. The Antimicrobial Activity of Essential Oils and Essential Oil Components Towards Oral Bacteria

Author: S. Shapiro, A. Meier, B. Guggenheim

Journal: Oral Microbiology and Immunology 1994: 202-208 (Copyright Munksgaard 1994)

Location: University of Zurich, Switzerland

Conclusion: Essential oils of tea tree, peppermint, and sage showed potent antimicrobial action against anaerobic oral activity.

Abstract: Antimicrobial activity of some essential oils on anaerobic oral bacteria was analyzed. The most potent essential oils tested were Australian tea tree oil, peppermint oil, and sage oil. Thymol and eugenol were the most potent oil components.

9. Anticarcinogenic Effects of the Essential Oils From Cumin, Poppy and Basil

Author: K. Aruna, V. M. Sivaramakrishnan

Journal: Phytotherapy Research, Vol. 10, 577-580 (1996)

Location: Cancer Institute (W.I.A.) Adyar Madras, India

Conclusion: Essential oils of cumin, poppy, and basil all possess potent anticarcinogenic properties.

Abstract: Essential oils of cumin, poppy, and basil were assessed for anticarcinogenic properties. The activity of glutathione-S-transferase, a carcinogen-detoxifying enzyme, was increased by over 78 percent in the stomach, liver, and esophagus of Swiss mice when they were treated with cumin, poppy, and basil essential oils.

10. Effects of Essential Oil on Lipid Peroxidation and Lipid Metabolism in Patients with Chronic Bronchitis

Author: S. A. Siurin

Journal: Klinicheskaia Meditsina, 75(10):43-5 (1997)

Location: Scientific Group NII of Pulmonology, Monchegorsk, Russia.

Conclusion: Lavender essential oil aids in normalizing lipid levels.

Abstract: Essential oils were tested in 150 patients with chronic bronchitis for their effects on lipid peroxidation and lipid metabolism. Essential oils of rosemary, basil, fir, eucalyptus, and lavender were found to have antioxidant effect and lavender was found to normalize lipid levels.

11. Effect of Essential Oils on the Course of Experimental Atherosclerosis

Author: V. V. Nikolaevskii, N. S. Kononova, A. I. Pertsoviskii, I.F. Shinkarchuk

Journal: Patologicheskaia Fiziologiia i Eksperimentalnaia Terapiia (5):52-3 (Sep-Oct 1990)

Conclusion: Inhalation of lavender and monarda essential oils reduces cholesterol content in the aorta of rabbits, providing an angioprotective effect.

Abstract: Lavender, monarda, and basil essential oils were tested in rabbits for their effect on atherosclerosis. When inhaled, lavender and monarda essential oils did not affect blood cholesterol content, but reduced cholesterol content in the aorta. These oils provide a heart-protective effect.

12. Inhibition of Growth and Aflatoxin Production in Aspergillus parasiticus by Essential Oils of Selected Plant Materials

Author: A. Tantaoui-Elaraki, L. Beraoud

Journal: Journal of Environmental Pathology, Toxicology and Oncology;13(1):67-72 (1994)

Location: Hassan II Institute for Agriculture and Veterinary Medicine, Rabat-Instituts, Morocco

Conclusion: Several essential oils (cinnamon, thyme, oregano, and cumin) were shown to have strong antifungal properties.

Abstract: Essential oils of cinnamon, thyme, oregano, cumin, curcumin, ginger, lemon, and orange were tested on *Aspergillus parasiticus* for antifungal properties. The most inhibitory essential oils were cinnamon, thyme, oregano, and cumin.

13. Odors and Learning

Author: A. R. Hirsch, M.D., L. H. Johnston, M.D.

Journal: J. Neurol Orthop Med Surg 17:119-126 (1996)

Location: Smell & Taste Research Foundation, Chicago, Illinois, USA

Conclusion: Pleasant odors increased performance of individuals on cognitive tasks.

Abstract: This study assessed the effects of hedonically positive odors on performance of cognitive tasks. Results indicate that normally performing subjects completed a cognitive task an average 17 percent faster on subsequent trials when a pleasing odor was present. Further studies are desirable to determine if odors would be useful in general education and education of those with learning disabilities.

14. Weight Reduction through Inhalation of Odorants

Author: A. R. Hirsch, M.D., R. Gomez

Journal: Annals of Clinical and Laboratory Science (Official Journal of the Association of Clinical Scientists) Volume 24 September-October Number 5

Location: Smell & Taste Research Foundation, Chicago, Illinois, USA

Conclusion: Use of aroma inhalers aided study volunteers in weight loss over a 6-month period.

Abstract: To measure the role of olfaction in weight loss, odorant inhalers were given to 3,193 overweight volunteers. Study participants were instructed to inhale odorants 3 times in each nostril whenever hunger occurred. Average weight loss was 2.1 percent body weight per month. These results suggest inhalation of odorants may induce sustained weight loss over a 6-month period.

15. Anti-inflammatory Activity of Passiflora incarnata L. in Rats

Author: F. Borrelli, L. Pinto, A. A. Izzo, N. Mascolo, F. Capasso, V. Mercati, E. Toja, G. Autore

Journal: Phytotherapy Research, Vol. 10, S104-S106 (1996)

Location: University of Naples, Naples, Italy

Conclusion: *Passiflora incarnata* extract was found to have anti-inflammatory activity in rats.

Abstract: Ethanolic extract of *Passiflora incarnata* (passion flower) was tested for anti-inflammatory activity in rats. The extract significantly inhibited swelling and inflammation.

16. Medroxyprogesterone Interferes with Ovarian Steroid Protection Against Coronary Vasospasm

Author: K. Miyagawa, J. Rosch, F. Stanczyk, K. Hermsmeyer

Journal: Nature Medicine, Vol. 3 (3); (March 1997)

Location: Oregon Health Sciences University, Beaverton, Oregon

Conclusion: Progesterone was found to cause less risk of cardiovascular disease than medroxyprogesterone, a synthetic progesterone.

Abstract: Progesterone and medroxyprogesterone, a synthetic progesterone, were tested on rhesus monkeys. Medroxyprogesterone was found to cause an increased risk of cardiovascular disease compared to progesterone.

17. Methyl-Sulfonyl-Methane (M.S.M.) A Double-Blind Study of Its Use in Degenerative Arthritis

Author: R. M. Lawrence

Journal: Preliminary correspondence, not yet published

Location: UCLA School of Medicine, Los Angeles, CA

Conclusion: MSM helps patients with degenerative arthritis in pain management.

Abstract: A double-blind study was conducted on patients suffering from degenerative joint disease. After 6 weeks, patients given MSM showed an 82 percent improvement in pain on average. MSM is a safe, non-toxic method of managing pain.

18. Chemopreventive Effect of Perillyl Alcohol on 4-(methylnitrosamino)-1-(3-pyridyl)-1-butanone Induced Tumorigenesis in (C3H/HeJ X A/J)F1 Mouse Lung

Author: L. E. Lantry, Z. Zhang, F. Gao, K. A. Crist, Y. Wang, G. J. Kelloff, R. A. Lubet, M. You

Journal: Journal of Cellular Biochemistry Supplement; 27:20-5 (1997)

Location: Medical College of Ohio, Toledo, OH.

Conclusion: Perillyl alcohol possesses chemopreventive effects in a mouse lung tumor experiment.

Abstract: Perillyl alcohol, a naturally occurring monoterpene found in lavender, cherries, and mint was given to laboratory mice which were then exposed to carcinogens. Perillyl-treated mice had a 22 percent reduction in tumor incidence compared to non-treated mice. Perillyl alcohol is an effective chemopreventive compound in mouse lung tumors.

19. Chemoprevention of Colon Carcinogenesis by Dietary Perillyl Alcohol

Author: B. S. Reddy, C. X. Wang, H. Samaha, R. Lubet, V. E. Steele, G. J. Kelloff, C. V. Rao

Journal: Cancer Research 1;57(3): 420-5 (1997 Feb)

Location: American Health Foundation, Valhalla, NY

Conclusion: Perillyl alcohol is shown to have chemopreventive activity in colon cancer in lab rats.

Abstract: Perillyl alcohol, a monoterpene found in lavender, was administered to rats which were then given azoxymethane (AOM), an agent causing colon carcinogenesis. Perillyl alcohol inhibited the incidence of adenocarcinomas of the colon and small intestine as compared to the control.

Appendix G - Scientific Research: Supplement Ingredients

1. The Chinese Wolfberry: A Breakthrough in Anti-aging and Immunity

In the early 1980s, a group of researchers from the Natural Science Institute began studying a region on the West Elbow Plateau of the Yellow River in Inner Mongolia where people lived to be over 100 years old—10 to 20 years longer than the average person in the region. The inhabitants shared one trait that distinguished them from others. They were predominantly vegetarian and regularly consumed wolfberries. Moreover, the people who consumed this fruit lived free of common diseases like arthritis, cancer, and diabetes.

Both the Chinese wolfberry (also known as *Lycium barbarum* by botanists and as the goji berry by native Chinese) and ginseng *(Panax ginseng)* have been highly regarded for centuries as the foremost nutritional and therapeutic plants in China. In fact, the Chinese hold a strong belief that human life might be extended significantly by using either of these herbs for an extended period. Unfortunately, ginseng is considered too strong for continuous use, and large amounts may not be suitable for people with high blood pressure or heart disease. On the other hand, the wolfberry is much milder, with no known risk from continuous use.

18 Amino Acids and 21 Trace Minerals

In 1988, the Beijing Nutrition Research Institute conducted detailed chemical analyses and nutritional composition studies of the dried wolfberry fruit. What they discovered was stunning! The wolfberry contained over 18 amino acids, 21 trace minerals, more protein than bee pollen, more vitamin C than oranges, and nearly as much beta carotene as carrots.

Perhaps this is why the Chinese have traditionally attributed so many benefits to the wolfberry, claiming it protects liver function, replenishes vital essences, improves visual acuity, and lowers blood

A university in Japan experimented with diffusing different oils in the office. When they diffused lemon, there were 54 percent fewer errors, with jasmine there were 33 percent fewer errors, and with lavender there were 20 percent fewer errors. When oils were diffused while studying and taking a test, test scores increased by as much as 50 percent.

Diffusing an essential oil while studying may also improve memory while taking a test. By inhaling the same aroma, the smell of the oil may encourage recall of facts or figures learned previously by bringing back the memory of what was studied.

pressure and cholesterol. The wolfberry was also said to strengthen muscles and bones, stimulate the heart, and work as an aid to treat diabetes and impotence. The big question was: Could these results be substantiated in clinical studies?

Since the early 1980s, the Chinese wolfberry has been the subject of a number of important clinical studies—including several published by the State Scientific and Technological Commission in China. These studies have documented the antioxidant and immune-stimulating properties of the Chinese wolfberry.

From July 1982 to January 1984, the Ningxia Institute of Drug Inspection conducted a pharmacological experiment using multi-index screening (Register No. 870303). Their conclusion was:

> The fruits and pedicels of wolfberry were effective in increasing white blood cells, protecting the liver, and relieving hypertension. The alcoholic extract of wolfberry fruits inhibited tumor growth in mice by 58 percent, and the protein of wolfberry displayed an insulin-like action that was effective in promoting fat decomposition and reducing blood sugar.

Another clinical experiment by the Ningxia Institute (Register No. 870306, October 1982 to May 1985) studied the effects of wolfberry on the immune, physiological, and biochemical indexes of the blood of aged volunteers. The results indicated that the wolfberry caused the blood of older people to noticeably revert to a younger state.

Can the Wolfberry Boost Immune Function?

According to a report of the State Scientific and Technological Commission of China, the wolfberry contains compounds known as lycium polysaccharides, which appeared to be highly effective in promoting immunity. These results were supported in a number of clinical trials.

In one study on a group of cancer patients, the wolfberry triggered an increase in both lymphocyte transformation rate and white blood cell count (measures of immune function). In another study involving a group of 50 people with lower-limit white blood cell counts, the wolfberry increased phagocytosis and the titre of serum antibodies (another index of immune function). Unhealthy levels of titre of serum antibodies have long been associated with Chronic Fatigue Syndrome (also known as Epstein-Barr). Does this mean that the wolfberry could be used as a weapon against Epstein-Barr? The possibilities are intriguing.

In another study, consumption of wolfberry led to a strengthening of immunoglobulin A levels (an index of immune function). Because the decline of immunoglobulin A is one of the signs of aging, an increase in these levels suggests that the wolfberry may enable injured DNA to better repair itself and ward off tissue degeneration.

Is the Wolfberry a Powerful Antioxidant?

As we grow older, the levels of lipid peroxide in our blood increase, while levels of health-protecting antioxidants, like superoxide dismutase (SOD), decrease. In a clinical study of people who consumed doses of wolfberry, SOD in the blood increased by a remarkable 48 percent while hemoglobin increased by 12 percent. Even better, lipid peroxide levels dropped by an astonishing 65 percent.

Does the Wolfberry Protect Eyesight?

A test was conducted on the effects of wolfberry on eyesight. Twenty-seven people were tested and showed a dramatic improvement in both dark adaptation and vitamin A and carotene content of their serum (measures of eyesight acuity).

More recent studies in the 1990s have lent additional scientific support.

Abstracts

1. Use of Wolfberry (*Lycium barbarum polysaccharides*) to Treat Cancer

Author: G. W. Cao, W. G. Yang, P. Du

Journal: Chunghua Chung Lui Tsa Chih 16 (Nov. 1994): 428-31

Location: Second Military Medical University, Shanghai

Conclusion: *Lycium barbarum* polysaccharides can be used as an adjuvant in the treatment of cancer.

Abstract: Seventy-nine advanced cancer patients were treated with a combination of LAK/IL-2* and *Lycium barbarum* polysaccharides. Patients treated with only LAK/IL-2 showed a response rate of only 16 percent, while those treated with both LAK/IL-2 and *Lycium barbarum* polysaccharides showed a response rate of 40.9 percent. Moreover, the mean remission in the *Lycium barbarum* group lasted significantly longer. *Lymphokine-activated natural killer cells (LAK) and interleukin 2 (IL-2).

2. The Role of Lycium barbarum Polysaccharide as an Antioxidant

Author: X. Zhang

Journal: Chung Kuo Chung Yao Tsa Chih 18 (Feb. 1993): 110-2, 128

Location: Beijing Military Hospital

Conclusion: The effects of free radicals on cells can be prevented and reversed by incubation with either *Lycium barbarum* polysaccharide or superoxide dismutase.

Abstract: Researchers incubated cells (Xenopus Oocytes) in a solution containing a free-radical-producing system for 6 hours. The changes in the electrical profile of the cell membranes were determined using a microelectrode electrophysiological technique. The results showed that *Lycium barbarum* polysaccharide prevented and reversed free radical damage to the cells.

3. Protective Action of *Lycium barbarum* on Hydrogen Peroxide-induced Lipid Peroxidation

Author: B. Ren, Y. Ma, Y. Shen, B. Gao

Journal: Chung Kuo Chung Yao Tsa Chih 20 (May 1995): 303-4

Location: Ningxia Medical College, Yinchuan

Conclusion: *Lycium barbarum* protects red blood cell membranes against lipid peroxidation.

Abstract: Hydrogen peroxide (H_2O_2), a powerful promoter of oxidative damage, was used to promote lipid peroxidation of the red blood cell membranes of rats. Dried *Lycium* berries showed the greatest protective effect against H_2O_2 damage, followed by *Lycium barbarum* polysaccharide.

4. Effects of *Lycium barbarum* on the Attachment and Growth of Human Gingival Cells to Root Surfaces

Author: B. Liu

Journal: Chung Kuo Chung Yao Tsa Chih 27 (May 1992): 159-61, 190

Location: College of Stomatology, Fourth Medical University, Xian

Conclusion: *Lycium barbarum* improved the attachment and growth of human gingival cells to root surfaces.

Abstract: A dose of 1.25 mg/ml *Lycium barbarum* was used to stimulate the in vitro attachment of human gingival fibrobasts to the surfaces of dental roots. In response to *Lycium barbarum* exposure, cells on diseased root surfaces increased in quantity, exhibited better growth and distribution. *Drynaria* displayed similar effects but was not as potent as the *Lycium barbarum*.

2. Stevia: A New, Safe, Non-caloric Supplement with Health-giving Properties

For over 1600 years, the natives of Paraguay in South America have used this intensely sweet herb as a health agent and sweetener. Known as *Stevia rebaudiana* by botanists and yerba dulce (honey leaf) by the Guarani Indians, stevia has been incorporated into many native medicines, beverages, and foods for centuries. The Guarani used stevia separately or combined with herbs like yerba mate and lapacho.

Fifteen times sweeter than sugar, stevia was introduced to the West in 1899, when M. S. Bertoni discovered natives using it as a sweetener and medicinal herb. However, stevia never gained popularity in Europe or the United States and was only gradually adopted by several countries throughout Far East Asia.

With Japan's ban on the import of synthetic sweeteners in the 1960's, stevia began to be seriously researched by the Japanese National Institute of Health as a natural sugar substitute. After almost a decade of studies examining the safety and antidiabetic properties of the herb, Japan became a major producer, importer, and user of stevia. Hundreds of food products began including it, and eventually stevia use spread through Asia. Stevioside, the super sweet glycoside derived from stevia that is 300 times sweeter than sugar, was even used to sweeten Diet Coke sold in Japan.

Even though stevia is still relatively unknown in the United States, it has gained widespread popularity as a low-calorie sweetener throughout South America and Asia. Both the stevia leaf and stevioside are used in Taiwan, China, Korea, and Japan, with many of these same countries growing large amounts of the raw herb.

In 1994, the U.S. Food and Drug Administration permitted the importation and use of stevia as a dietary supplement. However, its adoption by American consumers as a noncaloric sweetener has been very slow because the FDA does not currently permit stevia to be marketed as a food additive. This means that stevia cannot be sold as a sweetener (all sweeteners are classified as food additives by the FDA). Moreover, stevia faces fierce opposition by both the artificial sweetener (aspartame) and sugar industry in the U.S.

Stevia, however, is more than just a non-caloric sweetener. Several modern clinical studies have documented the ability of stevia to lower and balance blood sugar levels, support the pancreas and digestive system, protect the liver, and combat infectious microorganisms. (Oviedo et al., 1971; Suzuki et al., 1977; Ishit et al., 1986; Boeckh, 1986; Alvarez, 1986.)

In one study, Oviedo et. al. showed that oral administration of a stevia leaf extract reduced blood sugar levels by over 35 percent. Another study conducted by Suzuki et al. documented similar results. Clearly, these and other clinical evaluations indicate that stevia holds significant promise for the treatment of diabetes.

3. MSM: A New Solution for Arthritis, Allergies, and Pain

MSM (Methylsulfonylmethane) is a natural sulfur-bearing nutrient that occurs widely in nature (found in everything from mother's breast milk to fresh vegetables). It is an exceptional source of nutritional sulfur—a mineral that is vital to protein synthesis and sound health.

Why is sulfur so important to the body? Because sulfur is a mineral which, like vitamin C, is constantly being used up and depleted. When we fail to replenish our reserves of nutritional sulfur, we become more vulnerable to disease and degenerative conditions. Some possible signs of sulfur deficiency are:

• Poor nail and hair growth
• Eczema
• Dermatitis
• Poor muscle tone
• Acne / Pimples
• Gout
• Rheumatism
• Arthritis
• Weakening of nervous system
• Constipation
• Impairment of mental faculties
• Lowered libido

MSM is more than just another essential nutrient. According to research compiled by Ronald Lawrence, Ph.D., M.D., and Stanley Jacob, M.D., MSM represents a safe, natural solution for chronic headaches, back pain, tendonitis, fibromyalgia, rheumatism, arthritis, athletic injuries, muscle spasms, asthma, and allergies.

In a book entitled, *The Miracle of MSM,* both Dr. Jacobs and Dr. Lawrence discuss how MSM has benefited hundred of patients. A UCLA neuro-psychiatrist, Dr. Lawrence is convinced that MSM will revolutionize how millions of people deal with inflammatory autoimmune diseases like rheumatism, asthma, bursitis, and tendonitis, as well as auto-immune diseases like arthritis, lupus, scleroderma, and allergies.

Other doctors have also seen their patients dramatically improve using 2 to 4 grams of MSM daily. According to David Blyweiss, M.D., of the Institute of Advanced Medicine in Lauderhill, Florida, many patients experience a 50 percent improvement in their arthritis symptoms, along with less fatigue, better sleep, and better ability to exercise.

Dr. Lawrence has also used MSM to improve the condition of patients who were virtually crippled with arthritis and back pain. One patient was able to get out of bed for the first time after just two weeks on MSM. And after two months of MSM use, he could walk to the grocery store.

Another of Dr. Lawrence's patients was a 70-year-old woman who was suffering from severe arthritis. In this case, MSM actually postponed the need for double knee replacement. In fact, after only two months on oral MSM, she was walking again with much less pain and stiffness.

Numerous other MSM users have experienced results equivalent to cortisone—but without side effects like immune suppression, fluid retention, and weakness.

According to Stanley Jacobs, M.D., there may be no pharmaceutical therapy better—or safer—than MSM. "MSM has an important role to play in the nonsurgical treatment of back pain," he said. "I have seen several hundred patients for back pain secondary to osteoarthritis, disc degeneration, spinal misalignments, or accidents. For such pain-related conditions, MSM is usually beneficial."

"I have been recommending MSM for more than six months," said Richard Shaefer, a chiropractor from Wheeling, Illinois. "The results have been excellent. I consistently see major reduction in pain and inflammation in the area of arthritis joints, along with improved range of motion. I can't think of a single individual who isn't getting some kind of positive effect."

MSM may have other benefits aside from its pain and inflammation-reducing properties. Numerous patients have reported a surge in energy levels along with thicker hair, nails, and skin. Some have even reported a softening or disappearance of scar tissue.

One user reported a marked increase in stamina and energy after starting on MSM. "For a long while I have had the blahs," complained Lou Salyer of Tucson, Arizona. "I had no stamina. I had to force myself to get things done around the house. After two days on MSM, it was like a blast of energy. I am amazed at how much I get done now."

MSM may also do much more than relieve pain. "Prior to taking MSM (30 grams a day for 20 years), I would have a cold or flu two or three times a year," stated Dr. Jacobs. "Since I've been taking MSM, I've not had a single cold or the flu. I can't say that MSM prevented my cold or the flu, but it is a fascinating observation."

MSM contains an exceptionally bioavailable source of sulfur, one of the most neglected minerals needed by the human body. Carl Pfeiffer, M.D., Ph.D., a world-renowned expert on nutritional medicine, agrees, "Sulfur is the forgotten essential element."

Found in such foods as garlic and asparagus, the sulfur within MSM is a critical part of the amino acids cysteine and methionine, which form the building blocks of the nails, hair, and skin. Sulfur is also found in therapeutic mineral baths and hot springs that have brought relief to arthritis sufferers for centuries.

MSM is very closely related to DMSO, a powerful pain reliever that was the subject of a *60 Minutes* report in April, 1980. DMSO has been approved by the FDA for interstitial cystitis, a painful urinary tract condition.

The Youth Nutrient

Of particular importance is MSM's ability to equalize water pressure inside the cells—a considerable benefit for those plagued with bursitis, arthritis, and tendonitis. These kinds of inflammatory outbreaks are created when the water pressure inside the cells jumps past the pressure outside the cells, creating pressure and pain. MSM acts as a sort of cellular safety valve, affecting the protein envelope of the cell so that water transfers freely in and out of the cell. The result: rapid relief and less damage to tissues. And because it elasticizes the hold between the cells, MSM can restore flexibility to inflamed tissues.

When our bodies grow older and are chronically shortchanged of key minerals like sulfur and MSM, the bonds between our cells become increasingly rigid and brittle—a condition that can lead to a loss in skin flexibility and contribute to skin wrinkles. The internal manifestations of this cellular brittleness are far less visible but have a far greater negative impact on the body. MSM's ability to reintroduce flexibility into cell structures, therefore, can have widespread restorative affects.

4. FOS: Supernutrient Documented to Rebuild Intestinal Flora and Combat Candida, Cancer, and Infections

FOS (Fructooligosaccharides) are one of the best-documented, natural nutrients for promoting the growth of *Lactobacilli* and *bifidobacteria* bacteria, a key to sound health. FOS has also been clinically studied for its ability to increase magnesium and calcium absorption, lower blood glucose, cholesterol, and LDL levels, and to inhibit production of the reductase enzymes that can contribute to cancer. Because FOS can increase magnesium absorption, it can also lead to lowered blood pressure and better cardiovascular health.

In addition, FOS also has another benefit: It has a naturally sweet taste. Consisting of undigestible sugars found in fruits, vegetables, and grains, FOS possesses a palate-pleasing sweetness with only a fraction of the calories of refined sugar.

However, gaining beneficial quantities of FOS as part of a normal diet is very difficult, since you would have to consume over 15 tomatoes, a dozen bananas, or over 350 cloves of garlic to obtain just a 1/4 teaspoon of FOS.

The subject of over 40 human studies and 60 animal studies throughout the world, FOS has been intensively researched in Japan, the United States, and Europe for over a decade. FOS provides an outstanding source of nourishment for the beneficial bacteria that are our front-line defense against disease, while at the same time reducing the populations of harmful putrefactive bacteria and pathogenic yeast and fungi that can contribute to candida, chronic fatigue syndrome, and other illnesses.

5. HMB: A Natural Immune-booster and Muscle-builder

Beta-hydroxy beta-methylbutyrate (HMB), a natural derivative of the amino acid L-leucine, has been shown to be one of the newest and most powerful supplements for promoting growth in lean muscle tissue. Studies have also documented the ability of HMB to improve immune function and increase life expectancy in animals.

According to noted researcher, Richard Passwater, Ph.D., "HMB showed that it lowered total and LDL cholesterol levels in blood and helped strengthen the immune system while building muscles and burning body fat. This news is certainly of interest to body builders and other athletes, but it may also become of interest to cancer, AIDS, and muscular dystrophy patients."

Other health and fitness professionals agree. "HMB is one of the most exciting natural nutrients for supporting muscle growth and immunity that I've seen in quite some time," stated Dr. Robert Delmonteque, an expert on fitness. "HMB will enable many people to attain new levels of health and fitness—especially when combined with regular exercise and sound nutrition."

Abstracts

1. Method of Promoting Nitrogen Retention in Humans

Author: Nissen, S. L., N. N. Abumrad, et al.

Source: U.S. Patent and Trademark Office, Patent #5,348,979

Conclusion: HMB promotes protein retention and body fat loss in middle-aged adult males.

Abstract: In a placebo-controlled random-designed crossover study, five adult men received a placebo for 2 weeks, followed by 2 grams of HMB daily for another two weeks. During the control period, body fat content decreased from 12.4 to 12 percent and urinary nitrogen loss (a measure of muscle and protein loss) increased from 14.5 to 16.1 grams per day. However, during the HMB supplementation period, body fat dropped from 12.5 to 11 percent, and urinary nitrogen loss decreased from 16.7 to 15.4 grams per day.

2. The Effect of Leucine Metabolite HMB on Muscle Metabolism During Resistance Exercise Training

Author: Nissen, S. L., J. C. Fuller, Jr., J. Shell, et al.

Journal: Journal of Applied Physiology 81 (1996): 2095-2104

Conclusion: HMB spares muscle-damaged, physically active adults.

Abstract: Forty volunteers participating in a supervised exercise program were divided into three group. The first group received a placebo, the second group received 1.5 grams of HMB daily, and the third group received 3 grams of HMB daily. Muscle damage was assessed by measuring the amount of creatine phosphokinase (CPK) and lactate dehydrogenase (LDH) in the blood. The group receiving the highest amount of HMB had the lowest blood levels of both CPK and LDH. This indicated that HMB had muscle and protein-sparing effects in humans.

7. The Effect of Leucine Metabolite HMB on Muscle Metabolism During Resistance Exercise Training (2)

Author: Nissen, S. L., J. C. Fuller, Jr., J. Shell, et al.

Journal: Journal of Applied Physiology 81 (1996): 2095-2104

Conclusion: HMB spares muscle-damaged, physically active adult volunteers.

Abstract: Thirty athletes from the Iowa State University football team were randomly divided into two groups. The first group received a placebo, while the second received 3 grams per day of HMB. After seven weeks the gain in muscle mass and strength of the two groups were assessed. The HMB group gained an average of 13 ounces of lean muscle mass, compared with no gain for the control group. Moreover, the HMB group gained an average of 15 pounds in bench-press strength, compared with a 5.4 pound gain in the control group.

8. The Effect of HMB Supplementation on Strength and Body Composition of Trained and Untrained Males Undergoing Intense Resistance Training

Author: Nissen, S. L., L. Panton, R. Wilhelm, et al.

Journal: FASEB 10 (1996): A287

Conclusion: HMB promotes muscle gain and body fat declines in both athletes and nonathletes who embark on an exercise program.

Abstract: In a double-blind, placebo-controlled study, 40 volunteers submitted to a four-week strenuous exercise program. Half received a placebo, while the remainder received 3 grams daily of HMB. Following the four-week regimen, the HMB group's gain in muscle mass was 57 percent greater than the control group. In addition, the HMB group lost a significant amount more in body fat.

9. Effect of HMB on Body Composition Changes Measured by Computerized Tomography in Older Adults Participating in an Exercise Program

Author: Vukovich, M.D., N. B. Stubbs, et al.

Journal: FASEB 12 (1998): A652

Conclusion: HMB can safely increase muscle mass and reduce body fat in older adults.

Abstract: In a double blind, placebo-controlled study, 15 men and 16 women (average age 70) participated in a three-day-a-week walking program and a two-day-a-week strength training program. After 8 weeks body composition analyses were conducted by skinfold measurements and computerized tomography. The HMB group gained significantly more muscle mass (+1.6 percent) than the control group (-0.2 percent). The HMB group also shed more body fat (-3.9 percent) than the control group (+0.7 percent).

10. Effect of HMB on Health of Calves

Author: Van Koevering, M. T., D. R. Gill, et al.

Journal: Oklahoma State Animal Science Research Report (1993)

Conclusion: HMB dramatically reduced both morbidity (sickness) and mortality of shipping-stressed calves.

Abstract: Three truckloads of cattle (158 animals) were randomly assigned to either a control diet or a diet supplemented with 4 g of HMB. After 28 days the morbidity and mortality of the HMB-supplemented calves was compared with the control group. The HMB group displayed 15 percent less sickness and 94 percent less mortality than the control group.

11. Enhancement of Immunity by HMB in Chickens

Author: A. L. Peterson, M. A. Qureshi, et al.

Journal: Poultry Science 75 (1997)

Conclusion: HMB increases the growth and function of macrophage immune cells in chickens.

Abstract: Macrophages from a chicken cell line were exposed to 0, 10, 20, 40, 80, 100 mcg of HMB per 5 x 10^4 cells in a 96 well culture plate. At 100 mcg HMB exposure, macrophages exhibited a 19 percent and 21 percent increase in growth compared with untreated cells.

Appendix H - Comparative Antimicrobial Activity of Essential Oils and Antibiotics

The following are test data comparing the antimicrobial ability between essential oils (cinnamon and oregano) and antibiotics (penicillin and ampicillin). The method is disk diffusion and the results are the mean value of three replicates.

These preliminary data indicate that essential oils of cinnamon and oregano are comparable with penicillin and ampicillin in inhibitory activity against *E. coli* and *Staphylococcus aureus*.

Material	Loading amount (µl)*	*Escherichia coli* zone of inhibition (cm)	*Staphylococcus aureus* zone of inhibition (cm)
Penicillin	3	0	3.2
	6	0	3.4
	8	0	3.6
	12	0	3.6
Ampicillin	3	1.9	2.6
	6	2.1	2.6
	8	2.5	2.7
	12	2.6	2.8
Cinnamon	3	2.4	2.4
	6	2.8	2.8
	8	-	3.0
	12	3.0	3.2
Oregano	3	2.6	3.2
	6	3.3	3.6
	8	-	3.6
	12	3.3	3.8

*The concentration of penicillin = 1.76 unit / μl
The concentration of ampicillin = 5 μg / μl

Index